THE INTRAOCULAR IMPLANT LENS DEVELOPMENT AND RESULTS WITH SPECIAL REFERENCE TO THE BINKHORST LENS

PROEFSCHRIFT

TER VERKRIJGING VAN DE GRAAD VAN

DOCTOR IN DE GENEESKUNDE,

AAN DE RIJKSUNIVERSITEIT TE LEIDEN,

OP GEZAG VAN DE RECTOR MAGNIFICUS DR. A. E. COHEN,

HOOGLERAAR IN DE FACULTEIT DER LETTEREN,

VOLGENS BESLUIT VAN HET COLLEGE VAN DEKANEN TE VERDEDIGEN

OP WOENSDAG 15 JANUARI 1975 TE KLOKKE 16.15 UUR

door
MARCEL EUGÈNE NORDLOHNE
geboren te Goes in 1927

SPRINGER-SCIENCE+BUSINESS MEDIA, B.V.

Promotor:	PROF. DR. J. A. OOSTERHUIS
Co-promotor:	PROF. DR. M. C. COLENBRANDER
Co-referenten:	DR. A. TH. M. VAN BALEN
	PROF. DR. G. J. TAMMELING

Additional material to this book can be downloaded from http://extra.springer.com.

© Springer Science+Business Media Dordrecht 1975
Originally published by Dr.W, Junk B.V. -The Hague in 1975

ISBN 978-90-6193-176-8   ISBN 978-94-010-2342-9 (eBook)
DOI 10.1007/978-94-010-2342-9

Whatsoever thy hand findeth to do,
do it with thy might.

Ecclesiastes 9 : 10

Aan mijn ouders
mijn vrouw
mijn dochters

CONTENTS

THE INTRAOCULAR IMPLANT LENS
DEVELOPMENT AND RESULTS, WITH SPECIAL REFERENCE
TO THE BINKHORST LENS

CHAPTER I

COMPARISON OF SPECTACLE LENS, CONTACT LENS
AND INTRAOCULAR LENS
ADVANTAGES AND DISADVANTAGES

> Aphakia is the first complication
> of cataract extraction.
> after F. H. THEODORE, 1964

This chapter deals with the various optical ways of correcting aphakia, with special reference to aniseikonia (Appendix).

Aphakia may be corrected by one of the following methods:
1. A lens in front of the eye: the spectacle lens.
2. A lens in contact with the eye: the contact lens.
3. A lens inside the eye: the intraocular lens.

1   SPECTACLE LENS

Since the 17th century, the spectacle lens has fulfilled the needs of many millions of aphakic patients. More and more, however, are becoming dissatisfied with this solution, partly because of the growing demand for greater physiological perception, and partly because a later operating age implies diminishing ability to adapt to the optical errors inherent in the use of an optical aid in front of the eye.

The critical patient's point of view has been advanced by two ophthalmologists who have themselves undergone bilateral cataract extraction:

a.   briefly by MCLEMORE (1965), who says: 'an ophthalmologist giving his patients cataract spectacles, is creating visual invalids'.

b.   at length, by WOODS in 'The adjustment to aphakia' (WOODS, 1952). The most important disadvantages mentioned by WOODS, are:

1.   the astonishing increase in the size of familiar objects;

2.   diplopia in monocular aphakia, rendering binocular vision impossible until the second eye has been operated upon;

3.   lack of co-ordination between eye and hand due to the new visual imagery created by false spatial orientation which is even present in bilateral aphakia. Everything seems much closer than before. This can be overcome after several weeks of constant exercise and adjustment. During this period tumblers are overturned, ink is spilled and similar minor domestic tragedies occur;

4.   all straight lines are transformed into curves: the world becomes parabolic, and ocular movement causes this parabolic world to squirm like a writhing snake. This can be overcome by the simple trick of holding the eyes still, the gaze fixed through the optical centres of the correcting lenses, while moving the head slowly to look at a new object;

5.   a portion of the peripheral visual field, from about 35 to 55 degrees, depending on the size of the spectacle lens, is blotted out (area b in Fig. 1);

in addition, objects observed in the peripheral field may disappear if the gaze is moved towards them. This is particularly tiresome at distances between 0.5 and 3 m: 'faces and objects pop in and out of the blind area with the annoying insolence of a jack-in-the-box, leading to constant collision with chairs or individuals. This social handicap cannot be cured, it must be endured.'

The optical causes of these complaints are:

re 1, 2, 3   image magnification: about 25%.

re 4   spherical aberration giving rise to blurring of the periphery of the image, and pincushion distortion. Moreover, this distortion is asymmetrical if the eye is not looking through the optical centre of the correcting lens. Both can be partially rectified by an aspherical spectacle lens.

re 5 a   ring scotoma inherent in high dioptre convex lenses and causing the Jack-in-the-box phenomenon of moving objects (area b in Fig. 1).

re 5 b   roving ring scotoma (WELSH phenomenon), i.e. an aperture scotoma elicited by the movement of the eye, especially of the nodal point, behind an aperture of absolute limits, resulting in the apparent jumping of an object from

2

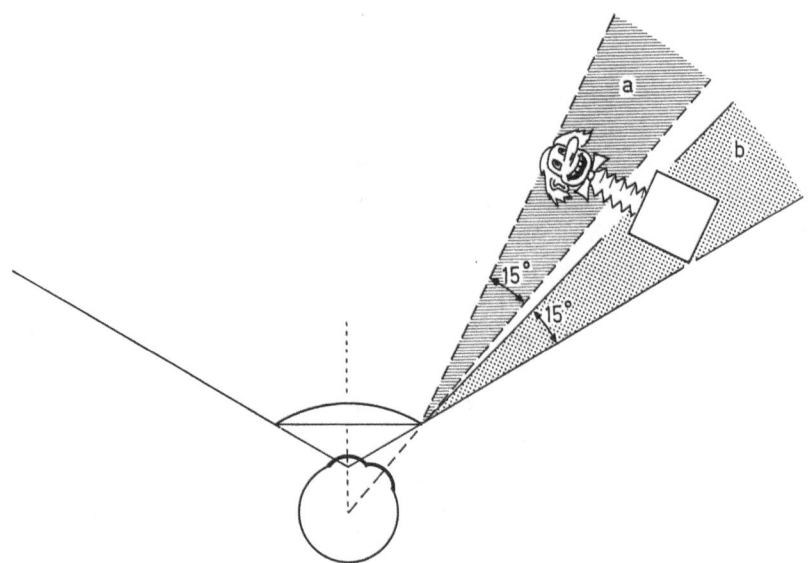

Fig. 1   (After R. C. WELSH, 1961b)

The roving ring scotoma with its Jack-in-the-box phenomenon of high positive spectacle lenses (spheric or aspheric). Area b is the ring scotoma of a spectacle corrected aphakic eye fixing centrally: Jack is observed with peripheral vision. If the eye turns towards Jack he is hidden in the area a: the ring scotoma has moved towards the centre.

one edge of the scotoma to the other which is caused by the refraction of rays passing through the edge of a powerful convex lens. This is the Jack-in-the-box phenomenon caused by the moving of the eye (WELSH, 1961b). See Fig. 1. 'It is obviously the eye rather than the scotoma which does the roving' (LINKSZ, 1964).

Thus it seems that adjustment to aphakia is not as easy as ophthalmologists often think. That may be the reason why patients with unilateral aphakia frequently prefer to use the fellow-eye, especially for distance vision, even if this eye has a less visual acuity (RIDLEY, 1951, 1952abc, 1953b, 1954; SLOANE, 1962), or even is actually amblyopic (see case F 1 on page 136).

According to COLENBRANDER the best solution in case of anisometropia of x dioptres is the full correction of the one eye and a modification of the correction of the fellow-eye by $\frac{1}{2}(x - 1)$ dioptres (COLENBRANDER, 1971).

Ophthalmologists who wish to obtain some insight into spectacle-corrected aphakic vision might like to try WELSH's suggestion and simulate aphakia by means of a combination of a contact lens of –14 D and a spectacle lens of +12 D (WELSH, 1965). The unadjusted binocular experience of this author during a long-lasting hour remains ineffable in his memory.

3

A contact lens for the correction of unilateral aphakia was first used by LITTLE in 1933 (cit. TROUTMAN, 1962a). Many disadvantages inherent in spectacle lenses do not exist with contact lenses (LINKSZ, 1964):

1. no significant magnification (only about 7%);
2. no appreciable spherical aberration: no pincushion distortion;
3. no ring scotoma: no Jack-in-the-box phenomenon and no roving ring scotoma, and therefore full peripheral vision.

Consequently, the contact lens gives hardly any false spatial orientation. Moreover, it is relatively safe since, in contrast to an intraocular lens, it can be removed if necessary. It is especially useful in cases of astigmatism caused by superficial corneal scarring (VAN BALEN, 1970, 1972a in the discussion; BINK-HORST & GOBIN, 1964ab, 1967d). The reduced corneal sensitivity in aphakia favours the tolerance by the cornea of a contact lens but is also dangerous, as it fails to warn the wearer of an impending complication.

The contact lens, however, has some disadvantages. These may be divided into:

a. general disadvantages as set out in the appropriate textbooks, and
b. those specifically related to aphakia:

1. Very few elderly aphakic patients possess the dexterity to insert or remove contact lenses and the perseverance to continue wearing them (RIDLEY, 1951, 1952abc, 1953a, 1958).

By chance, the author witnessed a case reported by BINKHORST (1962a). Having had one iris clip lens fitted, the patient was given the choice of another iris clip lens or a contact lens for his other aphakic eye: after prolonged trial of a contact lens the patient remarked: 'Just do it in the old-fashioned way, doctor!'

2. Very few children are able to wear contact lenses. As a rule, therefore, a contact lens does not prevent the loss of binocular vision in children with unilateral traumatic aphakia (BINKHORST & GOBIN, 1967d, 1969a in the discussion).

VAN BALEN (1970, 1972a) found that only 3 out of 15 unilaterally aphakic children under the age of 14 could be treated adequately with a contact lens.

BINKHORST & GOBIN (1967d) reported on the fitting of 10 out of 22 unilaterally aphakic children with contact lenses: suppression or diplopia developed in all cases (see also CHOYCE, 1959, 1960; BINKHORST & GOBIN, 1964ab; BINKHORST, GOBIN & LÉONARD, 1969bcd; BIERLAAGH, VAN DER WEE, KATS, LÉONARD & BINK-HORST, 1971).

3. A strong positive, i.e. a relatively heavy contact lens, may easily decentre downwards giving rise to a prismatic effect which might impair fusion (BINK-HORST, 1964ab; VAN BALEN, 1973).

4. When both eyes are aphakic or when the only useful eye is aphakic, even a patient with a well-fitting contact lens needs spectacles at some time – for example, to go to the bathroom at night or to find his contact lens(es) (WELSH, 1961a; MANN, 1961; MCLEMORE, 1963; LINKSZ, 1964).

5. The motivation of the unilaterally aphakic patient to keep wearing a contact lens is not always sufficiently strong and such motivation (MANN, 1961), as anyone who has prescribed contact lenses for teenage girls knows, is absolutely vital: once married, they tend to give up wearing them. However, there is an important difference between this category and aphakics: the eyes of young ladies can be better seen, and the aphakic eye can see better. Thus, practical experience reveals that the restoration of binocular vision is not the strongest motivation (see also below).

DIJKSTRA et al. (1958, page 29) found that only 12 out of 1100 (1.1 %) unilaterally traumatic aphakics were wearing a contact lens longer than 6 hours a day.

BONNET, GERHARD & MASSIN (1966) found that after 10 years 68 % of 308 unilateral aphakics had abandoned their contact lens (see Fig. 2). The reasons for abandoning them were diplopia (61 %), local irritation (31 %) and complications related to previous trauma or surgery (8 %). There was, statistically, no significant difference between traumatic and non-traumatic aphakics.

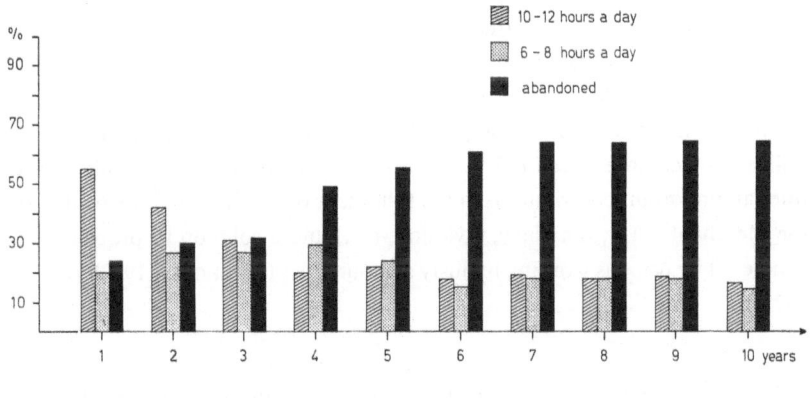

Fig. 2

Periods during which contact lenses were worn in 308 unilateral aphakics. Observation period 10 years. (From BONNET, GERHARD & MASSIN, 1966, page 166).

Many of the disadvantages associated with contact lenses (see page 4) do not apply to the intraocular lens. The advantages are mainly the same as those of contact lenses. To these should be added:

1.   An intraocular lens produces even less change in the size of the image, and, consequently, the maintenance of the binocular function is less difficult.

GIRARD, BINKHORST, GOBIN et al. (1962) compared 30 unilaterally aphakic adult patients wearing a contact lens (average age 49.6 years) with 30 unilaterally aphakic adult patients having an intraocular lens, in fact, an iris clip lens. Their average age was 67.7 years. A similar distribution of refractive errors and an average visual acuity of the operated eyes of 0.8 was found in both groups. On examination with the AO Space Eikonometer, the operated eye, as compared with its fellow eye, showed an average retinal image size increase of 6.99% (range 2–12%) in the group wearing a contact lens, and an average decrease of 0.20% in the group wearing an iris clip lens*.

Using the WIRT stereopsis test, the contact lens group showed an average of 45.7% WIRT stereopsis and the iris clip lens group an average of 81.8% (BINK-HORST & GOBIN, 1964ab). An additional handicap for the iris clip lens group was its age: the members of this group were, on average, 18.1 years older than those of the other group (VAN BALEN, 1970, 1973).

2.   An intraocular lens can be used at any age. With up-to-date techniques, no after-care is required. Instillation of pilocarpine hydrochloride 2% is only necessary in iris clip lens cases without a suture around the superior loops or through the iris. Bearing in mind the almost insurmountable difficulties with contact lenses in children (see page 4), *the intraocular lens in unilaterally aphakic children has made amblyopia prevention much easier, and has even made restoration of their binocular vision possible.*

3.   Since an intraocular lens is permanently present, it cannot be lost, and, unlike contact lenses, need not be removed before going to sleep. This constitutes an important contribution to the fulfilment of statutory requirements (for the Merchant Navy, the Navy, Aviation, etc.) and a solution to problems encountered by persons working in dusty surroundings (BINKHORST, 1959b, 1962a, 1972e).

---

* The original figure of 1.92% aniseikonia (GIRARD, BINKHORST, GOBIN et al., 1962) was later corrected by COLENBRANDER to 0.20% minification (BINKHORST & GOBIN, 1964ab). The difficulty arose over computing the average of cases with magnification and of cases with minification.

Disadvantages of intraocular lens types associated with complications related to the implant or the surgical techniques will be discussed extensively in Chapters II and III.

APPENDIX

ANISEIKONIA

A very important difference between the use of spectacle lens, contact lens and intraocular lens in connection with cases of unilateral aphakia is the average amount of aniseikonia produced.

The central question is the degree of aniseikonia with which binocular vision is still possible. Most authors consider 5–8% to be the limit (OGLE et al., 1958; LINKSZ, 1959; CHOYCE, 1961b; TROUTMAN, 1962a; CRONE & LEURIDAN, 1973ab).

OGLE et al. (1958) suggest that 1% aniseikonia may give rise to symptoms, and calculated that it was theoretically impossible to achieve binocular vision in the presence of aniseikonia of more than 5%.

LINKSZ (1959) found imperfect binocular vision in aniseikonia of 5% and more, and eye strain in cases exhibiting a lower percentage.

CHOYCE (1961b, 1964) studied people without aniseikonia after fitting them with iseikonic lenses. They did not notice aniseikonia of up to about 5%, but over 5% aniseikonia started to elicit complaints. Most of them agreed that 7 or 8% was the limit of tolerance.

TROUTMAN (1962a, 1963a) stated that aniseikonia within the range of 1 to 5% produces faulty spatial localisation and constriction of the field of stereopsis in everyday surroundings.

CRONE & LEURIDAN (1973ab), having found that cyclofusion and aniseikonia make the same demands on binocular vision, determined the range of cyclofusion by means of the synoptophore for 8 normal subjects. The limit of tolerance was found to lie between 5 and 8%.

Within this limit, however, the patient may be subject to considerable eye strain due to the efforts made to maintain simultaneous perception, fusion and stereopsis (LINKSZ, 1959).

Differences between spectacle lens, contact lens and intraocular lens in unilateral aphakia

1. Patients wearing a *spectacle lens* may be dissatisfied (see page 2) but their complaint is not due to aniseikonia, the degree of which is too large (approx. 25%) for fusional effort to have any chance of success.

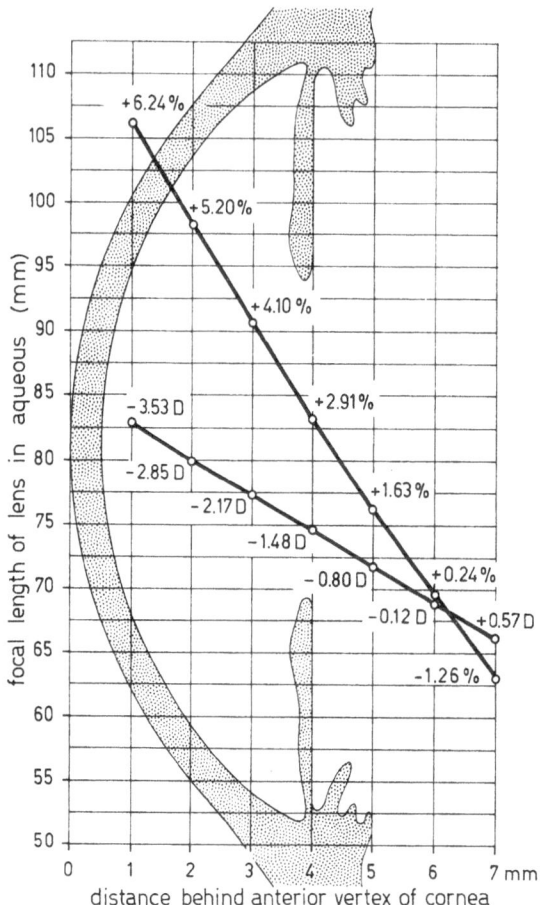

Fig. 3

Relationship in the schematic eye between the location of an infinitely thin intraocular lens producing emmetropia resp. iseikonia, its focal length in aqueous, and the size of the image resp. the refractive error in the anterior focal plane. In this drawing the emmetropic line shows at 1 mm behind the anterior vertex of the cornea an image magnification of 6.24%. The iseikonic line shows at 1 mm behind the anterior vertex of the cornea a myopia of –3.53 dioptres in the anterior focal plane (Courtesy R. C. TROUTMAN M.D.).

2. Patients wearing a *contact lens* exhibit aniseikonia of 2–12% (GIRARD, BINKHORST, GOBIN et al., 1962), with or without binocular vision. The percentage of aniseikonia depends largely on the pre-operative state of refraction. Conditions for the elimination of aniseikonia by means of a contact lens correction are most favourable in eyes with a pre-operative axial hyperopia of over 4 D or so (OGLE et al., 1958).

3. Theoretically, patients fitted with an *intraocular lens* stand the best chance of having iseikonia. In practice however, this depends on the dioptric power and the position of the implant in the eye as well as on the pre-operative retinal image size in each eye of the patient. TROUTMAN (1962a, 1963a) calculated for GULLSTRAND's schematic (aphakic) eye the relationship between the location of an infinitely thin intraocular lens producing emmetropia, its focal length in aqueous and the size of the image (the emmetropic line in Fig. 3). He also calculated this relationship for an infinitely thin intraocular lens producing iseikonia, its focal length in aqueous as well as the refractive error in the anterior focal plane (the iseikonic line in Fig. 3).

Emmetropia and iseikonia are only present at the point of intersection of both lines, i.e. at the point 6.2 mm behind the anterior vertex of the cornea where the second principal point of the crystalline lens is situated. Any other point along these lines gives either emmetropia *or* iseikonia. Any point not situated on either line gives ametropia *and* aniseikonia (as compared with GULLSTRAND's schematic *phakic* eye).

CHOYCE was the first to publish a report about residual aniseikonia after introduction of an anterior chamber implant, a CHOYCE Mark I (see page 22), for the correction of unilateral aphakia. Using the AO Space Eikonometer in 35 patients (CHOYCE, 1961b) and, later, in 70 patients (CHOYCE, 1964), which showed consistent readings, he found an average aniseikonia of 2% (range 0 to 9%) with an average residual anisometropia of –0.45 D (ranging from –1.25 to + 1.00 D). For his Mark VIII (see page 22) the average aniseikonia dropped to zero (CHOYCE, 1966b).

TROUTMAN (1962a, 1963a) measured the average amount of aniseikonia with the AO Space Eikonometer for the intraocular lenses in use in 1961: the RIDLEY lens, various types of rigid angle-fixated anterior chamber lenses, the DANNHEIM type lenses and BINKHORST's iris clip lens. His findings are tabulated below.

The measurements of GIRARD, BINKHORST, GOBIN et al. (1962) on 30 iris clip lens patients were mentioned on page 6. Their findings (average minification 0.20%) differ from those of TROUTMAN (average magnification 1.52%). This is due to differences in computation (see footnote on page 6).

	number	aniseikonia (%)			anisometropia (D)		
		lower limit	average	upper limit	lower limit	average	upper limit
1. RIDLEY lens	15	−7.00	− 2.84	+1.00	−5.75	−2.86	− 0.75
2. rigid angle-fixated anterior chamber lenses (various types)	14	−1.25	+1.96	+5.00	−5.00	−0.55	+3.00
3. DANNHEIM type lenses	6	−1.00	+2.17	+4.25	−2.75	−0.37	+1.75
4. BINKHORST's iris clip lens	21	−4.00	+1.52	+6.00	−3.75	−0.81	+3.00

Negative aniseikonia = magnification required for pseudophakic eye (= eye with lens implant).
Positive aniseikonia = magnification required for fellow-eye.

Planned iseikonia

As large as life and quite as natural.

The amount of residual aniseikonia produced by an intraocular lens of standard power for a given age group depends on the eye's individual deviation from the average power of the crystalline lenses of that group upon which the standard power of the artificial lens has been based.

STENSTRÖM (1946) found an average dioptric power of the crystalline lens of +17.35 D for 1000 eyes in the age group of 20 to 35 years.

GERNET & OSTHOLT (1973) calculated an average dioptric power of the crystalline lens of about +41 D for 66 eyes of newly born babies, of +32.2 D for 15 eyes of one year old children, and of +23.7 D for 446 adult eyes (age not mentioned).

BINKHORST determined empirically the following powers for the iris clip lens and its modifications (BINKHORST, 1972ab, 1973):

1 – 3 years	+22.5 D
3 – 10 years	20.5 D
10 – 20 years	19 D
20 – 35 years	18 D
35 – 50 years	19 D
> 50 years	19.5 D

These figures require further confirmation (BINKHORST, pers. comm.). They 'were meant to make the eye one to two dioptres myopic as compared with the fellow-eye since this was supposed to be the ideal situation in order to obtain as good an iseikonia as possible' (BINKHORST, 1973). This supposition was based on calculations for GULLSTRAND's schematic iseikonic pseudophakic eye: it has a myopia of 1.69 D at the anterior focal point (BINKHORST, 1972a). The difference between the values of GERNET & OSTHOLT, and of BINKHORST may be explained by the difference in the position in the eye of the crystalline lens and of the iris clip lens.

The advantage of implants of standard power is that ultrasonographic equipment need not be used to calculate the power of the lens. However, individually-planned iseikonia is indicated in cases where the standard power implant would fail to achieve iseikonia.

In recent years it has become possible to *aim* at iseikonia in the individual case by using exact clinical oculometry of both eyes to determine the implant power required.

The oculometric data necessary for calculating the implant power that would produce iseikonia, are:

a.   refractive power of the cornea. This can be determined by means of keratometry.

b.   axial length. This can be determined from ultrasonographic measurements.

c.   post-implant anterior chamber depth (in case of the iris-fixated lens implants). This can only be estimated from the pre-operative anterior chamber depth and the thickness of the crystalline lens. Extraction of a thick lens may increase the anterior chamber depth by 1 mm or more (GERNET, OSTHOLT & WERNER, 1971a).

d.   refractive power of cornea and crystalline lens as well as the axial length of the fellow-eye.

In 1969, at BINKHORST's request and using the above parameters, COLEN-BRANDER (1973) developed the following formula for calculating the implant power that would produce *emmetropia*:

$$D_L = \frac{1.336}{L - v - 0.000\ 052} - \frac{1.336}{\dfrac{1.336}{D_c} - v - 0.000\ 05}$$

where

D_L = equivalent refractive power in air of the Lens implant measured in Dioptres

L = axial Length measured in metres

v = Vertex distance of implant measured in metres

D_c = refractive power of Cornea measured in Dioptres

On the basis of this formula BINKHORST produced a diagram (BINKHORST, 1972b, 1973) from which, for a value of v = 0.0035 m (= 3.5 mm), the emmetropia-giving implant power may be read for every combination of D_c and L.

For every +/- 0.0003 m (= +/- 0.3 mm) difference in v, the implant power should be modified by +/- 0.5 D. In addition, a slight increase in power seems to be justified in view of a possible post-operative flattening of the cornea for which the surgeon and the techniques used may be responsible (BINKHORST, 1972a).

The whole procedure of planned implant power is subject to errors in calculation, keratometry, predicted anterior chamber depth, effect of surgery on corneal power, and the ultrasonographic determination of the axial length.

This is another reason for aiming at a slight myopia instead of emmetropia: the hypermetropic part of the post-implant refractive error distribution, useless in an eye without accommodation, is then eliminated. This can also be read from the diagram by adjusting the corneal parameter to include the required residual spectacle correction.

The *iseikonia*-giving implant power can also be read from BINKHORST's diagram. It is then a matter of equating the posterior focal length of the uncorrected pseudophakic eye with that of its uncorrected fellow eye.

In bilateral implants the surgeon has the additional freedom of making the second eye iseikonic *and* introducing 1 to 3 D of myopia in one or both eyes, e.g. for people who do a lot of close work.

For the evaluation of the results of planned iseikonia it should be borne in mind that, as time goes by, even iseikonia in unilateral pseudophakia may turn into aniseikonia due to swelling of the crystalline lens at an early stage of cataract formation, associated with increasing myopia (BINKHORST, 1972a).

SUMMARY

1. Spectacle lenses for the correction of aphakia have considerable disadvantages. Optically they are only adequate for vision along the optical axis, and consequently, the patient tries to look along the optical axis by turning his head instead of his eyes. Image magnification and ring scotoma, however, cannot be overcome and blurring of the periphery of the image only partially.

Binocular vision can only be present in binocular aphakics.

2. The contact lens has far better optical properties than the spectacle lens. Irregular corneal astigmatism is a strong indication.

Binocular vision is reportedly present in unilateral aphakics with an average of 46% WIRT stereopsis. However, successful use does not last in children, and decreases in adults over the years, especially in unilateral aphakics.

3. The intraocular lens has the best optical properties. It has rendered amblyopia prevention much easier in unilateral aphakic children, and has even made it possible to restore binocular vision.

Binocular vision is present in unilateral aphakics with an average of 82% WIRT stereopsis.

Iseikonia or only minimal aniseikonia may be achieved with a standard power implant lens or, in special cases, with an implant of individually-computed power.

We may thus conclude that, compared with the spectacle lens and the contact lens, the intraocular lens offers far the best theoretical and practical possibilities for both the optical correction of aphakia and the restoration of binocular vision.

CHAPTER II

HISTORY OF INTRAOCULAR LENS IMPLANTS

Quod natura relinquit imperfectum, ars perficit.

The history of intraocular lens implants can be divided into the following sections depending on the method of fixation, namely in the

A. posterior chamber
B. anterior chamber
   1. with angle-fixation
   2. with iris and/or capsular fixation

A POSTERIOR CHAMBER LENS OF RIDLEY

In the autumn of 1949 a Spirit of our Time placed an undergraduate student in the operating theatre of Harold RIDLEY (1951, 1952b) at St. Thomas's Hospital, London. This unknown student, seeing that RIDLEY was closing the wound after an intracapsular cataract extraction, exclaimed that he had forgotten to replace the diseased lens by a new one.

When destiny is ripe, few words are needed: this question inspired RIDLEY to consider the possibility of using an intraocular lens for the correction of aphakia.

The concept of an intraocular lens had occurred before. TAIEB (1955), MÜNCHOW (1964), and ASCHER (1965) found that CASANOVA (1725–1798) had referred in his memoirs to the Italian 'oculist' TADINI who had mentioned to him the idea of implanting an artificial lens after a cataract operation, in 1764/1765. It is fairly certain that CASANOVA passed on the idea to the Dresden court ophthalmologist CASAAMATA ($\pm$ 1742–1807) after 1774. Around 1795 SCHIFERLI saw CASAAMATA try to introduce a glass lens into the eye after a cataract operation: the lens immediately slid back towards the fundus of the eye.

The English ophthalmologist FOSTER (1940, cit. RIDLEY, 1951) wrote a fantasy about an intraocular glass lens replacing a cataractous lens. In this story 'An Englishman would wake up one morning with this idea but drop it because it had never been considered at Moorfields and the boy's school bill was due next week'. Three Americans, however, MCCLUSKY, ZINZINHEIMER and O'HARA, with large financial resources, produced after years of research a paper showing that, except for a limited period, the idea was impracticable. These invented names were considered completely seriously by both SCHRECK (1958a) and MÜNCHOW (1964)!

STRAMPELLI (1962) mentioned the unpublished fruitless attempts of MARCHI (1940) to fixate quartz lenses with platinum wires in the anterior chambers of animals.

14

RIDLEY (1951, 1952abc, 1953ab, 1954) made a biconvex perspex lens of about the same shape as the normal human lens. The diameter, however, was 8.35 mm, approximately 1 mm smaller than the normal human lens, to facilitate insertion and avoid undue pressure on the ciliary body.

Its weight in air was 112 mg.

With this lens RIDLEY carried out the first implant operation on 29th November 1949 after a short period of preparation. Following an extracapsular cataract operation under local anaesthesia without any sutures having been used, it was fitted in the posterior chamber of the left eye of a 45-year old female patient. Unfortunately the patient became rather myopic: visual acuity was 6/18 with – 18.00 DS / – 6.00 DC × 120. This was due to an error in the optical calculation. The second implant operation on 23rd August 1950 led to a similar result. Appropriate changes were made in the design (see Fig. 4). This lens could only be used after extracapsular extraction, and the operation had to be carried out as a one-stage procedure, because adhesions developing between the iris and the posterior capsule would otherwise have prevented insertion (RIDLEY, 1952a; CHOYCE, 1964).

After RIDLEY's first report at the Oxford Ophthalmological Congress in July 1951, many ophthalmic surgeons followed his example, some with good results initially (among others ARRUGA, BARRAQUER, EPSTEIN, PAUFIQUE and REESE) and some with less favourable results (among others FRANÇOIS, JONKERS and WEVE).

The many disappointing results were largely due to unsuitable preparation and techniques. However, this does not apply to all the surgeons mentioned above (BINKHORST, 1956a, 1957).

EPSTEIN (1957) inserted 84 RIDLEY lenses between November 1951 and December 1955. The complications encountered were: severe hyphaema (6), downward decentration (many cases), anterior dislocation (5), and posterior dislocation (2).

Needling of an 'anterior occlusio pupillae membrane' was necessary in 15 cases and of a posterior membrane in 24 cases. He suggested a flattened form of the implant to facilitate centration (EPSTEIN, 1957, 1959).

BINKHORST (1956a, 1957) studied RIDLEY's method in London. *He noted the contaminated state in which the lenses were delivered by the manufacturer, and the use of potentially dangerous disinfectants.*

He suggested several improvements, e.g. the thorough cleansing of the implants and the use of ultra-violet radiation to sterilise them (BINKHORST & FLU, 1956b; BINKHORST, 1956a, 1957). He inserted 16 of these lenses between 31st October 1955 and 18th January 1957. One eye was lost, due to an accidental infection. After 21–36 months, 10 out of 13 eyes had a visual acuity of 6/12 and over, and 12 performed well on the Worth four dot test (BINKHORST, 1959b). Nevertheless, BINKHORST (1959a) came to the conclusion 'that this technique is too much of a strain on the surgeon and especially

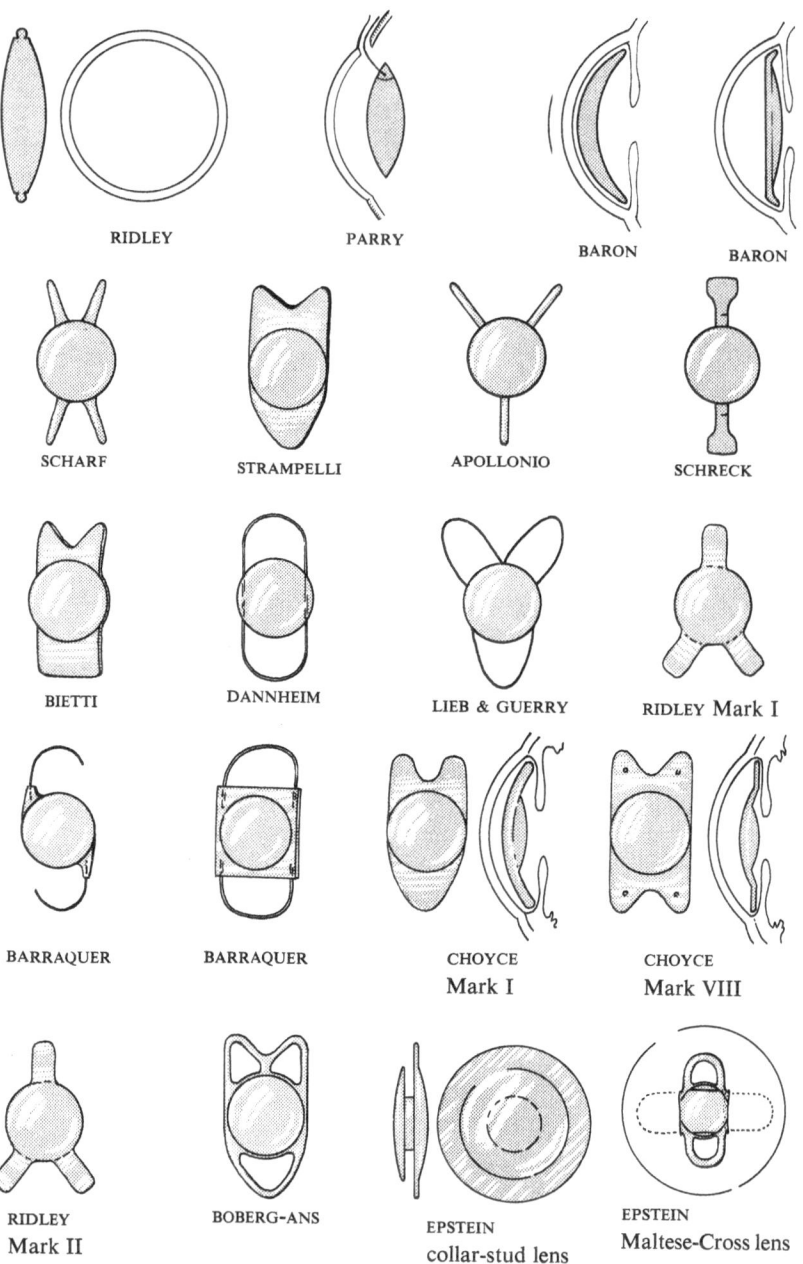

Fig. 4

Posterior chamber and anterior chamber lenses, as discussed in this chapter.

that it is asking too much of the human hand never to fail in completely sparing the delicate suspension system of the zonule and posterior capsule'.

RIDLEY himself primarily inserted 'approximately 1000 of these lenses, and many of his cases are still successful today' (CHOYCE, 1966a).

The RIDLEY lens procedure, however, has been abandoned completely in view of the number and frequency of the complications that occurred.

These complications, summarized by RIDLEY (1953b, 1954, 1958, 1960), were:
1. some degree of iritis, due mainly to residual lens material in the eye, and partly to inadequate removal of implant sterilizing solution.
2. occlusion of the pupil by a dense inflammatory membrane.
3. late thickening of the posterior capsule in young subjects whose lens cells were still in a state of active growth necessitating a technically most difficult needling (GUERRY, 1960).
4. loss of the anterior chamber for reasons unknown.
5. secondary glaucoma due to shallowness of the anterior chamber and a narrow filtration angle.
6. iris atrophy from pressure by the rim of a badly-centred lens was a late complication that might lead to anterior dislocation.
7. posterior dislocation, occurring in about 6% of cases, was a major catastrophe. Intracapsular extraction and attacks of coughing were especially dangerous in this respect.
   PARRY (1954) tried to anchor the RIDLEY lens by means of a tantalum thread with the ends left loose beneath the conjunctiva (see Fig. 4).
8. extraction of the implant was necessary in 15% of cases (RIDLEY pers. comm. to WORST, March 1970).

B ANTERIOR CHAMBER LENSES

1 *Anterior chamber lenses with angle-fixation*

The technical difficulties and complications associated with the RIDLEY lens led to the positioning of the artificial lens in the eye being changed. The place first chosen was the anterior chamber, the chamber angle being used for fixation purposes. There are several advantages:

1. implantation may be performed after both intracapsular and extracapsular cataract extraction.

2. secondary implantation may be performed. This has several advantages, such as the pre-implant knowledge of the refraction, visual acuity, pupillary function, as well as the possibility of examining the media and fundus.

3. dislocation, due to disintegration of the supramide of DANNHEIM's lenses, may occur but remains exceptional (see page 127).

While the development of the posterior chamber lens had been the work of one man using one model, anterior chamber lenses were designed by many investigators using many variations on the angle-fixation theme. The first designs (see Fig. 4) were put into practice by BARON, SCHARF, STRAMPELLI, APOLLONIO, SCHRECK, BIETTI, DANNHEIM, LIEB & GUERRY, BARRAQUER and RIDLEY.

BARON (1953) was the first to implant an anterior chamber lens, on 13th May 1952. It had the shape of a bent disc, bent towards the cornea to such an extent that it came into contact with the corneal endothelium (see Fig. 4). This resulted in corneal dystrophy. BARON (1954) tried without success to avoid these corneal lesions, using various models including one with a square section.

On 26th September 1953 SCHARF (1956, 1957) implanted the first anterior chamber lens of his own design in the shape of a shark's egg (see Fig. 4). During the discussion following the demonstration of 5 of SCHARF's patients on 5th December 1954, HALLERMAN predicted that corneal dystrophy would be the major complication with anterior chamber lenses of the angle-fixation type.

Moreover, even at that early stage one could notice the blemish that would mar so many discussions on artificial lenses: objections are voiced about a certain lens while the lens actually under discussion is quite a different one. This confusion of different types of lenses during discussion and in processes of thought has remained to the present day.

On 28th September 1953 STRAMPELLI (1954, 1955) implanted the first anterior chamber lens of his own design in the form of a meniscus ending in a dovetail (see Fig. 4). He made the first announcement about his experiences at the Congress of the Societas Lombardo di Oftalmologica in Pavia on 8th December 1953. This was the first public report about anterior chamber lenses. At the same time he demonstrated three of his patients.

At the same meeting APOLLONIO (cit. STRAMPELLI, 1962) also demonstrated three patients fitted with an anterior chamber lens of his own tripod type (see Fig. 4). Later he reduced the curvature and lengthened the supports in order to overcome post-operative torsion and dislocation. From 1st July 1954 onwards, BARRAQUER (1956, 1958, 1962) carried out 342 implant operations employing the STRAMPELLI lens, part of these in phakic eyes suffering from high myopia. He stressed the importance of the implant having an optimal length, minimal weight, and a radius which would avoid contact with DESCEMET's membrane and the iris.

After trials on animal eyes, and human eyes that were to be enucleated, SCHRECK (1954, 1955, 1956ab, 1958 ab) constructed a bipod lens having wider ends and a radius of 10 mm (see Fig. 4). With this lens he carried out several hundred implants in a relatively short time.

BIETTI (1955) commenced his work using a quadripod lens similar to that of APOLLONIO. He continued with STRAMPELLI-like lenses (see Fig. 4) but, in 1958, after 20 implant operations he discontinued that work pending further clarification of the problem of endothelial contact (GUERRY, 1960).

Since 1952 DANNHEIM (1956) tried to solve the problem of centring the lens in the anterior chamber (see below) by means of elastic supporting loops of 0.1 mm supramide thread. These stabilise the optical portion by means of pressure in the chamber angle (see Fig. 4).

After experiments on the eyes of dogs, LIEB & GUERRY (1957) implanted 40 lenses (GUERRY & GEERAETS, 1962). They closely resembled DANNHEIM lenses but the supramide loops were affixed tangentially by means of peripheral grooves, thus sparing a greater area of the refracting lens surface. If necessary the loops were made slightly curved, and the optical portion was made convex-concave (see Fig. 4).

BARRAQUER (1962) modified the DANNHEIM lens by cutting away half the loops, thus giving them an S-shape (see Fig. 4). In another modification he reduced the loops by enlarging the optical portion (see Fig. 4). It was thought that this would decrease the danger of forward displacement of the optical portion.

CHOYCE (1960) stated the following objections against the DANNHEIM lens and its variations:
1. the danger of irritation from the supramide.
2. the danger of the lens constituents coming apart.
3. the uncertainty of its actual position in the eye for the purpose of optical calculations.

RIDLEY (1957) made a one-piece tripod lens in the form of an inverted Y (Mark I) (see Fig. 4).

The length of the implant is of the utmost importance when fitting angle-fixated lenses.

Too large a lens produces deformation of the pupil by pushing the iris up, a slight hypotony due to the small goniodialysis, a retarded disappearance of loose pigment and, finally, corneal dystrophy (BARRAQUER, 1956, 1962; SCHRECK, 1958ab).

Too small a lens leads to decentring during eye movements causing irritation of the ciliary body and the angle structures. This results in goniosynechiae, secondary glaucoma and corneal dystrophy (CHOYCE, 1958; SCHRECK, 1958ab; BARRAQUER, 1962).

Different rules of thumb have been suggested for the accurate determination of the implant's total length. This, however, is a very difficult matter.

		corneal diameter	
RIDLEY	1957	vertical	+ 0.5 mm
STRAMPELLI	1958a	horizontal	+ 2.0 mm
		(to make an intentional goniodialysis with the haptic!)	
SCHRECK	1958ab	horizontal	+ 0.25 to 0.75 mm
CHOYCE	1958	horizontal	+ 1.0 mm
RIDLEY	1960	horizontal	+ 1.0 to 1.25 mm
CAUDELL	1962	a) horizontal	+ 1.0 mm
		b) measurement of the iridic angle diameter after transillumination of the sclera (BARRAQUER, 1956).	

1*The first reports of complications*

pn May 1958, in Paris, STRAMPELLI gave an extensive review of all possible comlications during surgery as well as early and late complications after surgery (27 items!). Out of 500 cases he had 25 failures (STRAMPELLI, 1958a).

In September 1958, in Brussels, he added that during recent months a new type of late complication had presented itself: after five years' quiescence, two-thirds of the eyes operated upon in 1953 now showed bullous keratitis. Following late necrosis due to compression of an extreme peripheral part of DESCEMET's membrane, imbibition occurred due to infiltration of aqueous into the corneal parenchyma. This led to endothelial corneal dystrophy (ECD). He suggested various ways of preventing ECD, by modifying the haptic portion which was the cause of the trouble.

These modifications were:
1. making the blunted ends come to rest against the sclera by means of an inverted cyclodialysis, i.e. without any contact at all with the cornea or with the trabecular meshwork.
2. the use of DANNHEIM loops. However, these may also cause ECD unless they are of the correct length.
3. external fixation by means of supramide loops perforating the corneo-scleral limbus and fixated subconjunctivally (STRAMPELLI, 1957, 1958b, 1961, 1962).* See Fig. 5.

The first lens with external fixation was described by STRAMPELLI in Madrid in 1956 (STRAMPELLI, 1957, 1961, 1963, 1968). The implant had a 5 mm diameter optic portion, and was suspended top and bottom by loops of 0.12 mm thick perlon. These perforated the sclera at 12 and 6 o'clock, and were buried subconjunctivally (see Fig. 5). The most difficult part of the operation was the determination of the correct amount of tension to be exerted on the loops before suturing (CHOYCE, 1964).
4. interposition of autoplastic auricular cartilage between the haptic ends and the trabecular meshwork.

* FEDOROV (1972) used fibres from the patient's Achilles tendon instead of supramide material.

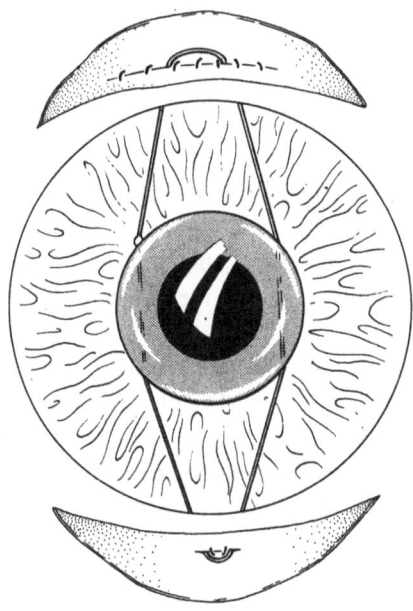

Fig. 5

Anterior chamber implant with external fixation (STRAMPELLI). The loop tips are buried subconjunctivally.

During the discussion with STRAMPELLI in Brussels in 1958 BINKHORST mentioned that he had seen corneal oedema 6 to 12 months post-operatively in 9 out of 35 cases fitted with an anterior chamber lens with rigid supports. These cases resisted all therapy (BINKHORST in the discussion with STRAMPELLI, STRAMPELLI, 1958b; BINKHORST, 1960ab).

On these grounds he warned against the further use of anterior chamber lenses with rigid supports in the chamber angle (BINKHORST in the discussion with STRAMPELLI, STRAMPELLI, 1958b; BINKHORST, 1959abc). According to him the corneal oedema must have been provoked by an intraocular traumatic insult, because

1. almost all patients had experienced sensitivity or pain in the eye at the slightest touch for months after the operation.

2. on histopathological examination, MANSCHOT found pressure atrophy in the chamber angle.

3. 4 out of the 9 cases showed trauma on the internal surface of the centre of the cornea in the form of a line-shaped scar parallel to the equator of the lens.

SCHRECK reported 12 extractions of his implant, out of 156 cases. Five of these were due to ECD (SCHRECK, 1958b). Later he reported 14 cases of ECD out of 178 (cit. KÜPER, 1962).

Later designs (see Fig. 4)

Since 1956 CHOYCE (1958, 1960, 1964, 1965, 1970ab) has designed eight modifications of the STRAMPELLI lens (see Fig. 4). These are known as CHOYCE anterior chamber implants, Marks I to VIII. The modifications apply mainly to the curvature of the optical portion and to the form of the feet and of the tips of the haptic portion.

Mark I (100 cases) caused intraocular iris prolapse in 8% of cases during the immediate post-operative period, and ECD in 22% after 13 years. Mark VIII (225 cases) produced no ECD and 95.5% were satisfactory up to 6 years afterwards or at death. CHOYCE (1970a) considered the Mark VIII lens to be 'the ultimate refinement of the STRAMPELLI concept upon which it is based'. An independent investigation of his patients has been carried out by PEARCE (to be published).

RIDLEY (1960, 1962) modified his Mark I into Mark II (see Fig. 4) as follows: it was made thinner, and the tips of the haptic legs were flattened in order to lessen the danger of pressure on the corneal periphery and to keep the lens close to, but just clear of, the iris.

He inserted 59 of these lenses between January 1960 and 1969, with only one case of ECD in an eye operated on in 1961 (RIDLEY, 1969).

BOBERG-ANS (1961, 1964b, 1965) modified the STRAMPELLI lens by fenestrating it (to avoid pupillary blockage), thus producing a rigid or semi-rigid fenestrated lens (see Fig. 4). The semi-rigid variety was, in turn, modified by BARRAQUER (BOBERG-ANS, 1964b, 1965).

Later reports of complications

BARRAQUER (in the discussion with STRAMPELLI, STRAMPELLI, 1958a) commenced implant operations on 1st July 1954 but discontinued them around 1960, having inserted 342 STRAMPELLI lenses, 140 DANNHEIM lenses, 9 BARRAQUER lenses, and 2 BOBERG-ANS lenses, after intracapsular or extracapsular extraction or in phakic eyes with high myopia. Details of these operations to be found in the literature, are:

25-11-1956 [1])	> 100 cases	0	ECD	0	implant extractions
31- 1-1959 [2])	411 cases	9	ECD	19	implant extractions
1- 5-1961 [3])	493 cases	30	ECD	55	implant extractions:
					37 STRAMPELLI lenses
					16 DANNHEIM lenses
					2 BARRAQUER lenses
1970 [4])	493 cases		approx.	250	implant extractions

[1]) BARRAQUER, 1956
[2]) GUERRY, 1960, KÜPER, 1962
[3]) BARRAQUER, 1962
[4]) BARRAQUER, pers. comm. 28-9-1973

BARRAQUER has now ceased implanting intraocular lenses entirely (pers. comm. 3–4–1971).

After 5 years KÜPER (1962) found one case of retinal detachment and 5 cases of ECD, out of 30 patients mostly suffering from traumatic cataract (26 SCHRECK lenses, 4 DANNHEIM lenses).

DANNHEIM (1962) mentioned incompatibility in about 5% of 650 DANNHEIM lens implants, ECD ranking highest amongst the causes.

GUERRY & GEERAETS (1962) examined 27 of the 40 original patients fitted 5 years previously with LIEB-GUERRY-type DANNHEIM lenses. No major complication had occurred. However, in 5 cases the optical lenticulus had tilted, presumably through loss of tensile strength and elasticity due to slow degradation of either the methylmethacrylate lenticulus, the supramide support, or both.

The CHOYCE anterior chamber implant Mark VIII is still in use today, but the other designs discussed above, have been abandoned: they were complete failures, mainly due to a high percentage of ECD. Like old soldiers, these lenses never died, they just faded away.

2. Anterior chamber lenses with iris fixation and/or capsular fixation

The next step in anterior chamber implant design was to avoid the chamber angle completely by fixation of the implant to the iris and, later on, to the capsular membrane, or to both.

EPSTEIN (1959) designed the 'collar-stud lens' (see Fig. 4), his own home-made modification of the RIDLEY lens with a deep equatorial groove as a safeguard against posterior dislocation. He inserted 24 of these lenses after June 1953 (15 after 1959). 'None of them developed ECD, but some developed glaucoma 8 to 12 years post-operatively, possibly by deposition of pigment in the trabecular system. In one case, however, the implant had to be removed because of a slight endothelial touch 17 days after implantation.' (EPSTEIN, pers. comm. 30–7–1971).

23

After an interlude with 24 anterior chamber implants (type not mentioned; 8 had to be removed due to imminent or manifest ECD), EPSTEIN (1962) proceeded with the one-piece Maltese-Cross lens, with iris cross fixation (see Fig. 4):

'a central optic portion is supported by four arms or limbs, two of which being solid lie behind the iris, and two fenestrated ones in front of it, so that the iris is gripped or clipped by the implant much more than by the iris clip lens.' (CHOYCE, 1964).

Since 1961 he has inserted 40 of these lenses. Three eyes developed ECD without any endothelial touch 4, 6, and 8 years respectively after implantation (EPSTEIN, pers. comm. 30–7–1971).

In the USA the same lens with all haptics solid, was called the COPELAND-BINKHORST* lens, and later the iris-plane lens. It has the shape of an aeroplane propeller.

---

* After R. D. BINKHORST, the younger brother of C. D. BINKHORST.

THE IRIS CLIP LENS

The iris clip lens was developed by BINKHORST in 1957 and was used for the first time on 11th August 1958 (case 1, page 89).

Up to 1st January 1972, approx. 2192 implant operations had been carried out by himself and other Dutch ophthalmic surgeons in the Netherlands alone.

BINKHORST arrived at this new design as a result of the sad records in the literature and by his own experience with 16 RIDLEY lenses (from 31-10-1955 to 18-1-1957), 35 angle-fixated lenses with rigid extremities (28-6-1956 to 31-10-1957) and (some of) 38 DANNHEIM lenses (28-11-1957 to 9-8-1962). He was the only Dutch ophthalmic surgeon who had experience with a variety of lens implants. Because of this background he was in a unique position to introduce a new development in lens implant design.

He proceeded on the basis of the following considerations:
1. acrylic material is well tolerated in the eye provided it has been properly cleansed and sterilised.
2. posterior chamber lenses have proved to have a strong tendency to dislocate.
3. most anterior chamber lenses with angle-fixation have a strong tendency to produce ECD.
4. the results with the RIDLEY lens indicate that contact of the implant with the posterior surface of the iris does not itself give rise to any complications (BINKHORST, 1959a, 1960a). Iris atrophy and its consequences (see page 17) are caused by uveitis, not by contact.
5. the results with the DANNHEIM lens indicate that contact of the implant with the anterior surface of the iris does not do any harm to the eye either (BINKHORST, 1959a).

On the basis of these data, BINKHORST conceived the idea of fixation to the iris diaphragm. He thus avoided fixation in the posterior chamber and in the chamber angle. In this way the most important complication arising from positioning the implant behind the iris, namely dislocation, was circumvented. So was the most important complication arising from positioning the implant in front of the iris, namely ECD. Medio tutissimus ibis (OVIDIUS).

BINKHORST's new lens was 'baptised' in Middelburg on the Isle of Walcheren, 5 miles from Flushing, on 3rd October 1958, at the 10th Members' Congress of the Royal Netherlands Society for the Advancement of Medical Science (BINKHORST, 1959b), just about seven years (VOS, 1971)* after RIDLEY had presented his first lens.

* The first use of the iridocapsular lens on 16th September 1965 suggests a biological rhythm of seven years in lens implant design, the idea apparently coming of age in 1972.

BINKHORST called this lens the 'iris clip lens'*, because of its resemblance to the fixation system of the paper-clip. Objections might be felt against this name since the loops of a paper-clip are located in one plane, while those of the iris clip lens are in two parallel planes. The paper is clipped: the iris is admitted, and that is quite a difference.

BINKHORST therefore changed the name to 'pupillary lens', but this name was later abandoned, because he maintains that lens implants should be classified according to their mode of fixation and not according to their location. Moreover, the optical portion of the iris clip lens is located in the anterior chamber and not in the pupillary area (BINKHORST, 1967abc, 1968a). With a view to tradition and for lack of a better alternative, the former name was retained.

The term 'pseudophakia' to indicate the presence of an artificial lens in the eye, was inaugurated by BINKHORST at Oxford in 1959 (BINKHORST, 1959a).

BINKHORST described the construction of the original implant as follows:

'The optical portion was identical with that of DANNHEIM's lens, i.e. an acrylic biconvex lens with a diameter of 5 mm and a thickness of about 0.6 mm. The haptic portion consisted of two pairs of supramide wire loops. The posterior pair of loops was drilled into the posterior surface of the optic portion and bent at right angles. These wire loops were inserted through the pupil and came to lie against the posterior surface of the iris, but did not touch the ciliary body. The distance between the ends of these loops was about 7 mm. The attachments of the posterior loops were 0.5 mm from the equator and thus formed a square, the diagonals of which were about 4 mm long. The posterior loops prevented a forward displacement of the lens. When the pupil was constricted around the attachments of these loops its shape became more or less square. However, in order to prevent posterior dislocation of the lens when the pupil was dilated, two flat wire loops had been mounted on the equator of the lens thus increasing the greatest diameter of the portion in front of the pupil to about 8 mm. These anterior loops were adjacent to the anterior surface of the iris, at a safe distance from the anterior chamber angle. The clearance between the anterior and posterior loops was about 0.75 mm, just enough to enable the iris to be slid in between. The loops consisted of supramide wire, 0.1 mm thick. These wire loops were chosen for the fixation of the lens, because it was considered most essential to keep the total weight as low as possible, about 6 mg in air, and to limit the contact with the iris to a minimum.' (BINKHORST, 1959a).

According to BINKHORST (1959a), the iris clip lens had the following advantages over the angle-fixated anterior chamber lenses:

1. the iris clip lens is not in contact with the anterior chamber angle and, therefore, cannot cause decubitus.

* The iris clip lens is manufactured by:

a) K. MORCHER, 7 Stuttgart – Bad Cannstatt, Ebitzweg 35, Western Germany. This manufacturer uses materials supplied by RÖHM and HAAS, Darmstadt, Western Germany. After much effort he managed to overcome the technical difficulties and is the largest supplier to date.

b) RAYNER & KEELER Ltd., Sheraton House, Lower Road, Chorleywood, Herts., England. This firm uses materials supplied by I.C.I. and has been actively engaged in the manufacture of intraocular implants since 1948.

2. knowledge of the diameter of the anterior chamber is not very important in iris clip lens implantation. Difficulties similar to those encountered in determining the so-called ideal length of the angle-fixated anterior chamber lenses, do not arise. The iris clip lens can even be implanted in the growing eye.

3. iris clip lens fitting is independent of the configuration of the anterior chamber as for example in the presence of peripheral anterior synechiae.

4. the action of the sphincter muscle gives exact centring of the lens when fitting an iris clip lens.

The iris clip lens has additional advantages in common with the angle-fixated lenses. These are:

5. choice of either one-stage or two-stage operation.

6. choice of either intracapsular or extracapsular cataract extraction.

7. adaptation of the dioptric power to suit the individual specification.

BINKHORST (1959a, 1960abcd) mentioned the following limitations during the initial period:

1. pupils that do not allow insertion of the posterior loops.

2. pupils that might cause dislocation of the loops at a later stage.

At present (1974) a variety of measures can be used to overcome nearly all the conditions mentioned below in this connection.

a) excessive rigidity of the iris sphincter muscle.
This can be overcome by radial iridotomy, followed by suturing with preplaced sutures (see page 62 and Fig. 69 on page 192).

b) adhesions of the posterior surface of the iris to the anterior vitreous membrane, as may result from intracapsular extraction. This is no longer a problem, since secondary implantation has been abandoned in these cases.

c) capsular remnants after extracapsular extraction.
This may be dealt with by needling.

d) an extremely wide pupil (special consideration should be given to the size of the pupil in darkness!).
This may be overcome by suturing the implant upon the iris by a loop suture (see page 56 ff.) or by instillation of pilocarpine twice daily.

e) large or total colobomata of the iris.
Sutures can be employed in the majority of cases.

PERMANENT AND TEMPORARY CHANGES IN THE DESIGN (1958–1973)

A. *Modifications*

In chronological order:

1. In May 1961, after 54 implant operations, the thickness of the posterior loops was altered from 0.1 to 0.2 mm. This was done for two reasons:

a) it became technically easier to produce the right angle in the posterior loop;

b) the difference between anterior and posterior loops was enhanced which was also a visual advantage during the operation.

For ease of recognition, the posterior loops were also made slightly pointed (BINKHORST, 1962b). The total weight was thus increased from 6 to 10 mg in air.

Other suggestions for increasing the visibility of the loops during the operation were made and put into practice by:

a. LURIE: the posterior loops were coloured black with a carbon pigment (I.C.I.) which is innocuous to the inner eye (BINKHORST, pers. comm.).

b. LÉONARD: the anterior loops were placed at an angle of 20° to the posterior loops, by rotation in the frontal plane (implant in situ). This modification, suitable for the beginner since insertion was thought to be easier that way (LÉONARD, pers. comm.), has been abandoned because it disorientates the surgeon (BINKHORST, pers. comm.).

c. FEDOROV: the angle between anterior and posterior loops at 90° (FEDOROV, 1965). The anterior loops were inserted vertically. 'This design may be slightly easier to insert in case of absolute absence of the anterior chamber' (BINKHORST, 1969d). See also page 136.

2. Initially, the dioptric power of the lens was made to suit the individual requirements. For this purpose the back vertex power of the spherical lens at 12 mm back vertex distance had to be calculated. In September 1962, when the primary fitting of implants became a routine practice, this procedure was no longer possible. The iris clip lens was given a standard power equivalent to a spectacle correction of + 13 DS at 12 mm back vertex distance (after April 1966 it was made equivalent to a spectacle correction of + 12 DS).

3. In June 1965 the length of the anterior loops was altered from 7.5 to 8 mm to 9 to 9.5 mm, which is the maximum for comfortable insertion. This was done in order to reduce the number of dislocations (24, or 11.54%) that had occurred amongst the first 208 implants (BINKHORST & LÉONARD, 1967e, 1968b). However this produced a marked increase of ECD (see page 104). And so the original length of 7.5 to 8 mm was restored on 1st January 1970 (see also page 104).

4. In 1967, at the suggestion of R. D. BINKHORST, brother of C. D. BINKHORST, the optic portion was changed from a biconvex to a simple convexo-plano acrylic lens, because

a) aqueous flowing through the pupillary aperture, would not be obstructed so easily.

b) optical computations would be easier and more accurate.

c) spherical aberration would, theoretically, be less.

The radius of curvature of the anterior surface of the standard power lens became 7.6 mm and its central thickness about 0.5 mm. The power of this lens in aqueous may be calculated as follows:

$$D_L = (n_2 - n_1) \frac{r_2 - r_1}{r_1 r_2}$$

where: $r_1 = 7.6$ mm $= 0.007\ 6$ m $\qquad n_1 = 1.336$ (aqueous)

$\qquad\quad r_2 = \infty \qquad\qquad\qquad\qquad\quad n_2 = 1.490$ (acrylate)

Thus $D_L = (1.490 - 1.336)\ (\frac{1}{0.007\ 6} - \frac{1}{\infty}) = 0.154 \times \frac{1}{0.007\ 6} = 20.26$ D.

5.   On 1st January 1971, the power was reduced from 20.26 DS to 19.5 DS in aqueous since the average residual anisometropia was found to be a little too high. For this, the radius of curvature of the anterior surface had to be changed to $\frac{0.154}{19.5} = 0.007\ 9$ m $= 7.9$ mm.

6.   In November 1971, all loops were manufactured bent backwards at a radius of about 30 mm in order to reduce the risk of corneal touch. For technical reasons the thickness of the anterior loops had therefore to be altered from 0.1 to 0.15 mm*.

7.   Early in 1972 the length of the diagonals of the square formed by the posterior loop attachments was reduced from 4 to 3 mm. This made it possible for the pupil to constrict to a diameter of 3 mm thus reducing the photophobia which occurred rather often with 4 mm diameter pupils** (see Figs. 6 and 8).

As a result of all these modifications, the standard iris clip lens weighs 9.35 mg measured in air, and 1.41 mg in aqueous.

Two temporary modifications were made, and another only considered:

8.   The biconvex optic portion was temporarily made in concave-convex form (BINK- HORST, 1962ac), because according to calculations by DUDRAGNE based on the schema- tic eye, the anterior and posterior principal planes would be situated at their physiolo- gical positions only under these conditions. Iseikonia would thus be achieved, admitted- ly at the expense of increased spherical aberration. Together with the loops, however, this lens with its relatively strongly-curved posterior surface was pushed forward by the vitreous, which resulted in corneal touch. The bending of the optic portion was not a practical proposition because of the anatomy of the eye. Only two patients were fitted with this lens (BINKHORST, cases 75 and 76), one of whom ended up with total ECD (see case 76 on page 109).

9.   Coloured admixtures to the acrylic material may diminish the sensitivity to visible and invisible radiation and protect the macula against radiation damage (BINKHORST,

---

* A preliminary experiment with depressed loops had already been made on 6th November 1969 in a case where the anterior loops in the fellow-eye were approaching the cornea (BINKHORST, case 422).

** BINKHORST had mentioned this possibility as early as 1962 (BINKHORST, 1962b, 1967ac).

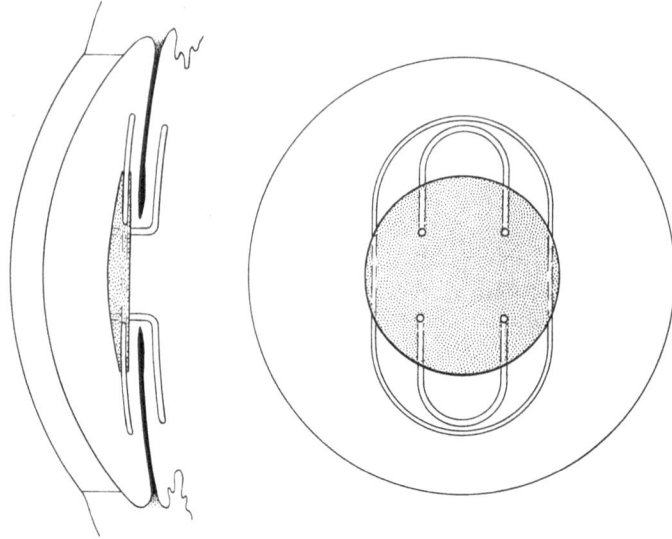

Fig. 6

Iris clip lens in 1972; sectional (L) and frontal view.

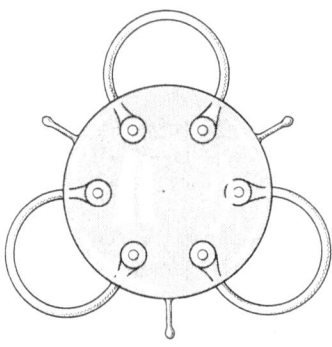

Fig. 7

FEDOROV's modification of the iris clip lens (1968), the so-called 'Sputnik lens'.

1967c). However, the real danger is situated in irritation caused by diffusion of these substances into the eye. BINKHORST carried out two experiments in August 1969 and another in January 1970, with carbon black coloured iris clip lenses. Absorption was too high, however, and it were these three eyes that showed temporary precipitates on the anterior vitreous membrane. These do not normally occur.

10.   Another modification considered by BINKHORST in 1967 but not introduced, was the construction of triple or quadruple loops, which might have produced rounder

30

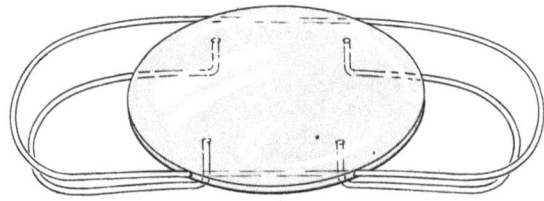

Fig. 8

Iris clip lens in 1972. The radius of curvature of the anterior surface of the convexo-plano optic portion is 7.9 mm to give a standard power in aqueous of + 19.5 D. Loop length $\dfrac{8.00}{8.00}$ mm.

pupils and a little more stability. 'It has to be borne in mind, however, that the weight of the iris clip lens is critical: even the use of metal instead of supramide wire loops makes it too heavy, and the same applies to glass as opposed to acrylic material for the optical lens' (BINKHORST, 1967ac).

11. It was for these same reasons that, in 1968, FEDOROV replaced the anterior loops by little prongs situated between the three posterior loops of a triple loop design (FEDOROV, 1972, pers. comm. 1973). Because of the prongs, his lens was nicknamed the 'Sputnik lens'. See Fig. 7.

12. A modification that would have made permanent miosis unnecessary, the so-called coloboma clip lens, was thought of by LÉONARD (pers. comm. 3-2-1972). In this modification there was a small notch at the top of the anterior superior loop. This notch would touch the top of the posterior superior loop. The point of contact could be in either a small opening in the iris, or in an enlarged coloboma. The increasing use of the iridocapsular lens (see below) in cases of senile cataract meant that the coloboma clip lens was never fitted in practice.

B.   FURTHER DEVELOPMENTS OF THE IMPLANT

Two other designs in current use derived from the iris clip lens, namely the iridocapsular lens (BINKHORST in 1965) and the iris medallion lens (WORST in 1970) were developed specifically to prevent dislocation and ECD. Since they do not possess anterior loops the principle of clip fixation does not apply to either modification.

1   Iridocapsular lens

The iridocapsular lens (see Figs. 9 and 10) was originally designed in 1965, especially for children (BINKHORST & GOBIN, 1967d). At present it is used for

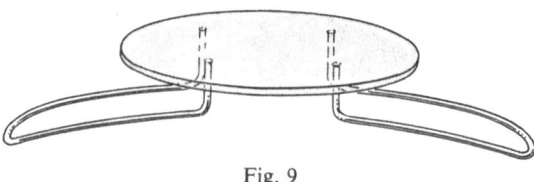

Fig. 9

Iridocapsular lens in 1972.

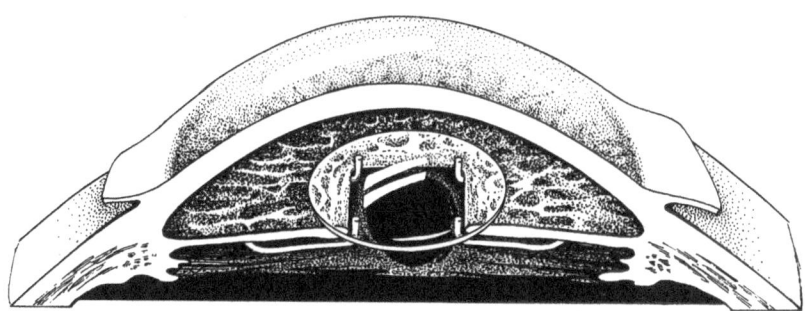

Fig. 10

Iridocapsular lens in situ 1972.

patients of any age, after extracapsular cataract surgery in one-stage as well as in two-stage procedures (BINKHORST, 1972e).

The optic portion is the same as in the iris clip lens and it is also located in the anterior chamber, immediately in front of the pupil and hardly touching the iris. It permits the free flow of aqueous through the pupillary aperture. There is only one pair of wire loops. These loops, bent slightly backwards, lie behind the lens and are buried in the iridocapsular cleft. Because they are in intimate contact with the inner eye they are made of 0.15 mm platinum-iridium wire, a most inert alloy. The increased weight of the implant is of no consequence: this is easily tolerated with iridocapsular fixation. The usual distance between the tips of the loops is 8 mm (9 mm before 1968; BINKHORST, GOBIN & LÉONARD, 1969c), but this may be slightly modified by the surgeon, where necessary (BINKHORST, 1967ac, 1969cd).

The weight is 15.10 mg in air, and 7.98 mg in aqueous.

The fixation mechanism is quite different from that of the iris clip lens, and requires a relatively strong circular capsular membrane behind the iris and some adhesions between this membrane and the iris. Whereas the central area of the membrane consisting of the posterior lens capsule only should be as clear as possible, it is advisable to leave a few cortical remnants of the lens at the periphery behind the iris. This promotes the development of iridocapsular adhesions embedding parts of the wire loops and giving extra stability to the pseudophakos as well as preventing undesirable mydriasis. To avoid vitreous complications, it is a sine qua non that the posterior capsule be intact.

On 16th September 1965 an iridocapsular lens in the form of an iris clip lens from which the anterior loops had been removed, was inserted for the first time. The first iridocapsular lens proper, having platinum-iridium loops, was inserted on 27th October 1965.

The iridocapsular lens has the following advantages over the iris clip lens:

1. the implantation is easier to perform;
2. the absence of anterior loops

a) reduces the risk of corneal touch to practically nil. It is possible for the optic portion to touch the cornea, but only when the eye is rubbed hard (BINK-HORST, pers. comm.).

b) renders implantation largely independent of the dimensions of the anterior chamber and the presence of iris colobomata and peripheral synechiae. After 1959 the implantation of *iris clip lenses* proved to depend more upon the dimensions of the anterior chamber than had been initially assumed (see below and page 27).

3. the fixation of the posterior loops by iridocapsular adhesions

a) reduces the risk of dislocation to a minimum.

Dislocation will occur only if these adhesions have not formed, e.g. after a milky cataract or if too much lens material has been removed.

b) allows mydriasis without any risk of dislocation since the iris sphincter muscle is not used for fixation.

c) improves stabilisation of implant and vitreous (see page 231 ff.).

Consequently, the iridocapsular lens may be used in cases where the iris clip lens is contra-indicated, such as:

1. a corneal diameter of 10.50 mm or less (microphthalmia, not fully grown eyes).
2. a shallow anterior chamber.
3. an eccentric pupil.

Disadvantages of the iridocapsular lens are:

1. insertion is possible only after *extracapsular* cataract extraction because fixation depends entirely on the presence of the posterior capsule.
2. complete removal of the implant will be difficult in the event of good fixation, but surgical experience has, so far, not been obtained.

Separate dissection of the optic portion is relatively easy.

3. the relatively heavy weight (7.98 mg in aqueous) may cause the iridocapsular lens to dislocate behind the iris if the lens has not been sufficiently fixated in the iridocapsular cleft.

4. needling is necessary in a number of cases, because of secondary cataract. The regaining of good visual acuity may, therefore, demand some fortitude on the part of the patient (slow method).

As a result the iridocapsular lens cannot be used when:

1. the crystalline lens is dislocated.

2. fixation in the iridocapsular cleft cannot be expected to take place, e.g. in cases of:

a)   milky cataract.

b)   aphakia after intracapsular lens extraction.

c)   secondary implantation without synechiae.

3. the patient prefers intracapsular extraction because restoration of visual acuity is usually more rapid (quick method).

In these cases the iris clip lens or the iris medallion lens (see below) may be used.

2   *Iris medallion lens*

The iris medallion lens, designed by WORST, was a logical sequel to his method of loop-iris-suturing (see page 56 ff.). Having first adapted this suture to the construction of the iris clip lens, he then conceived the idea of adapting the construction of the lens to the suture.

This led to the design of the so-called iris medallion lens, or M.W. iris clip lens*.

The iris medallion lens (see Fig. 11) consists of an optic portion of 5 mm diameter surrounded by an eccentric haptic portion of 8 mm diameter. The whole lens is made of one piece of material. Two perforations in the eccentric haptic portion (one on the nasal and one on the temporal side) are made to take the perlon iris suture.

This modification has only the usual two posterior loops. The weight is 11.00 mg in air, and 1.70 mg in aqueous.

The standard power of this lens is + 20 D in aqueous, but any power is available*. The iris medallion lens was inserted for the first time on 18th December 1970.

---

* The iris medallion lens is manufactured by Medical Workshop, Heresingel 28, Groningen, Holland.

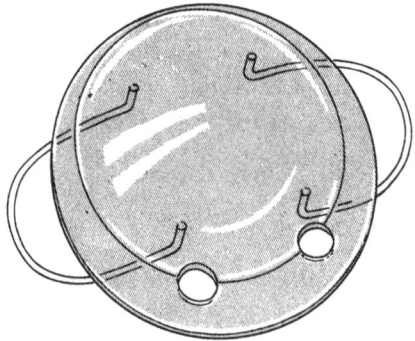

Fig. 11

Iris medallion lens in 1972, observed from about one o'clock.

The advantages of the iris medallion lens are mainly the same as those of the iridocapsular lens. In addition, it is possible:
1. to insert the lens after intracapsular cataract extraction.
2. to remove the lens easily (see case 460 on page 144 and case 508 on page 159).

A possible disadvantage may turn out to be its dependence on the perlon suture and its iris bite.

CHANGES IN SURGICAL TECHNIQUES (1958–1973)

Recent surgical techniques will be dealt with extensively in the next chapter, but two earlier turning points are mentioned below:

1 *The change from secondary to primary implantation in 1961*

Primary implantation was initially only performed on older patients with only moderate general health and with senile cataract.

Later on, the change from secondary to primary implantation turned out to be a fortunate one when the advantages of primary implantation such as the sparing of the corneal endothelium by one-stage surgery, and the rapid restoration of visual acuity, proved to be greater than those of secondary implantation (see page 17). Its disadvantages were the necessity of determining an implant standard power, and the unknown reaction of the eye (BINKHORST & LÉONARD, 1967e, 1968b). A useful aspect was that if there were vitreous problems after the cataract extraction, the insertion of the implant could be cancelled. The preference for primary implantation as a routine procedure was later underlined in an interim report of BINKHORST & LÉONARD (1967e, 1968b), who found 5 cases (7.14%) of ECD in 70 secondary implantations and none in 124 primary implantations. Five years later, after a total of 694 iris clip lens implant operations, these percentages were 4.46 and 6.36 respectively, the latter being due mainly to the temporary $\frac{\text{anterior}}{\text{posterior}}$ loop length of $\frac{9.00}{9.00}$ mm (see page 102).

2. *The change from intracapsular iris clip lens implant to extracapsular iridocapsular lens implant around 1971*

The main objective (BINKHORST, 1972e, 1973) of this change was to establish absolute security for the corneal endothelium, even in unfavourable circumstances, by combining the advantages of the iridocapsular lens (see page 33) with those of extracapsular cataract extraction. These advantages include: small incision with fewer cases of striate keratitis and less astigmatism; safer surgery due to less bulging of the vitreous and, moreover, fewer cases of ECD; better stability of vitreous and implant; fewer cases of maculopathy. One disadvantage of extracapsular surgery was found to be the occurrence of secondary cataract. The frequency of needling may, however, decrease considerably with increasing experience, especially as regards the group of patients with senile cataract (BINKHORST, 1972b, 1973).

SUMMARY

The characteristics of the principal implants are summarised in Fig. 12.

type of implant	RIDLEY	STRAMPELLI, CHOYCE and others	BINKHORST iris clip lens	BINKHORST iridocapsular lens	WORST iris medallion lens
determination of size	easy (standard)	difficult measurement	easy (standard)	easy (standard)	easy (standard)
insertion	difficult	easy	easy	easy	easy
removal	difficult	easy	easy	difficult	easy
one-stage	most preferable	possible	preferable	preferable	preferable
two-stage	less preferable (iridocapsular adhesions!)	preferable	preferable after extracapsular surgery	possible	less preferable
intracapsular	prohibited (dislocation!)	advisable	possible	prohibited	possible
extracapsular	obligatory	possible	possible	obligatory	possible
monocular case	ideal indication	ideal indication	ideal indication	ideal indication	ideal indication
binocular case	possible	possible	possible	possible	possible
traumatic case	not always possible	ideal indication	not always possible	ideal indication	possible
anterior dislocation	unusual	—	1.00% } last 300 cases (see page 105)	0.59% } out of 170 cases (see page 137)	1.73% } out of 173 cases (see page 173)
posterior dislocation	6%	—	3.33%	4.70%	
ECD	RIDLEY 0% EPSTEIN 4.76%	STRAMPELLI 0–10% BARRAQUER 30–50% CHOYCE Mark VIII, 1970 0%	3.33%	0.59% (one special case)	2.89% (mainly suture contact)

Fig. 12

Comparison of the principal implants discussed in this chapter.

37

CHAPTER III

TECHNIQUES

This chapter deals with three technical aspects of the iris clip lens and its modifications, namely:

The materials and sterilisation of the implant.

The surgical techniques used for the implant operation.

The treatment of post-operative complications.

THE MATERIALS AND STERILISATION OF THE IMPLANT

Perspectives in perspex.

1 *Materials used for the implant*

a. Polymethylmethacrylate, generally known as Perspex or Plexiglass is a plastic formed by polymerisation of many single molecules of methylmethacrylate. Its refractive index is 1.49, and its specific gravity is 1.19.

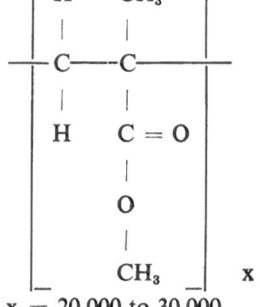

x = 20 000 to 30 000

During the Battle of Britain, many plastic canopies of Spitfire aeroplanes were shattered by enemy gun fire, and occasionally pieces of plastic material (polymethylmethacrylate) became lodged inside the eyes of pilots. It was noted that in many cases, despite the fact that several fragments had entered and become embedded in the globe, there was little, if any, reaction to the plastic material, provided these fragments did not move about inside the eye.

In 1949, it occurred to RIDLEY that such a plastic substance might be utilised to replace the human lens (TROUTMAN, 1962a). In his very first lecture on lens implantation RIDLEY (1951) said: 'plastic compounds have been widely used in surgery, especially for filling gaps in bones, not only of the skull, but also in joint cavities where movement and the presence of synovial fluid resembles to some degree conditions inside the eye' (RIDLEY, 1951, 1952ac).

Other materials, for instance silicate glass, were also considered (SCHRECK, 1958b).

Glass and acrylic compounds have much in common in addition to being inert to body fluids. Both are almost perfectly transparent, have constant optical properties, and can be worked mechanically to a high degree of accuracy. Though less hard and, therefore, more easily scratched, methacrylate has the enormous advantage of being light-weight, its specific gravity (1.19) being only half that of glass (approx. 3) and not much in excess of that of the aqueous fluid (1.004) (RIDLEY, 1952abc).

Polymethylmethacrylate transmits 90 to 92% of light. It is light, strong, and can be polished to a smooth finish, although nowadays all intraocular lenses are cast. It contains occasional air bubbles of 30 to 40 μ in diameter. These are not interconnected and do not promote bacterial penetration. Owing to the numerous methyl groups, it is hydrophobic. Intraocular and contact lenses, however, may absorb water up to 1.5% of their weight, due to the high surface area to mass ratio. This is important in connection with sterilising fluids (EASTERBROOK et al., 1969).

Today every manufacturer claims that no filler, plasticiser, ultraviolet light absorber or other ingredient, has been added to his fully polymerised product, and that degeneration and depolymerisation of his product is impossible. This is an important factor since the monomer used is highly irritant to the eye.

b. *Supramide (or Ultramide)* is a partly crystalline polymer of caprolactam, dicarbonic acids (adipic acid, sebacic acid) and diamines (hexamethylendiamine). Its specific gravity is 1.13.

$$\left[\begin{array}{cc} H & H \\ | & | \\ C & C \\ | & | \\ H & C=O \\ & | \\ & NH_2 \end{array}\right]_x$$

It has a certain flexibility which, in the past, made it useful for haptic purposes in lens implant design. This flexibility, however, is of no avail for the iris clip lens and its modifications.

Disintegration of supramide loop tips was observed by BINKHORST in three implanted DANNHEIM lenses (see cases IC 14 and IC 77 on page 128).

It has never been observed in iris clip lenses, not even after 15 years of use (BINKHORST, 1968b, 1973).

c. *Platinum-iridium* is a very inert metal aloy. It is, therefore, useful for haptic parts that are in intimate contact with the inner eye. Its specific gravity is 21.55 (9 parts platinum, 1 part iridium).

2 *Sterilisation of the implant*

Acrylate cannot be boiled without risk of distortion. It is affected by certain organic solvents including alcohols and formaldehyde (RIDLEY, 1952a).

As a sterilising agent, RIDLEY (1952ac, 1953b) chose 1 % cetrimide for at least one hour, after which the implant was thoroughly rinsed in distilled water. Cetrimide (tetra-decyltrimethylammoniumbromide) does not affect perspex, but since it belongs to the group of quaternary ammonium compounds, it is a highly surface-active substance. It adheres strongly to the hydrophobic surface of a perspex object, e.g. a lens implant, to the extent of 1 % of its weight (GOLDMANN, cit. SAUBERMANN, 1955). In the course of time it disengages itself from the perspex and can cause irritation of the eye.

On the following grounds it seems probable that the inflammatory response observed initially (THEOBALD, 1953; WOLLENSAK, 1960; GUERRY & GEERAETS, 1962) was not caused by the perspex material:

1. the observed inertness of the perspex fragments in the eyes of Spitfire pilots.
2. histopathologically SMITH (1956) found no increase of fibrous tissue formation in long-term cases. This is suggestive of a stimulus by a noxious substance becoming expended.
3. SCHRECK (1958b) implanted lenses that, by accident, had been sterilised several times with 1, 2 or 3 % cetrimide. The more frequent the sterilisation with the higher percentage of cetrimide, the greater the production of precipitates in the anterior chamber.
4. better methods of sterilisation produced far less irritation or none at all.

CHOYCE (1970a) concluded: the use of cetrimide was disastrous.

STRAMPELLI (1958ab) advocated the 'humanisation' of lens implants by depositing them in the lobe of the ear for 3 or 4 months. With this method, precipitates on the implant did not occur.

BINKHORST & FLU (1956b) used the bactericidal action of ultraviolet rays of 253.7 nm wavelength. The lens implant was irradiated for 30 minutes. Room temperature was maintained by means of a ventilator.

Frederick RIDLEY (1957) introduced a method of implant sterilisation which has been in use ever since. It has been used for BINKHORST lenses since mid-1968. The lens implant is sterilised in 10% NaOH for one hour at 30°C, killing even the spores of B. subtilis. It is subsequently stored on 0.1% NaOH. Immediately before implantation, the NaOH is replaced by 0.5% $NaHCO_3$ to neutralise it. Finally, the lens implant is rinsed in RINGER solution or saline.

WORST (pers. comm.) found that it took between 5 and 10 minutes for all traces of NaOH to disappear. Thus $NaHCO_3$, and saline do not overcome the surface-bonding effect as quickly as is generally believed. Nevertheless, this method of sterilisation has proved to be reliable, easy, and cheap.

THE SURGICAL TECHNIQUES USED FOR THE IMPLANT OPERATION

A little learning is a dangerous thing.

It should be pointed out that the surgical techniques have altered many times in the course of the years. Even slight modifications turned out to have a most important effect upon the results. The current procedure for the lens implant operation may be divided into pre-operative measures, surgery, and post-operative care. For the sake of conciseness, surgery and post-operative care have been grouped in one section.

1. *Pre-operative measures*

a. Mental and physical preparation of the surgeon. (This can easily be neglected!)

It stands to reason that the surgeon who plans to insert a BINKHORST lens or one of its modifications in an aphakic eye, should have made a thorough *theoretical* study of lens implantations in general. If he is unaware of the calamities that have occurred in the history of lens implant operations, he works like a sleep-walker who considers his performance excellent, but when consciousness returns the results of his ignorance are revealed. The well-prepared surgeon, however, is *consciously* able to avoid mishaps.

The surgeon who inserts artificial lenses should have extensive *practical* experience of cataract operations in general. His suturing technique should have reached a sufficiently high level to produce an absolutely watertight wound closure. He should have witnessed a sufficient number of implant operations performed by experts, so that he will be familiar with the handling of the common major and minor difficulties of lens implantations (bulging vitreous, seeing the loops during the insertion, etc.).

It is highly desirable that during his first implant operation he be assisted by an expert, since many of the finer points can only be learned under personal guidance.

An implant operation *can* be postponed. It *should* be postponed if the surgeon is not in good condition. Better to lose time than to lose eyes.

b. Instruction of the theatre staff. (This too, can easily be neglected!)

The sterile nurse should also have an accurate knowledge of the implantation technique. She should have a steady hand.

The other nurses should protect the surgeon against external influences that might disturb his concentration. During the implant operation his attention should be confined to the anterior chamber. All telephone bells, alarm clocks, and staff locating systems should be inactivated, doors should preferably be kept locked. Talk, not directly related to the operation, should be avoided.

Good theatre nurses are a blessing to the eye!

c. Preparation of the artificial lens.

The lens, packed in a sealed pyrex vial filled with 0.1 % NaOH, should be checked by the surgeon in advance. After all, he remains responsible, even if it is a question of a defective lens. In the case of the iris clip lens, the overall length of the anterior loops is most important: 8 mm is the maximum length tolerable in the average eye. In addition, the loops of all BINKHORST type lenses must be properly bent back (see page 29).

d. Examination, instruction and preparation of the patient.

The pre-operative ophthalmological examination is the same as that for cataract extraction without implantation. But since it is intended to fit an implant, special attention should be paid to the corneal endothelium (FUCHS' corneal dystrophy, deposits), the aqueous (TYNDALL effect, cell clumps), the iris (coloboma, stromal atrophy), anterior and posterior synechiae, the response of the sphincter muscle to short acting mydriatics, and to miotics and possibly to the corneal radius, anterior chamber depth, and the axial length.

The patient should be informed that the operation will be performed under general anaesthesia, and that a new lens will be inserted only if surgical conditions permit.

The patient is admitted several days before surgery, for a general check-up by the physician. The actual pre-operative measures may be commenced only if the latter gives his permission. This procedure facilitates the adaptation of the patient to hospitalisation.

The day prior to surgery

The author's routine, which differs only in detail from the current routine of BINKHORST, is as follows:
a. decadron drops every 3 hours. Decadron = dexamethasone sodium phosphate.
b. globenicol drops every 8 hours.
c. 500 mg penbritin (capsules) four times a day.
  1 tablet vit. B complex twice a day to maintain vit. B absorption, otherwise taken care of by the intestinal flora which is killed by the penbritin.
d. bowel regularity with natrium-lauryl-sulfo-acetate (Microlax) suppositories.
e. cutting eye lashes and shaving eyebrow.
f. an eye shield is fitted to prevent contamination of the eye by 'dirty' fingers.
  Antibiotics and decadron are administered to minimise intraocular reaction.

Omitting them may lead to extensive cellular reaction of the anterior uvea with deposits of cell clumps in the anterior chamber, on the lens surface, and sometimes in the anterior part of the vitreous during the post-operative period. This is frequently accompanied by a hypopyon of varying height (BINKHORST, 1962be).

Acetazolamide (Diamox) is given by most surgeons, including BINKHORST, on the assumption that:

a) it prevents a precipitate lowering of the intraocular pressure at the moment the eye is opened.

b) it reduces the volume of the vitreous and helps to prevent the vitreous from bulging.

However, in the author's opinion this is doubtful since the hypotensive effect in normal eyes is only very slight (BLEEKER, 1963). For that reason he stopped using Diamox after his first 84 implant operations.

Day of the operation.

a) the patient is not allowed to have any food or drink.

b) two hours prior to surgery: two drops of homatropine hydrobromide 0.5 % are instilled into the conjunctival sac.

c) one hour prior to surgery: premedication as ordered by the anaesthetist. intramuscular injection of one vial ($=6.5$ mg) thiethylperazine (Torecan) as an anti-emetic.

Anaesthesia

General anaesthesia during lens implant operations should produce complete muscle relaxation with hypotony of the eye. Post-operative vomiting should be eliminated.

General anaesthesia is preferred to retrobulbar anaesthesia, because:

a) the duration of the operation is not restricted.

b) sudden movements by the patient are avoided.

c) it has an additional tension-lowering effect on the eye.

d) retrobulbar anaesthesia interferes with the control of the pupillary size because of the prolonged action of novocaine.

e) occasionally, retrobulbar anaesthesia gives rise to retrobulbar haemorrhage.

2. *Surgery*

The special instruments used in the lens implant operation, are depicted in Fig. 13.

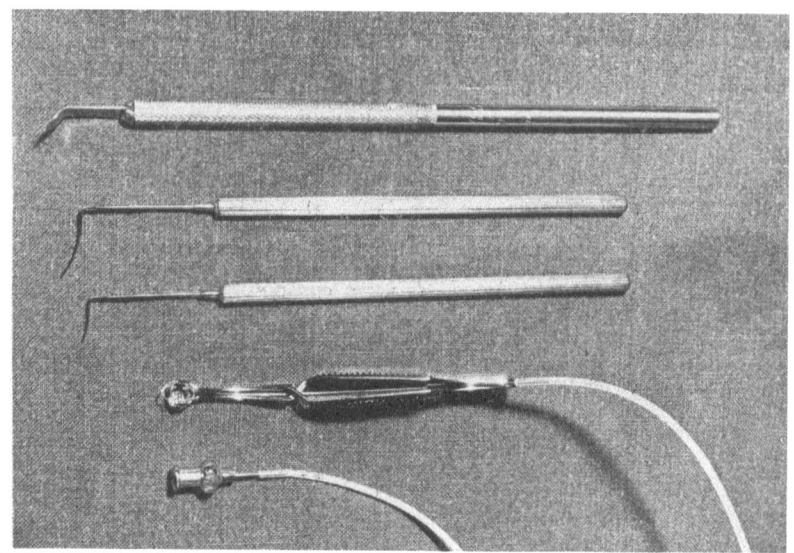

Fig. 13

a) BEAVER knife no. 66, b) iris repositors, two sizes, c) special lens forceps with polyvinyl-chloride tubes for intracameral irrigation.

Cataract extraction in lens implant surgery

The following preparations, which form part of BINKHORST's routine, are considered to be very useful in cataract surgery and particularly in lens implant surgery:

1.   brushing all instruments with a marten hair brush, in order to prevent flues being inserted into the eye.

2.   extensive conjunctival lavage with saline through a wide blunt canula, and mechanical cleaning of the lid margins with a piece of cotton wool soaked in saline.

3.   covering the area adjacent to the field of surgery with 'steridrape'.

4.   one or two preplaced perlon sutures in the keratome incision.

This is not meant as a safety measure in case of vitreous prolapse, but to prevent unnecessary astigmatism and to allow the anterior chamber to contain air as soon after the implantation as possible.

5.   lateral illumination with a hammer lamp, especially during implantation, when maximum visibility is required.

6.   iris repositioning with the iris repositor. Any adhesion of the iris to the cornea should be corrected.

7.   use of warm fluids (28°C).

Features of the author's technique are:

1. colibri lid speculum of BARRAQUER.
2. bridle suture through the superior rectus muscle insertion. FLIERINGA's scleral ring is not used.
3. the conjunctiva is incised with scissors 2 to 3 mm behind the corneal limbus, and parallel to it. This incision and the intended corneo-scleral incision are concentric. The conjunctiva is then dissected anteriorly with scissors and with a BEAVER knife no. 66 to provide room for more exact corneo-scleral suturing. The resulting conjunctival flap is folded down over the cornea (BINKHORST et al., 1966).
4. keratome incision enlarged with CASTROVIEJO scissors.
5. cryoextraction if intracapsular extraction is intended.

If extracapsular extraction is intended, the anterior lens capsule is extracted with toothed forceps, a DAVIEL's spoon is pressed on the posterior wound edge and the nucleus is delivered by external pressure.

All intraocular manipulations should be carried out with the utmost care. The eye, and in particular the corneal endothelium, has to be spared as much as possible. Therefore, unnecessary movements of instruments in the anterior chamber must be avoided altogether.

As good visibility is a sine qua non, the following points must be stressed:

1. any haemorrhage should be stopped or, better still, avoided, for its prevention is much more important in implant surgery than in plain cataract surgery.
a. bleeding conjunctival and episcleral vessels should be cauterised, and the author uses the DIXEY cautery for this purpose. This applies particularly to the temporal region, where the dissection of the conjunctival flap may be more difficult.
b. when approaching the 3 o'clock – 9 o'clock line with the corneo-scleral scissors, the original circular course should not be continued, nor should there be any deviation outwards, for this leads to difficulties in haemostasis at the ends of the incision and may cause peripheral synechiae later on. It is the author's experience that it is preferable to curve the ends of the incision slightly inwards, thereby increasing the curvature, as suggested by WORST.

If, however, a haemorrhage does occur at the end of the incision, a safe procedure is to place a microsponge at the bleeding point and wait for a while. Some other measures against haemorrhage, such as a local corneo-scleral suture or filling the anterior chamber with air, are also relatively safe, bur repeated irrigation of the anterior chamber or even removal of the blood clots with a blunt iris hook or with untoothed forceps, are manipulations to which the corneal endothelium may react unfavourably at a much later stage.

2.   the corneal flap should be held gently and preferably without folding the cornea. The latter leads to the development of folds in DESCEMET's membrane, stromal oedema and poor visibility during the implantation; post-operatively, it entails more corneal striae and more chance of endothelial decompensation afterwards (see page 68).

External irrigation with saline helps to eliminate poor visibility caused by corneal folds (BINKHORST, 1973).

3.   lateral illumination with a hammer lamp may improve visibility considerably, especially during iris clip lens implantation in eyes with brown irides.

4.   the use of a microscope may make it easier to observe more details of the implant operation but a drawback is that the perlon suture tends to float against it (ALKEMADE, pers. comm.), and that the surgeon's field of view is restricted.

PRIMARY INSERTION OF AN IRIS CLIP LENS AFTER INTRACAPSULAR EXTRACTION

I   Cataract extraction

The following conditions should be fulfilled:

1.   The corneo-scleral incision must be sufficiently large and clean to enable
a.   extraction and insertion without damage to the corneal endothelium. In general, an incision of 170 to 180° will suffice.
b.   exact corneo-scleral suturing, i.e. absolutely watertight and without any risk of iris incarceration.

2.   After the extraction, the pupil should be 3 to 4 mm in diameter, round and central, and the sphincter muscle should be intact. If the sphincter is ruptured, it will react poorly to miotics and will not have a firm grip on the lens, which increases the risk of dislocation. In the event that the sphincter ruptures during cataract extraction, the iris clip lens should be sutured to the iris or the implantation abandoned. If the pupil remains wide with an intact sphincter, pupillary constriction is most probably prevented by a vitreous bulge. In any case, the pupil should never have been dilated with extra mydriatics, because this can cause a mydriasis which is not reversible during the time of the operation (BINKHORST, 1973). See also case 19 (page 189) and case 64 (page 49).

3.   Vitreous strands should not enter the wound. Even after a 'vitreous sweep' with a repositor (see page 54), the chance of vitreous strands inducing a decentration of the pupil upwards, possibly causing corneal touch and ECD, is too

46

great to perform an implantation. Where vitreous reaches the anterior chamber, it can be pushed back with the lens, if the surgeon considers his skill sufficient, but surgeons of only moderate experience should, in these cases, refrain from implantation (BINKHORST, 1973).

II Implantation

> I venture bravely through the Gate,
> My intention is noble and pure and chaste.
> The Magic Flute.
> Act I, Scene 15.

If, after cataract extraction, the eye is in a suitable condition for a lens implantation (see above), the unsterile nurse is asked to open the vial containing the implant. The 0.1 % NaOH solution is aspirated with a syringe and replaced by the neutralising 0.5 % NaHCO$_3$ solution from the second vial. The lens is removed from the vial by the surgeon with untoothed forceps, without touching the rim of the vial. The latter is kept at an angle by the unsterile nurse. The lens is put down, grasped anew with the special lens forceps, inspected once more against a dark background, and rinsed in RINGER's solution or saline. It should never be touched by fingers, gloved or ungloved. When held by the special lens forceps, it is advisable to steady the lens with another pair of forceps in case it jumps away because the surgeon's grasp is not sufficiently firm. If this does occur, the lens should be returned to the manufacturer for resterilisation, and a spare lens should be inserted.

The implantation may be performed with the loops horizontal, vertical or in any other position.

However, vertical implantation has the following advantages:

1. the technique is easier.

2. the stability of the lens is better. The reason for this is the fact that the horizontal movements of the human eye are definitely more frequent than the vertical movements.

Horizontal movements of the eye cause a *horizontal* lens to swing. In some cases this may lead to periodical corneal touch and in the long run to ECD.

The same applies during sleep, but to a lesser degree:

a) rapid eye movements occur during dreams.

b) the head may lie on its side.

A disadvantage of vertical implantation may be the increased chance of vitreous interposition at 6 o'clock (BINKHORST, pers. comm.).

The optic portion of the lens is grasped by the special lens forceps in such a way that the loops lie parallel with the forceps, and that one pair of them may be inserted at 6 o'clock. The sterile nurse squirts saline through the polyvinyl-chloride tubes attached to the special lens forceps in order to expel the air. The whole system of lens, special lens forceps, polyvinylchloride tubes and syringe is then moved towards the eye by the surgeon in co-ordination with the sterile nurse assisting him. At the very last moment, before entering the eye, the lens is held above the eye and the sterile nurse puts a few drops of saline on the cornea to improve visibility. With toothed forceps held in his left hand the surgeon lifts the cornea by the conjunctival flap just enough to enable him to introduce the lens into the anterior chamber with his right hand, without touching the corneal endothelium or the anterior vitreous membrane. The attention of the surgeon is directed towards the tips of the inferior loops. When these loops are close to the pupillary margin at 6 o'clock, visibility should be maximal (wet cornea, intracamerular irrigation by the sterile nurse, lateral illumination). The insertion continues in the same direction until the iris slides between the two inferior loops. It is a sure sign that the iris is *between* the loops and not anterior or posterior when the pupillary margin is stretched by the posterior loop attachments. The procedure should be repeated if this does not occur.

Simultaneous irrigation may be of some help.

There are various methods of inserting the superior loops:

1.   In the case of a *rather wide pupil* the insertion is continued until the tip of the superior posterior loop enters the pupillary area. The lens is then moved backwards to bring the superior posterior loop behind the iris. When both posterior loops are in position behind the iris, a freshly prepared 1 : 100 solution of acetylcholine is introduced into the anterior chamber through the special lens forceps. This results in an immediate constriction of the pupil. The special lens forceps are then removed with the utmost care.

The wide pupil method has the following disadvantages:

a.   one has to wait and see whether the pupil will constrict after implantation.

b.   there is a greater chance that the corneal endothelium may become damaged at 6 o'clock.

c.   if the pupil is not wide enough, it may prove impossible to manoeuvre the superior posterior loop behind the iris, because the inferior loops cannot be moved any nearer to 6 o'clock.

In that case, a narrow pupil manoeuvre has to be performed. According to BINKHORST, irrigation with epinephrine solution is absolutely contra-indicated since this may damage the corneal endothelium, most probably because of the reducing additive (BINKHORST, pers. comm.).

Case history.
Case 64 (BINKHORST). Female, born 1891.
  6–7–61 intracapsular cataract extraction with iris clip lens implantation OS. Chymotrypsin proved to be necessary because of a strong zonular resistance and epinephrine because of too narrow a pupil. The epinephrine, however, caused wide dilatation of the pupil resulting in dislocation of the implant. This required instrumental repositioning.
13–7–61 striate keratitis.
20–7–61 central corneal oedema which subsided after some months.
  1–2–62 corrected visual acuity 0.63 (NORDLOHNE).
14–8–67 incipient ECD.
  5–70 bullous keratopathy. Visual acuity 0.02 (PEARCE, 1972).

2. In the case of a *rather narrow pupil* the special lens forceps are removed with the utmost care. The curved end of an iris repositor, introduced sideways, is placed between the two proximal loops, to keep them in place while pushing the implant slightly towards 6 o'clock. The iris is caught at the pupillary margin with a blunt iris hook and is placed between the loops with a gentle swing. The iris repositor and the blunt iris hook are removed slowly and with the utmost care. The whole manoeuvre may be performed with the corneal flap replaced, or in the open with it held up by the sterile nurse. Irrigation of the anterior chamber with acetylcholine is not then necessary.

The same manoeuvre can also be performed with toothed forceps (OOSTINGH, pers. comm.) or colibri forceps (MELLES, pers. comm.) grasping the iris halfway, pulling it proximally until it can slide between the loops.

The pupil is more or less square when one of these manoeuvres has been successful. Exact centring, if still necessary, may be performed by careful internal manipulation with an iris repositor. External manipulation should be avoided, because it endangers the corneal endothelium.

The narrow pupil method has the disadvantage of possible vitreous incarceration in the area where the iris is raised with a blunt iris hook. The surgeon should co-ordinate his hand movements very carefully to minimise its occurrence.

In general, the narrow pupil method is preferable because the surgeon can be sure that the pupil will maintain adequate miosis post-operatively.

B Horizontal implantation

The pupil needs to be rather wide. If this is not the case, the vertical implantation technique is preferable.

The optic portion of the lens is grasped by the special lens forceps in such a way that the loops, perpendicular to the forceps, can easily be inserted at 3 and 9 o'clock. The lens is introduced into the eye and with the same uninterrupted transverse motion the first pair of loops is inserted. Then, continuing that motion, the lens is moved along until sufficient room is created to insert the second pair of loops. It depends on the surgeon's preference which pair of loops is inserted first. Some prefer to start with the loops on the same side as the hand used for insertion, making an abduction movement. This leaves the other hand free to manipulate the forceps (WORST, pers. comm.). When the pupil has become square with – or preferably without – the use of acetylcholine irrigation, the special lens forceps are removed.

III Iridotomies and iridectomy

Free communication between posterior and anterior chamber is an essential requirement for the prevention of pupillary block. Consequently, one or two peripheral iridectomies have to be made.

An alternative is to perform peripheral iridotomies and this gives a cosmetically more satisfactory result. Since iridotomies may become blocked more easily than iridectomies, three should be made, e.g. at 11, 12 and 1 o'clock, and not too peripheral, because the further in the periphery they are, the more easily they become blocked (see case 97 on page 87). It is necessary to check their patency by mechanically opening them with an iris repositor. After iridectomy or iridotomies, careful repositioning of the iris and centring of the implant with an iris repositor has to be performed.

Haemorrhage caused by the iridectomy or iridotomies should be washed out of the anterior chamber so that blood cannot block the chamber angle.

IV Suturing and air insufflation

The preplaced corneo-scleral perlon suture(s) is (are) tied with at least two knots, and the loose ends are burnt off with a DIXEY cautery.

As soon as possible, i.e. sometimes even before the knotting of the preplaced suture(s), the anterior chamber is filled completely with sterile air from a sterilised syringe.

Air is used for several reasons:

1. it protects the corneal endothelium from contact with the implant lens during suturing.

2. it detaches the iris from the chamber angle, thus preventing the develop-

ment of gonio-synechiae. PEARCE found some degree of gonio-synechiae present in only 19% of 72 BINKHORST patients, as opposed to 35% of 115 of his own intracapsular aphakics operated on without air insufflation (PEARCE, 1972; BINKHORST, 1973).

3. during suturing air does not escape as easily as a liquid.

4. it improves visibility by keeping out blood from haemorrhages after iridectomies or iridotomies, and from other sources.

5. it facilitates the checking of the patency of the iridotomies by inspection from below through the cornea. If they are closed they should be opened up with an iris repositor.

Air should be introduced only when the tip of the canula is clearly visible in the anterior chamber. At the same time, the lens should be tilted by external pressure on the cornea so as to prevent air from penetrating behind the lens – thus pushing it forward – or even behind the iris. Air in the wrong place should be aspirated.

Subsequently, the corneo-scleral wound is closed with between 8 and 13 perlon sutures which are not removed later as this material does not cause any foreign-body reaction in the tissues. Since 1971, the suture ends have not been cut but are cauterised as short as possible with the DIXEY cautery. The sterile nurse can see better when using the cautery than when using the scissors. Furthermore, the suture ends are blunted by the heat.

The following points must be stressed:

1. during suturing, circulation of air in the operating theatre should be kept to a minimum, to prevent the 0.025 mm thread blowing against the operating microscope, for example. The unsterile nurses are sometimes unaware of this since they are unable to see the suture at all! For them the whole performance of suturing resembles the work done by the tailors in ANDERSEN's fairy tale 'The Emperor's New Clothes'!

2. the sutures should be placed a little deeper than halfway in, so as to be sure of obtaining a well-closed wound.

3. to prevent irritation by the loose ends, each suture may be rotated in its track in order to bury the ends in the sclera.

After suturing, almost all the air in the anterior chamber is replaced by RINGER's solution or saline, since too much air in the anterior chamber can give rise to air blockage of the pupil and/or the iridotomies. Subsequently, the corneo-scleral wound and its sutures are buried under the conjunctival flap. This flap has to be sutured too, using the same type of perlon suture as for the corneo-scleral wound.

Next, pilocarpine hydrochloride 2% drops and eserine salicylate 0.25%

ointment are instilled in the eye which is not padded but just covered by an eye shield with a central hole in it. The perforation in the shield is meant to enable:

a. the nurses to instil eye drops without having to remove any adhesive tape.

b. the surgeon to inspect the eye without having to remove any adhesive tape.

c. the patient to enjoy the improved acuity of his operated eye soon after the operation.

Complications during the implantation and how to handle them

1   Bulging vitreous is the most difficult complication

If the bulge is excessive, the lens should not be inserted. If the bulge is moderate, the pupil should be made as narrow as possible for safety's sake. Only the experienced surgeon may then proceed. He can choose either of two methods of insertion:

a   vertical implantation. Author's method.

The distal loops are introduced across one side of the iris, along the slope of the herniating vitreous, with a slow, horizontal, semicircular, movement, towards their 6 o'clock position and insertion. When the special lens forceps are removed, the proximal loops will point slightly upwards. The iris repositor is placed between the proximal loops, pressed down and the insertion completed routinely (see case 40 on page 182). The final adjusting and centring may be effected when the wound is almost completely sutured and there is still sufficient saline in the anterior chamber. Air insufflation would impair vision at this moment.

b.   horizontal implantation. WORST's method.

The lens is placed on the slope of the vitreous bulge in the 9 o'clock – 3 o'clock position, with or without inserting the loops, and close enough to the 6 o'clock position to be able to suture the corneo-scleral wound watertight. When the wound is partly closed, the vitreous bulge is pressed back by filling the anterior chamber either with air if the loops are already in place, or with saline if the loops are still to be inserted. If necessary, the loops are inserted by manipulating the lens with a iris repositor or a blunt iris hook. Having obtained a horizontal insertion, it is still possible to change one's mind and effect a vertical insertion: the lens is given a quarter turn by means of two instruments used simultaneously (see Fig. 17 on page 69).

52

2   Incarceration of the vitreous between the loops or between iris and lens.

a)   at 6 o'clock.

During insertion of the inferior loops a slight resistance is felt when the vitreous is caught.

The best way of handling this is to withdraw the lens a little and start anew with the insertion, at the same place, or to try at the 5 o'clock or 7 o'clock position. Dislocation may occur within the first 24 hours if this is not done (see case 65 on page 186).

The lens may spring back when the special lens forceps are released (see case 485 on page 92 and the 1st case history on page 176).

b)   at 12 o'clock.

One may try to cover a small incarceration with the iris, using toothed forceps to manipulate the latter. If this fails it is usually best to do nothing at all and proceed with the operation (see case 71 on page 184).

However, a large incarceration is a serious complication, nearly as serious as vitreous loss. Depending on the extent of the surgeon's experience, this may be dealt with either by repeatedly cutting off the vitreous bulge, or, which is probaby better, by removing the implant (see 2nd case history on page 176).

c.   at 3 o'clock or 9 o'clock.

The principles are the same as for the 6 o'clock insertion.

3   Vitreous loss

The only moderately-experienced surgeon should refrain from inserting an iris clip lens. Only the fully experienced surgeon may proceed as follows:

a.   the vitreous prolapse is drawn out with microsponges and cut with DE WECKER scissors as often as necessary until there is no longer any vitreous left in the wound or in front of the anterior surface of the iris. This is a well-known way of dealing with vitreous prolapse.

b.   the iris clip lens is inserted.

c.   the corneo-scleral wound is completely and carefully closed.

d.   air is injected.

e.   another microsponge is drawn across the sutured wound with centrifugal movements, thus picking up any vitreous strands. Their presence is betrayed by the simultaneous movements of the iris. Any strands encountered in this way are severed.

f.　a 'vitreous sweep' with the long iris repositor along the internal wound helps to detach any vitreous strands that may still be incarcerated in the corneoscleral wound.

4.　Loss of watery vitreous due to degenerative liquefaction of the vitreous may result in a funnel-shaped iris with a retroplaced pupil. This makes insertion of the loops difficult or impossible. In these cases the iris may be brought back into the frontal plane by irrigation or external pressure.

Post-operative care.

1　Routine medication

a.　one drop of dexamethasone sodium phosphate (Decadron) four times a day until the patient is discharged.

b.　one drop of pilocarpine hydrochloride 2% twice daily for the rest of the patient's life. These drops should be instilled first thing in the morning and last thing at night. Pilocarpine medication is superfluous if the iris clip lens is iris-fixated by a suture.

c.　250 mg acetazolamide (Diamox) orally three times a day for the five postoperative days, in order to prevent the IOP from rising during the early postoperative period.

d.　the penbritin capsules (see page 42) are discontinued on the 5th postoperative day.

e.　an intramuscular injection of 900 mg Tanderil is given on the 3rd, 4th and 5th day in order to reduce intraocular irritation.

f.　the patient is discharged on the 12th post-operative day.

2　Routine nursing

Blood congestion in the head should be prevented by

a.　a semi-upright position, three pillows being placed under the patient's head after surgery.

b.　easy defecation, ensured by an appropriate diet, for example. The patient should not strain during defecation. If necessary, a Microlax suppository is administered.

3　Routine refraction

a.　the first refraction and determination of visual acuity is carried out on discharge from the hospital. A check for macular oedema is carried out at the same time.

b. the first spectacles are prescribed 6 weeks after the operation.

c. the final spectacles are prescribed 6 months after the operation.

d. annual or biennial check-ups.

SECONDARY IMPLANTATION OF AN IRIS CLIP LENS AFTER INTRACAPSULAR EXTRACTION

Since this operation is no longer routinely performed (see page 35) it is only briefly described.

Secondary implantation should not be undertaken until the eye is completely quiet, i.e. until all signs of irritation have subsided, for example at least three months after cataract extraction. The surgical technique in secondary implantation is more difficult than in primary implantation, and there is a slightly-increased risk of complications during the operation (BINKHORST et al., 1966). The presence or absence of posterior synechiae should be checked in advance under mydriasis (BINKHORST, 1959ab, 1960c, 1962be).

A corneo-scleral incision of 120° is sufficient for the introduction of the implant. The incision is preferably made on the temporal side, because this partially avoids the incision of the first operation, gives more room for manoeuvring, and may have a favourable influence on corneal astigmatism. Prior to actual implantation, posterior synechiae are broken with a straight or bent spatula (BINKHORST, 1962b).

PRIMARY IMPLANTATION OF AN IRIS CLIP LENS AFTER EXTRACAPSULAR EXTRACTION

This operation is no longer routinely performed either. Its place has been taken by iridocapsular lens implantation. If, however, after extracapsular extraction, iridocapsular adhesions are not expected to form, e.g. in cases of milky cataract, an iris clip lens should be inserted instead of an iridocapsular lens.

The technique is essentially the same as for a primary iris clip lens implantation after intracapsular extraction (see page 46).

SECONDARY IMPLANTATION OF AN IRIS CLIP LENS AFTER EXTRACAPSULAR EXTRACTION

It may be necessary to employ this method in the case of an extracapsular aphakic eye without pre-existing posterior synechiae in which, after cutting, the loops of an iridocapsular lens can become embedded (see page 60).

The technique is essentially the same as for a secondary iris clip lens implantation after intracapsular extraction (see this page).

It had been estimated that, after intracapsular extraction, approximately 5 % of iris clip lenses would dislocate after discontinuation of the use of miotics (BINKHORST, 1969a, 1971a; WORST, 1972a in the discussion). This induced WORST to suture the anterior loops to the iris with perlon, since this is a stable material which does not cause any foreign-body reaction in the tissues (WORST, 1970, 1971bcde, 1972ab). This method of iris fixation makes the use of miotics not only superfluous, but even permits full dilatation of the pupil, thus facilitating ophthalmoscopy. Consequently, a main objection to the iris clip lens, namely the difficulties encountered during ophthalmoscopy, has been eliminated by the introduction of the iris suture (WORST, 1971de). However, if the pupil becomes too wide, monocular diplopia may occur (HENKES in the discussion with WORST, WORST, 1972a), but this can be prevented by pilocarpine drops or, in future, by the use of an implant with a larger optical portion (WORST, 1972a).

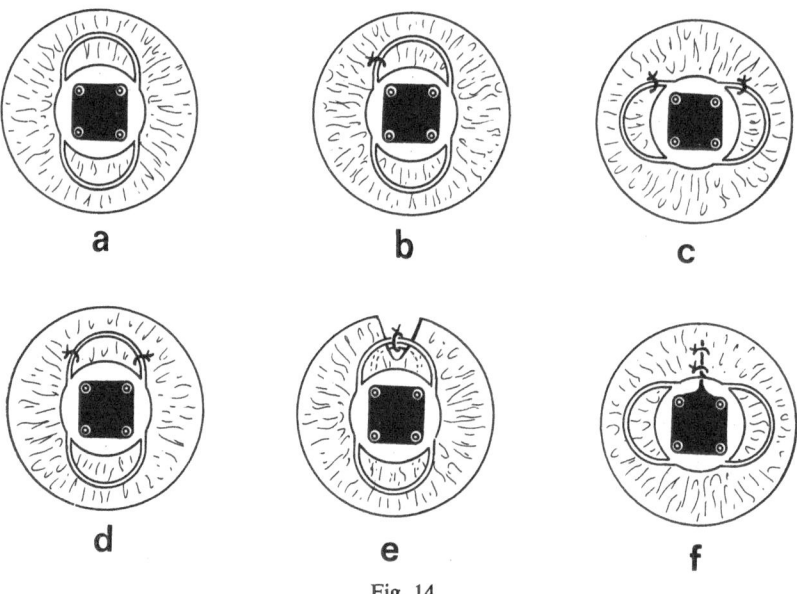

Fig. 14

Methods of fixation in iris clip lens implantation.
a) pilocarpine fixation in vertical implantation. No suture.
b) one post-placed loop suture in vertical implantation.
c) two preplaced loop sutures in horizontal implantation.
d) two preplaced loop sutures in vertical implantation (see also Fig. 15).
e) transiridectomy suture.
f) radial iridotomy with two preplaced iris sutures.

Case history.

Case 333 (WORST). Female, born 1908.

4–12–70 intracapsular cataract extraction followed by iris clip lens implantation OD. The implant was sutured to the iris.

19– 1–71 corrected visual acuity was 1.0.

Monocular double images were present when the pupil was wide.

Therapy: pilocarpine eye drops.

There are several technical alternatives for loop sutures:

*a. post-placed loop suture(s) after horizontal or vertical implantation (*WORST*)* See Fig. 14b.

One suture is usually sufficient to prevent dislocation, but two may be em-. ployed for greater security. Each suture is carefully placed, *through* the iris and *around* the loop. Because of the difficulty of suturing through the entire thickness of the iris, the suture may be passed through a peripheral iridectomy. It should be tied securely and cut as short as possible with scissors, to protect the corneal endothelium. Cauterisation of this suture could cause thermal damage to the implant. If the suture ends are too long they may scrape the corneal endothelium and cause ECD (see case 132 on page 160 and case 602 on page 161).

b. preplaced loop suture(s) in horizontal or vertical implantation (WORST).

1 horizontal implantation

Before extraction, a special 6 mm needle threaded with perlon* is passed through the iris just peripheral to the sphincter muscle. The two long suture ends are left outside the eye. Great care must be taken that no inadvertent snarling occurs. Before implantation, the needle is passed through the axilla of the upper branch of *both* anterior loops: after implantation, the knot will be formed *behind* the lens.

2 vertical implantation. See Figs. 14d and 15

The suture is passed through the iris in two places, just peripheral to the sphincter muscle. After implantation, the central part of the suture is pulled through the superior loop, and cut. The two separate loops of the suture are tied around the corresponding vertical parts of the superior loop.

* This needle may be obtained from Medical Workshop, Heresingel 28, Groningen, Holland.

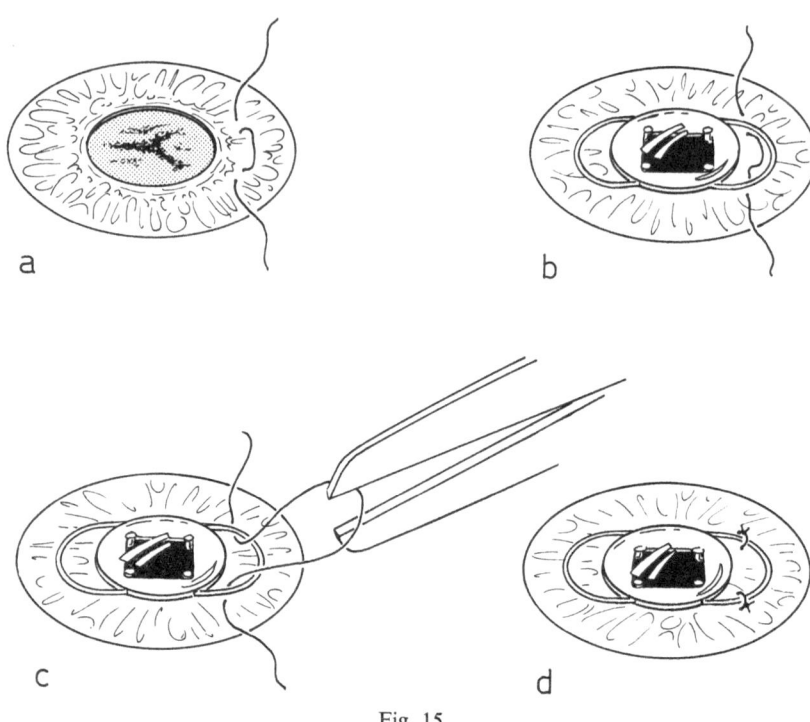

Fig. 15

Technique of preplaced loop suture in vertical iris clip lens implantation (Courtesy J. G. F. WORST, M.D.).

c. transiridectomy suture

This is the suturing together of both superior loops through the 12 o'clock iridectomy. See Fig. 14e. With the transiridectomy suture, the implant fixation is relatively independent of the iris (WORST, pers. comm.; BINKHORST, 1972bc, 1973). If the peripheral iridectomy at 12 o'clock is made as a radial cut and a little more centripetal than usual, the implant can move down in case of maximal mydriasis, without dislocation of the inferior loops.

The anterior loop is grasped with fine forceps whereupon the posterior loop appears in the coloboma. Both loops are tied together loosely over a fine repositor with one perlon suture which is cut short. For this suture it is advisable to use a 12 mm long completely blunt metal wire threaded with perlon* to prevent vitreous prolapse.

---

* Obtainable from Medical Workshop, Heresingel 28, Groningen, Holland.

This implantation can be performed only after extracapsular cataract extraction. The advantages and disadvantages of extracapsular, as opposed to intracapsular, extraction were mentioned on page 36 (BINKHORST, 1972be, 1973).

Attention should be paid to the following surgical details:

1. the incision can be limited to 120°, which is wide enough to facilitate the delivery of a hard lenticular nucleus and to introduce an implant.

2. partial removal of the anterior capsule with toothed forceps, to ensure good access to the lenticular substance.

3. aspiration of lens material in the young patient or expression of the hard nucleus in the old patient.

4. irrigation of the anterior chamber with both straight and sharply-bent canula, the latter being used for irrigation under the upper iris segment. A certain amount of lenticular material is, however, necessary to form iridocapsular adhesions (BINKHORST, 1967b, 1968a, 1969a, 1972e).

5. vertical insertion. As soon as the inferior loop is placed behind the lower iris segment, the forceps are removed and the upper iris segment is pulled over the superior loop with a blunt iris hook, while the implant is held down with a fine repositor.

6. two peripheral iridectomies. Particularly in extracapsular surgery, where two iridectomies are safer than one in case of blockage by lens material.

7. repositioning of the iris with an iris repositor.

8. excessive deepening of the anterior chamber with air, enabling inspection of the chamber angle. Any adhesion of the iris to the incision should be corrected with an iris repositor.

9. multiple corneo-scleral and conjunctival perlon sutures.

10. most of the air is replaced by saline: the iris is brought level with the chamber angle.

11. pilocarpine hydrochloride 2% eye drops are instilled and eserine salicylate 0.25% ointment is applied.

12. an eye shield with a central hole is placed over the eye.

Post-operative care

1. pilocarpine hydrochloride 2% drops twice daily, as long as there are no firm iridocapsular adhesions. The development of these adhesions should be studied carefully. Having discontinued pilocarpine medication on the 4th or 5th day, movement of the implant when the light of the slitlamp is switched on and

off, indicates that iridocapsular adhesions have not yet been formed. In the absence of such movements, a mydriatic test with mydriaticum ROCHE is performed at the end of the first week to check the iridocapsular adhesions and to prevent the development of posterior synechiae, particularly at the pupillary border (BINKHORST, 1969bcd, 1971a, 1972e, 1973).

2. dexamethasone sodium phosphate (Decadron) eye drops four times a day for 4 to 6 weeks.

3. needling of lens remnants is necessary in a number of cases.

Cloudy secondary cataract may be absorbed spontaneously. It can be assisted by hot fomentations and careful mydriasis.

Fibrillar secondary cataract can sometimes be swept away with a needle knife behind the lower iris segment, leaving the posterior capsule undamaged.

Membraneous secondary cataract has to be dissected with a needle knife. The position of the implant with respect to the pupil enables unrestricted access to the pupil with instruments (BINKHORST, 1973). The lens itself prevents herniation of the vitreous into the anterior chamber through a perforated posterior lens capsule.

SECONDARY IMPLANTATION OF AN IRIDOCAPSULAR LENS

The technique is largely the same as for primary implantation. However, to achieve fixation of the iridocapsular lens in an eye with extracapsular aphakia, it is absolutely essential to insert the loops at the site of freshly-cut capsular strands or posterior synechiae in order to facilitate the development of adhesions (BINKHORST, 1967ac, 1969acd, 1971a, 1972be, 1973).

The implantation of an iridocapsular lens after preliminary needling is the technique of choice in children with congenital or traumatic cataract, with the exception of infants under the age of about 12 months, in view of the surgical complications that tend to arise in the latter category. These are, for example, iris incarceration, iris bombé, iritis, and intractable pupillary membranes (BINKHORST, 1967ad, 1969bcd, 1970b, 1971b, 1972bcde, 1973).

Preliminary needling is recommended, a few days to a week prior to the removal of the cataract.

The advantage of this procedure is that it usually produces a satisfactory loosening of the lens fibres, enabling a more effective evacuation of the lens material.

Disadvantages:

a) irritation by lens material.

b) the risk of raised intraocular pressure.

60

c) increased risk of haemorrhage during the implant operation, because the eye has become hyperaemic.

The surgeon should therefore be ready to proceed with the implant operation whenever required.

Swollen lens material is removed by aspiration and irrigation only, and without using DAVIEL's spoons. This spares the corneal endothelium, since extensive manipulation in the anterior chamber is thereby avoided.

PRIMARY IMPLANTATION OF AN IRIS MEDALLION LENS

Surgical technique

1. Having opened the anterior chamber over 180°, a perlon suture is passed through the iris just peripheral to the sphincter at the 12 o'clock position. The iris needle* required for this purpose, is of a particular length and has a certain curvature to facilitate the placing of this suture. The suture ends are left long.
2. intracapsular or extracapsular cataract extraction.
3. the ends of the iris suture are passed through the corresponding holes in the iris medallion lens in such a way that the knot will come *behind* the lens. This prevents contact of the free suture ends with the corneal endothelium.
4. it is essential that the loops of the suture be kept away from the loops of the lens during the lens implantation which follows.
5. the lens is held in a pair of needle holders (special forceps* are now available).

The first loop is hooked behind the pupillary border, the second is inserted after withdrawing the iris slightly with forceps. The pupil is constricted with pilocarpine hydrochloride 2%.
6. the iris suture is tied behind the haptic portion. It is necessary to make *three* knots, to prevent it from loosening.
7. the anterior chamber is rinsed with saline.
8. the suture ends are cut short.
9. peripheral iridectomy at 12 o'clock.
10. wound closure.

Post-operative care

Dexamethasone sodium phosphate (Decadron) and neomycine eye drops are administered 6 times a day. This medication is continued for two to three weeks.

---

* Medical Workshop, Heresingel 28, Groningen, Holland.

1 *Suturing a coloboma, e.g. iridencleisis*

A sector coloboma is not a contra-indication for an iris clip lens implantation: it can be sutured with one or two preplaced perlon sutures. It must be stressed that in most cases the gap should be bridged, not closed. If the sutures are drawn too tight, they may eventually tear the iris (see case 108 on page 167). In case of a 12 o'clock coloboma the implantation will have to be of the horizontal variety.

2 *Suturing a radial iridotomy*

In cases with a small pupil due to iris rigidity or the prolonged use of miotics in glaucoma, it is sometimes a serious mistake to extract the lens without making a radial iridotomy. If this is not done, the sphincter could rupture at any point, after which the pupil will remain permanently wide.

The correct way to handle such a case is to perform a radial iridotomy prior to lens extraction. This can be started in a peripheral iridectomy (BINKHORST, WORST) or with an iridotomy in mid-iris (author's method). See Fig. 69 on page 192. The latter method preserves a little more of the normal anatomical structure of the iris tissue. The iris cleft can be closed with two preplaced perlon sutures, one of which will re-unite the sphincter.

The implantation will have to be of the horizontal variety.

3 *Use of the iris clip lens for the obturation of the pupil prior to extraction of a cataract* (FEDOROV) *or secondary membranes* (BINKHORST, *pers. comm.*) *through a basal coloboma*

FEDOROV (1969d) invented this method for cases where vitreous loss could be expected, such as in traumatic cataract. The iris clip lens or iridocapsular lens is inserted prior to cataract extraction in order to prevent vitreous loss through the pupil. As a result the pupil may become decentred upwards. Vitreous loss through a basal coloboma is less dangerous since it leaves the pupil central. See case IC 50 on page 126 and case IC 51 on page 131.

4 *Implantation of an iris clip lens or iridocapsular lens in an eye with a mutilated anterior segment*

Implant surgery in eyes with a mutilated anterior chamber is not impossible. 'For the inventive surgeon it is nearly always possible to find a solution, even in seemingly hopeless cases. With anterior and posterior synechiolysis and extraction of secondary cataract after cutting it out with VANNAS scissors through a peripheral iridectomy, corepraxis may be necessary before implantation. One-stage surgery, providing room and fixation for the implant, is to be preferred for understandable reasons, and, especially in children, for functional reasons. Two-stage surgery has to be considered if the depth of the perforation is not exactly known. It should be borne in mind, however, that needling of a capsular membrane for better ophthalmoscopy, would seriously reduce the chance of a successful implant operation later' (BINKHORST, 1972e).

POST-OPERATIVE COMPLICATIONS AND THEIR THERAPY

All's well that ends well.

1 *Early complications*

a. Pupillary block may be encountered where the peripheral colobomas are non-existent, only the stromal part of the iris having been cut, or where they are too small, blocked by air, blood, lens material or vitreous body, but only in those cases where the circulation through the pupil is blocked as well.

It is wise, therefore, to check the patency of the peripheral colobomas during operation. Iridotomies should not be made too peripherally because they then become more easily blocked. The symptoms of pupillary block are: pain, high intraocular pressure, iris bombé, and a flattened air bubble in a shallow anterior chamber.

Therapy:

1. laying the patient's head on its side may lead to a change in the position of the air bubble and, subsequently, to the reopening of an iridotomy. This only applies to cases where too much air is left.

2. discontinuation of miotics and careful administration of a mydriatic. If these measures do not have an early effect on the depth of the anterior chamber (depending on the cause!), the surgeon should not hesitate to perform:

3. an additional peripheral iridectomy

or

4. a transfixion of the iris.

b. Shallow anterior chamber with low intraocular pressure may be caused by:

1. a fistulating corneo-scleral wound.

Therapy: additional corneo-scleral sutures.

2. a choroidal detachment, which is rarely seen after an implantation.

Therapy: as after cataract extraction without implantation.

c. Transient striate keratitis may be seen after extensive manipulation in difficult implant operations, particularly secondary implantations.
No therapy.

d. Precipitates on the implant may be divided into:
1. pigmented precipitates caused by surgery or, in some cases, by the posterior loops touching the pigment epithelium of the iris. Visual acuity is usually undisturbed.
2. greyish-white precipitates caused by:
– lens material. These are only observed after extracapsular extractions and disappear in the course of a few weeks.
– infectious material. They remain or disappear with the infection itself.
In both cases visual acuity may be reduced. See also pages 87 and 154.

2. *Complications that may occur earlier or later*

a. Uveitis is occasionally seen, either soon after implant surgery or later on (see also pages 87 and 155).
Therapy: local administration of corticosteroids.

b. Dislocation.

Dislocation of an iris clip lens may be caused by:
1. too much air in the anterior chamber.
2. too wide a pupil, due to:
a. sphincter being ruptured during cataract extraction, or damaged by pressure of the posterior loop attachments.
b. pilocarpine being erroneously discontinued.
c. mydriatic being erroneously administered.
d. pupil dilatation at night.
1. darkness has an effect on the dilatation of the pupil that varies considerably from person to person. Its extent should be known prior to implantation.
2. orgasm may dilate some pupils excessively.

Case history.
Case 24 (worst). Female, born 1920.
1967 blunt trauma OS.
1968 mature cataract OS.
1969 intracapsular cataract extraction with iris clip lens implantation OS. No loop sutures, but pilocarpine medication twice daily.
The implant dislocated 3, 30 and 65 weeks after operation, due to orgasm on the same day of each week. Non-operative repositioning.
Further preventive measure: Phospholine iodide eye drops.

3. loop length of the implant being too short.

4. severe ocular trauma in pseudophakic eye (see pages 119 and 171).

For the distribution of the different types of dislocation, the reader is referred to page 93.

Repositioning of a dislocated iris clip lens

1. urination and defecation by the patient before treatment is started is a practical measure that prevents interruption of therapy at an unfavourable moment, for example when re-insertion has nearly succeeded after several hours of work (LÉONARD, pers. comm.).

2. exact location of the implant by slitlamp examination or ophthalmoscopy.

3. dilatation of the pupil with a mydriatic of short duration, e.g. mydriaticum ROCHE, since the pupil must be constricted rapidly after re-insertion of the loops.

4. the patient lies with his head hanging over the edge of the operating table either prone or supine, depending on the type of dislocation.

5. if both pairs of loops are dislocated, one of them can usually be re-inserted fairly easily by manipulating the patient's head, tapping it, and possibly the eye too. The second or solitary pair of dislocated loops must have a sufficiently-wide pupil for re-insertion. If this kind of manipulation brings the loop tips into proximity with the pupillary border, the pupil should be constricted as quickly as possible by instilling pilocarpine hydrochloride 4% eye drops. If the patient is lying prone, it will be necessary for the surgeon to sit or lie on the floor and work above his own head. The miotic should then be administered by means of a spray.

6. instrumental re-insertion with corneal anaesthesia is necessary if the above methods fails. If only one pair of loops is in the anterior chamber, it is usually relatively easy to re-insert the wandering implant with a needle knife. Simultaneous irrigation with saline through a contrapuncture may be considered, in order to ensure sufficient room for manipulation.

7. in difficult cases, e.g. when the lens has rotated back-to-front, extensive intraocular manipulations will be required. These will not be discussed in detail since the surgical technique varies from case to case.

8. recurrent dislocation may be treated by inserting a secondary loop suture (BINKHORST). The technique is as follows:

a. an incision of 3 to 4 mm is made in the cornea with a VON GRAEFE knife, a PEARCE knife, or a GILETTE blade, at the site of a loop tip and perpendicular to it. In addition, a contrapuncture may be made. When aqueous escapes, the loop tip approaches the incision.

65

b.   a perlon suture around the loop and through the iris, is loosely tied and cut as short as possible.

c.   the anterior chamber is refilled with air or saline, and anterior synechiae are swept away via the contrapuncture.

d.   the corneal incision is sutured.

Case history.
Case 59 (author's case). See page 186 and Fig. 65 opposite page 196.

Dislocation of an iridocapsular lens may occur if iridocapsular adhesions have not formed. Unless repositioning is spontaneous (see case IC 28 on page 133 and case IC 30 on page 129), therapy is always surgical, and consists of:

a.   instrumental repositioning, followed by:

1)   permanent use of pilocarpine eye drops

2)   loop iris suture, in case of relapse

b)   replacement by an iris clip lens (see case IC 6 on page 128).

c.   *Cystoid macular oedema* may be elicited by cataract surgery.

It is often associated with small haemorrhages and may appear as a pseudo-macular hole (BINKHORST, 1967e, 1968b). The aetiology of cystoid macular oedema is still unknown, but vitreous traction by forward displacement of the vitreous body has been considered a major cause of the macular changes (IRVINE, 1953). Its incidence is higher in cases with vitreous loss or vitreous incarceration (JAFFE, 1972b). Excessive uveal reaction has also been regarded as a factor promoting macular oedema (BINKHORST, 1960c, 1962bde, 1972b, 1973).

According to COLENBRANDER, there is a relationship with the duration of the operation. Progressive macular oedema starts to develop from the moment the eye has been opened until it is closed again. Complications, such as vitreous loss, increase the length of the operation and in the presence of a lot of oedema changes occur that are difficult or impossible to reverse (COLENBRANDER, pers. comm. 8-3-1974).

Despite the fact that forward displacement of the vitreous occurs less frequently in pseudophakia, than in aphakia, development of cystoid macular oedema does not seem to occur less frequently after cataract extraction with lens implantation than without it. On the contrary, its early occurrence *seems* to be more frequent in pseudophakia. Whether cystoid macular oedema is *significantly* more frequently encountered in pseudophakia than in aphakia, remains to be investigated. This, according to WORST (pers. comm. 13-2-1974) might be due to:

66

1. the damage incurred more frequently by the anterior vitreous membrane in cases fitted with a BINKHORST lens implant. WORST performed several binocular implant operations where cystoid macular oedema developed in the eye with a damaged anterior vitreous membrane but not in the other.

2. the flow of the aqueous back towards the vitreous, because the intraocular hydrodynamics have been changed by the presence of the implant in the pupil.

3. the over-exposure to light, because the square of the posterior loop attachments was relatively too large before 1972.

As regards therapy, the tendency to spontaneous recovery may be supported by local or systemic corticosteroids.

3 Late complications

a. Endothelial corneal dystrophy (ECD) is the most dreaded complication of lens implantation.

Its stages are:

1. local epithelial oedema near the incision or the anterior loop tips of the iris clip lens.

2. striate keratitis with incipient corneal oedema.

3. generalised corneal oedema.

4. 'bullous keratopathy', epithelial bullae.

MILLER & DOHLMAN (1970) described its aetiology as a decompensation of the aqueous pump function of the endothelium. In 38 of a series of 50 unilateral aphakic eyes with obviously healthy corneas they found a significant thickening of the cornea and concluded that this must have been caused by stromal oedema unaccompanied by epithelial oedema, i.e. a beginning of endothelial decompensation. Simple, uncomplicated, extraction itself, therefore, may actually have initiated the endothelial malfunction (BINKHORST, 1972b, 1973).

The later stages may manifest themselves if promoting factors were already present, e.g. FUCHS' endothelial dystrophy (see page 104). Serious operative and post-operative complications also play an important part in promoting this condition (see page 106). The main cause of ECD, however, is the intermittent or continuous contact of the implant with the corneal endothelium, brought about by incorrect size and shape of the implant, or its dislocation (see page 104).

Prevention of ECD

The chances of the patient developing ECD may be diminished by measures minimising surgical trauma, for example:

a. all instruments introduced into the anterior chamber should be perfectly polished on their superior corneal side, without any sharp edges, in order to avoid scraping the corneal endothelium if this is inadvertently touched.

b.   all intraocular movements should be made carefully, and never briskly; unnecessary movements should be avoided.

c.   the corneal flap should be lifted as gently as possible and preferably without any appreciable corneal folding (see also page 46).

d.   over-abundant irrigation should be avoided.

e.   only artificial aqueous at 28°C should be used for irrigation.

f.   the chamber angle should be inspected carefully and any gonio-adhesions should be broken.

g.   intraocular pressure should be restored as soon as possible and carefully controlled by palpation during recovery.

h.   any post-operative inflammation should be suppressed maximally by means of corticosteroids.

Unfortunately, the promotive factors may cause the patient's 'endothelial damage allowance' (BINKHORST, 1973) to be surpassed, and the signs of dystrophy will then become apparent. It is, therefore, of the utmost importance to examine the corneal endothelium by slitlamp biomicroscopy in order to asses endothelial vitality *before* subjecting the eye to surgery. In this connection it should be remembered that implant operations tend to be more traumatic than other surgery (BINKHORST, 1973).

Therapy of ECD

In the early stages, some degree of regeneration is possible if the causative factor is eliminated, e.g. removal of loop contact by surgical intervention at an early stage of ECD may clear the cornea.

The following techniques are currently used:

1.   Loop amputation of the iris clip lens (BINKHORST). See Fig. 16.

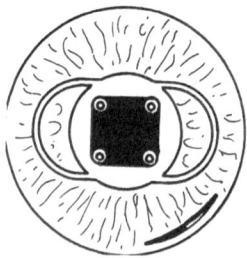

Fig. 16

Loop amputation through a corneal incision.

A 3 to 4 mm limbal or corneal incision is made with a keratome or PEARCE knife. VANNAS scissors are used to cut first the distal loop pillar, then the proximal loop pillar and, finally – as if they were forceps – to extract the loop. The incision is closed with one or two perlon corneal sutures.

2. Rotation of the iris clip lens (SETIAWAN ONG). See Fig. 17.

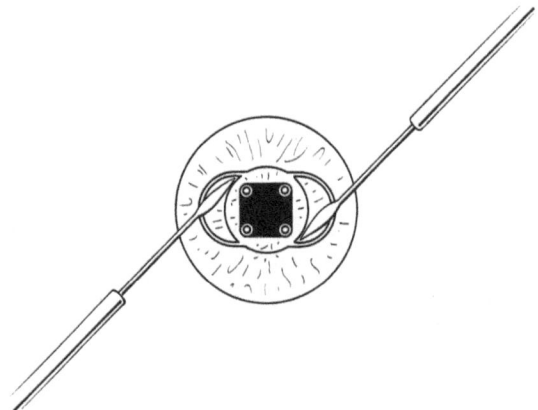

Fig. 17

Implant rotation with two needle knives.

The implant is rotated through 90° by the simultaneous use of two needle knives under mydriasis. However, the lens may spring back due to posterior synechiae, while the vitreous may also impede rotation.

3. Extraction of an iris clip lens may have the same result, but it puts an end to all prospect of pseudophakia and is a considerable additional trauma to the cornea that should be avoided if at all possible. The eye is incised over 120° with a keratome and scissors, near a loop tip. The iris is freed from the proximal loops and the implant is removed, pulling at the proximal posterior loop with a blunt iris hook. The surgeon must make sure that any synechiae attached to the implant have been broken beforehand.

ECD in its later stages is resistant to any therapy, including extraction of the implant. Penetrating keratoplasty is the only rational treatment to attempt, and this is even safer when the lens implant is in situ.

b. *Iris atrophy* (see page 227) may be present in the form of
– pressure atrophy of iris tissue showing as four deep grooves in the pupillary

margin of eyes with an iris clip lens under pilocarpine miosis. Late dislocation might thus be caused by interference with the sphincter's action.

– local atrophy of the pigment epithelium. In most cases, however, gonioscopy does not reveal any greater amount of pigmentation in the chamber angle of pseudophakic than of aphakic eyes. This means that pigmentation is mainly caused by loss of pigment during surgery, not by loop friction.

c. *Retinal detachment* is mainly seen in implantations after intracapsular extraction of senile cataracts (see page 110). Since the early years of iris clip lens implantation, one criticism has been that the observation of the ocular fundus prior to surgery for retinal detachment or photocoagulation in diabetic retinopathy is supposedly hampered by a narrow pupil. This is not true, because the pupil may be dilated in the supine patient without much risk, especially in cases with loop sutures. However, it would be better to keep the eye immobilised until the pupil is again constricted (JUNGSCHAFFER, 1972).

CHAPTER IV

RESULTS OBTAINED BY C. D. BINKHORST

> 'I've had plenty of practice', the Knight said
> very gravely: 'plenty of practice'.
> Lewis CARROLL: Through the Looking-
> Glass and What Alice Found There.
> Chapter VIII: 'It's My Own Invention'.

INTRODUCTION

This chapter deals with the results of BINKHORST lens implant operations performed by C. D. BINKHORST, the only surgeon with a post-operative follow-up period of up to 15 years.

For this purpose the author had free access to the case histories of all patients with BINKHORST lens implants, and was given the opportunity to examine 70 patients with 89 implants (NORDLOHNE, cited by BINKHORST, 1972b, 1973).

Until 1st January 1972 BINKHORST performed 864 BINKHORST lens implant operations subdivided into 694 iris clip lenses and 170 iridocapsular lenses. The closing date of 1st January 1972 was chosen by the author so that he would have sufficient time for a minimal follow-up period for the evaluation of the results of the most recent cases.

Of the 864 cases, and excluding the deceased patients, it was possible to trace all patients after 1st January 1970. This date was chosen by the author because all patients having been examined six months after the operation, a blank period of maximally 1½ years was considered acceptable by him.

A general review of numerical data is given in Fig. 18 at back of book. They are based on data from BINKHORST, KATS, LÉONARD, GOBIN, SETIAWAN ONG, ROMMEL and ophthalmologists who referred patients, and were collected by the author from records of operations, index cards, letters as well as by his own investigations (see below).

Occasionally, these ophthalmologists are mentioned in the case histories. The data of the investigation by PEARCE in May 1970 (PEARCE, 1972), though mentioned in the case histories, were not included, because they did not form part of BINKHORST's records.

71

The data of all cases were listed with respect to cause of cataract, sex of patient, left or right eye, binocular or monocular implantation, age at time of operation, observation period in days between date of operation and last date of refraction, and visual acuity at that date. 'Visual acuity' stands for the resolving power of the eye when the latter is corrected by a pre-corneal optical appliance. The 'age at operation' is taken in the present work to be the difference between the year of birth and the year in which the operation was carried out.

All cases were numbered consecutively by BINKHORST from 1 onwards (St. Elisabeth Hospital in Sluiskil) and from 1001 onwards (Juliana Hospital in Terneuzen). The first iris clip lens is indicated as C 1, the first iridocapsular lens as IC 1 (Sluiskil), or C 1001 and IC 1001 (Terneuzen). In this chapter, however, only IC is indicated while the C has been omitted.

Of these 864 eyes, 409 (47.3%) were from BINKHORST's own area (Zeeuwsch-Vlaanderen in the Province of Zeeland), 108 (12.5%) came from the remainder of Zeeland, 318 (36.8%) from the remainder of the Netherlands and 29 (3.4%) from abroad.

Two implantations of an iris clip lens of the FEDOROV type, are described separately on page 136 (cases F1 and F2).

The development of implant design, surgical technique and post-operative care was spread over 10 years. During this period the number of cases operated on annually was relatively low, as can be seen from Fig. 39 on page 122.

BINOCULAR IMPLANT OPERATIONS

The group of binocular implant operations consists of 130 patients (75 ♂ and 55 ♀) fitted with an iris clip lens in both eyes, 5 patients (3 ♂ and 2 ♀) fitted with an iris clip lens in one eye and an iridocapsular lens in the other as well as 12 patients (9 ♂ and 3 ♀) fitted with an iridocapsular lens in both eyes.

Of these 147 patients the first operation was carried out on the left eye in 57 (38.8%) cases, and on the right eye in 61 (41.5%) cases while 29 (19.7%) were operated upon in a single session.

The indication for implantation in both eyes in one session was the higher average age at operation of 79.68 years in 28 patients with senile cataract, and oligophreny in one child with congenital cataract. The interval between the two implant operations ranged from 0 to 3647 days, with an average of 515 days (for the iris clip lens it was 545 days). Fig. 19 shows the data and results of the iris clip lens implantations in binocular cases.

It is noteworthy that there is no significant difference in the average visual acuity of the eyes whether operated on first or last, even when the interval between operations was more than 4 years.

72

interval between implantations in binocular cases	number of patients	average age at operation in years		average observation period in days		average visual acuity	
		1st eye	2nd eye	1st eye	2nd eye	1st eye	2nd eye
0– 365 days	75	69.12	69.63	558	484	0.64	0.61
366– 730 days	26	64.85	66.11	900	523	0.71	0.80
731–1095 days	14	65.07	67.43	1379	920	0.78	0.76
1096–1461 days	9	67.67	71.22	2160	1123	0.54	0.56
>1461 days	11	63.91	70.73	3058	965	0.61	0.60
total	135	67.34	68.91	1027	612	0.66	0.66

Fig. 19

Data and results of iris clip lens implant operations performed by BINKHORST on binocular cases relative to the interval between the implant operations.

MONOCULAR IMPLANT OPERATIONS

The group of monocular implant operations consists of 429 patients (213 ♂ and 216 ♀) fitted with an iris clip lens, and 141 patients (85 ♂ and 56 ♀) fitted with an iridocapsular lens.

The number of 570 monocular cases as opposed to only 147 binocular cases is relatively high in view of the 71.5 % of senile cataract encountered (see Fig. 42 on page 124). This may be explained by BINKHORST's expectant attitude during the early days of operating mainly on monocular cataract cases. In addition, the average operation age was high, and many patients had died before a second operation had even been considered.

Causes of cataract

Data and results of iris clip lens implant operations, related to the cause of the cataract, are shown in Fig. 20.

cause of cataract	num-ber	♂	♀	L	R	average age at operation in years	average observation period in days	average visual acuity
senile	567	276	291	268	299	69.97	729	0.64
traumatic (15 perf.)	52	46	6	24	28	38.38	739	0.64
unknown	51	34	17	24	27	52.33	1064	0.75
complicated	14	5	9	5	9	57.64	904	0.56
heterochromic	4	2	2	3	1	62.00	1213	0.56
thermic	2	2	—	2	—	55.00	2533	0.95
radiation	1	—	1	1	—	81	1852	0.10
congenital	1	—	1	1	—	18	1086	?
juvenile	1	1	—	1	—	32	2930	1.00
diabetic	1	—	1	—	1	33	760	0.35
total	694	366	328	329	365	65.80	772	0.65

Fig. 20

Data and results of 694 iris clip lens implant operations performed by BINKHORST, relative to the cause of the cataract.

Exclusion of cases

Evaluation of the visual acuity results took place after exclusion of 17 cases for the following reasons:

1. 14 cases out of the rather homogeneous group of 505 primary implantations of an iris clip lens after intracapsular cataract extraction, because a normal implant was no longer in situ. These are subdivided as follows:

enucleation after severe ocular trauma (case 300 on page 113), extraction of implant because of high myopia (case 181 on page 112 and case 353 on page 99), or trauma (case 1004 on page 119), dislocation into the vitreous in high myopia (case 204 on page 99),

experimental implant model (case 76 on page 109) and absence of data because of death (8 cases).

2. 3 cases after extracapsular implantation consisting of:

extraction of implant due to inflammation (case 67 on page 112), mongolian idiocy with keratoconus and congenital cataract (case 343 on page 120),

central corneal degeneration with simultaneous autokeratoplasty (case 573 on page 120).

The latter two cases were excluded because of the exceptional procedure.

The data and results of the remaining 677 cases are:

a) The *age at operation* ranges from 5 to 92 years, with an average of 65.70 years. Fig. 40 on page 122 shows the frequency curves for the iris clip and iridocapsular lenses. Its highest frequency occurred at 71 years of age.

The relation between age at operation and visual acuity is shown in Fig. 21. The results calculated per 5 year age group, for the average visual acuity achieved as well as the percentage of eyes attaining a visual acuity of 1.0 and over, de·crease progressively after the age of 70. This is undoubtedly due to an increase in the frequency of senile macular changes.

b) The *observation period* ranges from 4 to 4498 days, with an average of 768 days. Fig. 22 shows the frequency curve. The highest frequency is at 184 days. The relationship between observation period, age at operation and visual acuity is also shown in Fig. 22.

The increase of the average visual acuity during the first 10 months, and especially during the first 3 months, is remarkable. To some extent this is promoted by the decrease in corneal astigmatism in the post-operative period. Fig. 23 shows, for primary intracapsular BINKHORST lens implantation, that average visual acuity decreases progressively in cases of residual spectacle astigmatism of more than one dioptre, both for the BINKHORST series and the WORST series.

The great variation in visual acuity in the course of the years, however, must be due to all the modifications of the implant mentioned on page 27 ff.

c) The *visual acuity* ranges from 0 to 1.25, with an average of 0.65. The relationship between visual acuity and surgical procedure is shown in Fig. 24. The relationship between visual acuity and age at operation in primary intracapsular iris clip lens implant operations is shown in Fig. 25.

The outstanding feature, namely the 58 cases (11.9%) of primary intracapsular iris clip lens implantation with a visual acuity of 0.10 or less, may be explained for the greater part by 27 cases of total ECD (see page 100 ff.) and 7 cases of retinal detachment (see page 110 ff.). Forty-two out of these 58 cases attained a visual acuity of 0.05 or less.

It would have been interesting to make a comparison with a series of aphakic patients operated on by BINKHORST during the same period, but this was impossible for administrative reasons.

76

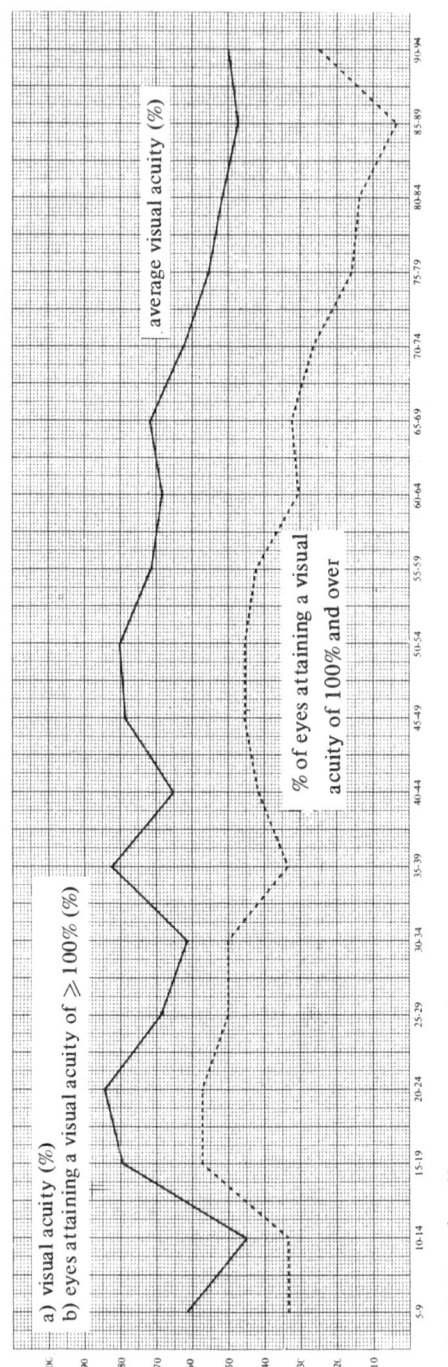

age at operation (5 year age groups)

Fig. 21. Relationship between age at operation and visual acuity in 677 iris clip lens implant operations performed by BINKHORST.

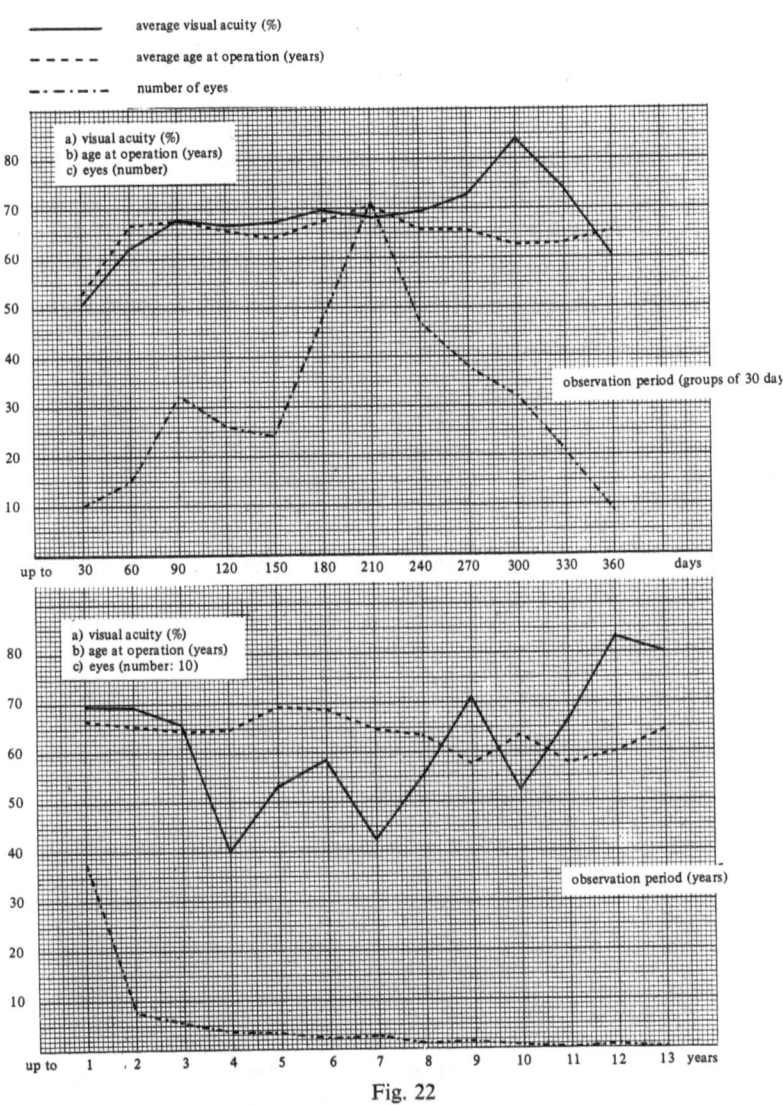

average visual acuity (%)

average age at operation (years)

number of eyes

a) visual acuity (%)
b) age at operation (years)
c) eyes (number)

observation period (groups of 30 days)

a) visual acuity (%)
b) age at operation (years)
c) eyes (number: 10)

observation period (years)

Fig. 22

Relationship between observation period, age at operation, and visual acuity in 675 iris clip lens implant operations performed by BINKHORST. In two cases the observation period was unknown.

The 373 cases with an observation period of up to 360 days are shown separately with a subdivision in groups of 30 days.

Therefore the main features of 675 iris clip lens implant operations by BINK-HORST were compared with those of a series of plain cataract extractions performed by other surgeons. In 1965/1966 MÜLLER & PAPASTYLIANOS (1968) re-examined 1879 eyes that had undergone plain cataract operations in the period 1955–1965. The percentage of eyes in this series achieving a visual acuity of 0.10 and less, was 6.8. This percentage would have been about 5.4 had the relative spectacle magnification (25 %) been taken into consideration. The average visual acuity with an aphakic correction for the whole series was calculated by the author to be 0.81 which is 24.6 % more than 0.65. This percentage is about

| residual spectacle astigmatism | BINKHORST | | | |
	number	average age at operation in years	average observation period in days	average visual acuity
—	67	68.91	495	0.73
until 1 D	98	66.28	697	0.79
until 2 D	141	67.72	632	0.78
until 3 D	64	70.00	557	0.74
until 4 D	16	70.75	460	0.55
until 5 D	5	63.00	667	0.54
total	391	68.00	606	0.76

	WORST			
—	54	69.83	195	0.75
until 1 D	92	69.66	186	0.80
until 2 D	126	70.31	209	0.74
until 3 D	109	71.44	189	0.67
until 4 D	55	73.62	139	0.63
until 5 D	39	74.33	145	0.61
total	475	71.10	185	0.71

Fig. 23

Data and results of primary intracapsular BINKHORST lens implant operations performed by BINKHORST and WORST, relative to residual spectacle astigmatism. Cases with visual acuity below 0.3 were omitted in order to be relatively sure that spectacle astigmatism had been reliably determined: knowledge of a cylindrical component is of no practical value when the visual acuity is only 0.02.

Cases with spectacle astigmatism over 5 D were omitted in view of their small number.

surgical procedure	number	percentage visual acuity													average visual acuity
		0–10	11–20	21–30	31–40	41–50	51–60	61–70	71–80	81–90	91–100	101–110	111–120	121–130	
primary intracapsular	489	58	22	20	40	35	29	93	22	41	110	3	6	10	0.62
secondary intracapsular	74	9	–	3	4	4	2	18	5	6	14	3	3	3	0.70
secondary extracapsular	35	3	5	1	2	3	4	1	–	1	13	2	–	–	0.64
primary extracapsular	77	1	4	3	3	7	1	20	3	6	24	1	2	2	0.75
total	675	71	31	27	49	49	36	132	30	54	161	9	11	15	0.65
%		10.5	4.6	4.0	7.3	7.3	5.3	19.6	4.4	8.0	23.9	1.3	1.6	2.2	

Fig. 24. Distribution of visual acuity in 675 iris clip lens implant operations performed by BINKHORST, relative to surgical procedure. In two cases the visual acuity is not known.

age at operation in 10 year age groups	number	percentage visual acuity													average visual acuity
		0–10	11–20	21–30	31–40	41–50	51–60	61–70	71–80	81–90	91–100	101–110	111–120	121–130	
15–24 years	1	—	—	—	—	—	—	1	—	—	—	—	—	—	0.66
25–34 years	2	—	—	—	—	—	—	—	—	—	1	1	—	—	1.02
35–44 years	6	2	—	—	—	1	—	1	1	—	1	—	—	—	0.49
45–54 years	43	2	1	1	1	2	1	11	—	4	15	—	3	2	0.80
55–64 years	108	12	6	2	6	7	8	14	7	10	30	1	1	4	0.68
65–74 years	172	20	6	5	13	13	5	37	8	17	42	1	2	3	0.65
75–84 years	128	20	6	9	17	9	12	21	5	8	20	—	—	1	0.53
85–94 years	29	2	3	3	3	3	3	8	1	2	1	—	—	—	0.50
total	489	58	22	20	40	35	29	93	22	41	110	3	6	10	0.63
%		11.9	4.5	4.1	8.2	7.2	5.9	19.0	4.5	8.4	22.5	0.6	1.2	2.0	

Fig. 25. Distribution of visual acuity results in 489 primary intracapsular iris clip lens implant operations performed by BINKHORST, relative to age at operation, in groups of 10 years. In two cases the visual acuity is not known.

equal to the relative spectacle magnification which applies only to patients corrected by spectacle lenses. We may thus conclude that the average visual acuity without relative spectacle magnification is essentially the same in both series. However, since both series differ in many aspects, definite conclusions should not be drawn from this comparison.

COMPLICATIONS DURING OPERATIONS

The operative complications in 694 iris clip lens implantations were

1. bulging vitreous,   10 cases (1.44 %)
2. vitreous in the anterior chamber,   21 cases (3.03 %)
3. vitreous loss,   5 cases (0.72 %)
4. minor accidents,   5 cases (0.72 %)

1. *Bulging vitreous* had no consequences for the final result in 7 out of 10 cases.

In 3 cases a relationship with the later occurrence of retinal detachment, macular degeneration or FUCHS' corneal dystrophy which increased in severity, could have been present.

Case histories.
Case 188. Female, born 1895.
23– 6–65 intracapsular cataract extraction with iris clip lens implantation OS. Bulging vitreous was present.
11–10–65 retinal detachment, not surgically treated because of its hopeless prognosis.
24– 1–72 visual acuity $1/\infty$.

Case 454. Female, born 1883.
14– 5–70 unintentional extracapsular cryoextraction OS. The vitreous which presented itself in the wound, was pushed back with the iris clip lens. The latter was inserted horizontally. Vitreous sweep. Some vitreous remained incarcerated at the lower side of the implant.
20– 5–70 the vitreous herniated nasally between iris and implant, and touched the cornea at 6 o'clock. This had no further consequences.
28–11–70 macular degeneration of the retina. Corrected visual acuity 0.15.
20–12–72 death of patient.

Case 1021. Female, born 1893. Syphilis (congenital?).
    Pre-operative FUCHS' corneal dystrophy.
11–10–68 intracapsular cataract extraction with heavy bulging of the vitreous and horizontal iris clip lens implantation. The pupil which was rather narrow initially, became extremely wide towards the end of the operation and did not react to miotics.
    Post-operatively a marked striate keratitis progressing to total ECD.

15–10–71 downward decentration of the implant due to wide paralytic pupil. Corrected
visual acuity 0.05.

2. *Vitreous in the anterior chamber*, present in 21 cases, had no effect on either
the transparency of the cornea or the IOP. It protruded through the pupil or
through the peripheral coloboma, with or without touching the cornea, adhered
to the wound causing slight decentration in some cases, was present in an
anterior loop, or herniated between pupillary border and implant (case 1076,
below).

Case histories.
Case 335. Male, born 1899. Pre-operative, slight cornea guttata.
22– 8–68 intracapsular cataract extraction OD with complications: after chymotrypsin
the lens capsule ruptured but was totally removed, iris prolapsed, the pupil
enlarged and injection of air dislocated the implant temporarily.
14–10–68 nasal decentration caused local corneal oedema.
24–10–68 amputation of the nasal loop.
17–11–71 vitreous in front of the implant, partly touching the cornea. Cornea was
clear, IOP normal.
16–11–72 corrected visual acuity 0.6.

Case 1044. Male, born 1882. Diabetes mellitus.
25– 4–69 intracapsular cataract extraction with horizontal iris clip implantation OD.
Capsular forceps accidentally ruptured the lower half of the sphincter muscle
over 180°.
30– 9–69 slight upward decentration.
11–10–69 corrected visual acuity 0.9.
17–11–71 vitreous in front of the implant, almost touching the cornea. Cornea was
clear, IOP normal (SETIAWAN ONG).

Case 1076. Female, born 1886.
16 - 1–70 intracapsular cataract extraction with iris clip lens implantation OS. The
operation was rather haemorrhagic, the ruptured capsule was completely
removed, some formed vitreous slid into the wound, the vitreous sweep
appeared to be successful, but a small vitreous hernia remained in the pupil
after lens implantation.
11– 7–70 corrected visual acuity 0.8.
18–11–71 cornea was clear, IOP normal (SETIAWAN ONG).

3. *Vitreous loss* had been observed in 5 cases. It requires the utmost care and is
a contra-indication for implantation for the beginner (see page 53), since
typical pseudophakic complications may arise. Examples are decentration and
dislocation entailing the danger of ECD due to corneal touch.

Out of 5 cases where BINKHORST thought that implantation was still justified,
one case showed prolonged irritation, and another developed a retinal detachment. The other 3 cases had no complications associated with vitreous loss.

Case histories.

Case 39. Male, born 1904. (BINKHORST, 1962b).

14– 8–44 straw in OS causing iridodialysis and cataract.

19– 7–45 fixation of the iris root.

25– 2–60 intracapsular cataract extraction. The anterior chamber filled with thin fluid vitreous.

29– 7–60 secondary horizontal iris clip lens implantation.

$$\frac{\text{Anterior}}{\text{Posterior}} \text{ loop length } \frac{8.00}{6.50} \text{ mm.}$$

14–10–60 total dislocation into the anterior chamber due to inadequate posterior loop length. The author replacing BINKHORST during his holiday, decided to wait for his return.

25–10–60 repositioning under mydriasis with a blunt iris hook. To the author's surprise it took only 10 seconds. Acetylcholine, air injection.

29–10–60 anterior dislocation of the superior loop (promoted by air in the posterior chamber?).

2–11–60 repositioning with a blunt iris hook. Acetylcholine, no air injection.

30– 5–61 corrected visual acuity 1.10.

11– 8–66 total ECD.

10–11–66 corneal inlay, design CHOYCE.

19–12–72 corrected visual acuity 0.10.

Case 135. Female, born 1895. Diabetes mellitus. Leg amputated in 1968.

7–11–63 intracapsular cataract extraction with iris clip lens implantation OD. At the moment the implant forceps were released, the vitreous membrane ruptured and vitreous presented itself in the wound. Extraction of about 1/2cc vitreous with air injection and vitreous sweep.

11– 6–65 corrected visual acuity 0.66.

2– 4–69 death of patient.

Case 282. Male, born 1907.

6– 7–67 intracapsular cataract extraction with iris clip lens implantation OS. The lens capsule and the vitreous membrane ruptured simultaneously. Extraction of about 1/2cc of vitreous. Vitreous sweep.
Prolonged irritation.

7–10–69 corrected visual acuity 0.65. Cornea clear, IOP normal.

Case 451. Male, born 1940. The right eye was hit by a stick in 1951.
Lens fragmentation, the anterior vitreous membrane has ruptured.

23– 4–70 some vitreous loss immediately after incision. Posterior synechiolysis, extraction of lens remnants, iris clip lens implantation, vitreous sweep.

9– 5–70 corrected visual acuity 0.10. Irregular corneal surface.

20– 7–70 retinal detachment with a hole.

23– 7–70 aspiration of subretinal fluid.

6– 8–70 ditto, with encircling procedure.

7– 9–70 retinal folds. Visual acuity $1/\infty$.

Case 493. Male, born 1954. In June 1968 the right eye was hit by a stone.

28– 1–71 extracapsular cataract extraction. Capsular and lens remnants were left intentionally at 6 o'clock.

4– 3–71 secondary iris clip lens implantation. Large vitreous loss.

7– 1–72 the implant adhered to the secondary cataract with good stabilisation. Corrected visual acuity 0.5.

4. *Minor accidents.*

In four cases one or more flues could be seen in the pupil.

In one case a small hole was cut in the iris in error, and a piece of metal (needle tip?) was left on the iris at 11 o'clock.

In another case, however, an expulsive haemorrhage at the end of the implantation remained incomplete, possibly due to the presence of the implant.

POST-OPERATIVE COMPLICATIONS AND THEIR SEQUELAE

Data and results of post-operative complications, implant extractions and one enucleation are shown in Fig. 26.

Post-operative complications and their sequelae will be discussed in the approximate order in which they developed after implantation. For their distribution with respect to surgical procedure the reader is referred to Fig. 45 on page 137.

1. *Pupillary block. Two cases (0.29%).*

In both cases the outcome was favourable.

Case histories.

Case 85. Female, born 1901. (BINKHORST & LÉONARD, 1967e, 1968b).

4– 1–62 intracapsular cataract extraction OD with one iridectomy (LEFFERTSTRA).

17– 5–62 secondary iris clip lens implantation.

18– 5–62 air block, treated by placing the patient on her side.

21–12–71 corrected visual acuity 0.75 (LEFFERTSTRA).

Case 183. Male, born 1941. (BINKHORST & LÉONARD, 1967e, 1968b).

9– 4–65 iron wire perforation of OS causing a cataract, with lens material in the anterior chamber.

10– 6–65 extracapsular cataract extraction with primary iris clip lens implantation. Chymotrypsin enabled secondary extraction of the lens capsule.

11– 6–65 pupillary block treated with transfixion of the iris.

23– 6–65 posterior capsulotomy.

1– 4–66 corrected visual acuity 1.0.

15–11–71 cornea and implant clear (SETIAWAN ONG).

	number	%	average age at operation in years	average observation period in days	average visual acuity
pupillary block	2	0.29	42.50	1900	0.90
choroidal detachment	2	0.29	77.50	215	0.55
unintentional corneo-scleral fistula	11	1.58	65.00	1338	0.49
uveitis (endogenous or exogenous)	11	1.58	63.00	1626	0.56
macular damage (oedema or pseudo-hole)	23	3.31	64.87	1369	0.24
decentration	24	3.46	63.62	728	0.62
dislocation	53	7.64	60.62	1562	0.64
ECD total	32	4.61	68.81	1843	0.04
partial	10	1.44	68.10	1494	0.29
retinal detachment	13	1.87	62.08	1020	0.22
extraction of implant	4	0.58	67.50	784	0.35
enucleation	1	0.14	74	225	0
cases with complications (total)	150	21.61	63.93	1380	0.45
cases without complications (total)	544	78.39	66.32	603	0.70

Fig. 26

Data and results of post-operative complications, implant extractions and one enucleation in 694 iris clip lens implant operations performed by BINKHORST. The total number is 186, but the actual number of cases is 150 since some of the patients showed more than one complication. The total number of cases without complications has been added for comparison.

2.   *Choroidal detachment. Two cases (0.29%).*

This type of complication was not investigated systematically. Resolution was spontaneous.

Case histories.
Case 24. Female, born 1881. (BINKHORST, 1962b).
22– 7-58 intracapsular cataract extraction OD.
 5-11-59 secondary iris clip lens implantation. Incision not sutured.
 9-11-59 resuturing because of wound leakage. Choroidal detachment nasally.
12-11-59 repositioning of dislocated nasal posterior loop with a blunt iris hook.
 5-11-60 corrected visual acuity 0.66.

Case 338. Male, born 1891.

29– 8–68 intracapsular cataract extraction with iris clip lens implantation OS.

9– 9–68 choroidal detachment nasally and temporally, with extremely shallow anterior chamber.

13– 9–68 anterior chamber at normal depth again.

1–11–68 corrected visual acuity 0.45. Probably no ill-effects.

19– 2–72 domiciliary visit: clear cornea.

Two other cases of choroidal detachment were related to the cataract extraction, but not to the implantation 4½ months later.

3. *Unintentional corneo-scleral fistula. Eleven cases (1.58%).*

Of these, 6 were secondary and 5 primary implantations and chymotrypsin was used in 3 of them. In two further cases a cystic scar was present. In the suturing technique of 8 to 13 corneo-scleral sutures at a little more than half the depth (see page 50 ff.), unintentional corneo-scleral leakage is a rather rare occurrence, even when using chymotrypsin in 17.43% of cases (see page 117).

This complication had an effect on the final result of only two cases: in one it caused an anterior dislocation of the nasal loop which contributed to the development of total ECD (case 28 on page 98), and in the other macular degeneration might have been promoted by the low IOP (case 250, below). In spite of this the risk of corneo-scleral leakage should be completely avoided in lens implant surgery.

Case histories.

Case 250. Female, born 1905.

16– 3–67 intracapsular cataract extraction with iris clip lens implantation OS. Eight corneo-scleral sutures.

20– 3–67 temporary corneal touch of the temporal loop.

10– 4–67 temporary filtering wound.

16– 9–67 macular degeneration of the retina.

19– 2–68 corrected visual acuity 0.02.

21– 5–73 situation stationary.

Case 262. suturing with only 3 MCLEAN's sutures by a visiting foreign surgeon resulted in a cystic scar.

Case 559. cataract extraction performed elesewhere, resulted in a cystic scar which had to be avoided: incision was made on the corneal side of the scar.

One special case will be mentioned here that could well have been mentioned under pupillary block: extensive iris incarceration was possibly caused by iridotomies that were located too near the periphery, or were too small.

Case history.

Case 97. Female, born 1891. (BINKHORST & LÉONARD, 1967e, 1968b).

3– 8–62 intracapsular cataract extraction with iris clip lens implantation OD. Chymotrypsin used. Nine corneo-scleral sutures.

4– 8–62 extremely shallow anterior chamber.

5– 8–62 iris incarceration between all sutures, i.e. in eight spaces. Removal of all sutures, enlarging the peripheral iridotomies, acetylcholine, air injection, nine corneo-scleral sutures.

29–10–62 corrected visual acuity 1.0.

5–70 epithelial corneal oedema in the upper third without visible signs of endothelial dystrophy. Corrected visual acuity 0.25 (PEARCE, 1972).

6– 7–70 macular changes. Corrected visual acuity 0.10.

4. Deposits on the implant were observed mainly after extracapsular extraction (see also page 64).

They gradually disappeared and impaired vision only temporarily. Fine dusting with iris pigment was not recorded systematically, because it did not interfere with vision.

5. Uveitis (endogenous or exogenous). Eleven cases (1.58%). Evidence of uveitis developed in two cases with a history of uveitis complicated by cataract.

Post-operative infection developed in two other cases.

After treatment 10 cases of early or late uveitis turned out to be of little or no consequence with respect to the final result. However, in one serious case the implant had to be removed, but 9 years later the eye appeared to have regained full aphakic visual acuity (see case 67 on page 112).

Case histories.

Case 8. Female, born 1895. (BINKHORST, 1962d).

18–11–58 intracapsular cataract extraction OS.

12– 3–59 secondary iris clip lens implantation.

14– 3–59 small hypopyon, treated with terracortril eye drops.

16– 3–69 hypopyon disappeared.

11–11–63 corrected visual acuity 1.0.

28– 6–65 corrected visual acuity 0.5.

7– 5–70 death of patient.

Case 16. Female, born 1905. Complicated cataract OS. (BINKHORST, 1962d).

21– 2–55 acute iridocyclitis OS of undetermined cause.

21–11–57 intracapsular cataract extraction.

25– 6–59 secondary iris clip lens implantation.

28– 6–59 early post-operative relapse of uveitis treated with penicillin and cortisone acetate (Adreson).

30– 7–59 needling of a pupillary membrane.

7– 1- 71 quiet eye, corrected visual acuity 0.5.

Case 23. Male, born 1877.

18– 6–59 extracapsular cataract extraction OS.

6– 8–59 needling of secondary cataract.

8– 9–59 secondary iris clip lens implantation.

10– 9–59 hypopyon, successfully treated with cortisone acetate (Adreson).

17– 9–62 corrected visual acuity 0.5.

1– 9–66 death of patient.

Case 62. Male, born 1885.

19– 6–61 recently resolved conjunctivitis OD.

22– 6–61 intracapsular cataract extraction with iris clip lens implantation OD.

3– 7–61 hypopyon, red reflex hardly visible. Probable incipient vitreous abscess. Penicillin, sulfonamide, later streptomycin.

9–10–61 pupil blocked by membranes; eye quiet.

12–10–61 needling.

2–11–61 corrected visual acuity 0.33.

5–12–61 death of patient.

Case 67. See page 112.

Severe infection, with massive exudates, necessitating implant extraction. However, the final aphakic corrected visual acuity was still 0.9!

Case 74. Male, born 1895.

10– 8–61 intracapsular cataract extraction with iris clip lens implantation OD.

23–10–61 post-operatively, a low-grade iritis persisted for 6 months, and was treated with atropine and decadron (PEARCE, 1972).

29– 6–71 corrected visual acuity 1.0.

Case 161. Female, born 1908. Complicated cataract OD.

8– 3–44 chronic uveitis OD.

19– 9–45 aqueous now clear. The keratic precipitates were disintegrating.

1–10–64 intracapsular cataract extraction with iris clip lens implantation OD.

4– 1–65 late uveitis of obscure origin, possibly relapse of earlier uveitis, and complicated by glaucoma.

9– 6–66 unfortunately the patient did not consent to a glaucoma operation.

12– 8–71 some ECD infero-temporally. Corrected visual acuity 0.12.

Case 230/371. Female, born 1909. Cataract ODS, cause unknown.

8– 9–**66** unintentional extracapsular cataract extraction with iris clip lens implantation OD. Epinephrine was instilled into the anterior chamber.

30– 9–68 an organised exudate covered part of the implant. The eye was quiet. Corrected visual acuity 1.0. This remained so until at least May 1970 (PEARCE, 1972).

20– 3–69 intracapsular cataract extraction with iris clip lens implantation OS. Chymotrypsin used.

21– 9–73 corrected visual acuity OD 0.66, OS 0.80.

A membrane was present only in the right eye, i.e. in the eye which had been treated with epinephrine.

Case 285. Male, born 1912.

7– 9–67 intracapsular cataract extraction with iris clip lens implantation OD. Chymo-trypsin and the erysiphake were used in view of the tense capsule.

11– 9–67 hypopyon, treated systematically with penicillin and streptomycin.

18– 9–67 blocked pupil, treated locally with atropine, glaucosan and dexamethasone sodium phosphate (Decadron).

25– 9–67 eye was quiet.

4– 4–68 corrected visual acuity 0.7.

Case 286. Female, born 1902.

14– 9–67 intracapsular cataract extraction with iris clip lens implantation OD. Chymo-trypsin and erysiphake were used in view of the tense capsule.

15– 9–67 posterior dislocation of nasal loop, possibly due to the air bubble being too large.

18– 9–67 repositioning with needle knife.

18– 9–67 small hypopyon which vanished spontaneously three days later.

17– 2–71 corrected visual acuity 1.0.

18–11–71 corneal oedema nasally, probably due to the nasal loop approaching and intermittently touching the cornea.

4– 5–72 rotation of the implant to a vertical position. Further data are absent.

6. *Macular oedema. Twenty-three cases (3.31%), all intracapsular.*

Seven of these cases (1.01%) showed a macular hole appearance. It is not certain whether there is a relationship between macular oedema and pseudopha-kia (see page 66). IRVINE (1953) mentioned an incidence of 2% after uneventful cataract extraction, but this percentage depends also on the zeal of the investiga-tor when tracing macular oedema: it is encountered more frequently when one specifically looks for it. JAFFE (1972b) estimated an incidence of at least 40% after normal cataract extraction.

The low average visual acuity of 0.24 in this group is only partly explained by the seven cases of total or partial ECD. The remaining 16 cases also showed a low average visual acuity, viz. 0.27. The possible relationship between the two conditions will be discussed on page 107.

Some case histories:

Case 1. Female, born 1879. (BINKHORST, 1962d).

20– 3–58 intracapsular cataract extraction OD. Choroidal detachment.

11– 8–58 secondary horizontal iris clip lens implantation. The temporal loop was adjusted with a blunt iris hook.

14– 8–58 corrected visual acuity 0.4.

5–11–58 many greyish spots noticed on the implant's surface. Cortisone acetate (Adreson) eye drops.

8–12–58 the spots had almost disappeared. Some cell clumps in the anterior chamber. Adreson was discontinued. Some macular oedema. Corrected visual acuity 0.3.

2– 2–59 corrected visual acuity 0.4. Less macular oedema.

5–11–60 corrected visual acuity 0.66.

20–11–60 death due to a cerebral haemorrhage.

Case 2. Male, born 1880. (BINKHORST, 1962d).

24– 4–58 intracapsular cataract extraction OD.

11– 8–58 secondary horizontal iris clip lens implantation. During the manoeuvre with the blunt iris hook the implant was held with an iris sonde.

4– 9–58 corrected visual acuity 0.66.

5–12–58 corrected visual acuity 0.33. Macular oedema and pseudo-hole.

17– 8–59 corrected visual acuity 0.5.

12– 7–60 corrected visual acuity 0.4.

11– 7–62 death of patient.

Case 63. See page 106.

Case 216. Female, born 1889.

24– 2–66 intracapsular cataract extraction with horizontal iris clip lens implantation OS.

2– 5–66 corrected visual acuity 1.0.

8– 1–68 corrected visual acuity 0.3. Oedema and pseudo-hole in the macula.

6– 5–68 corrected visual acuity 0.45. Macula 'dried out'.

14– 7–69 corrected visual acuity 0.33.

18– 8–71 corrected visual acuity 0.3. Peripheral epithelial corneal oedema from 11 to 3 o'clock (NORDLOHNE).

27– 9–71 the very mobile implant touched the cornea intermittently. Severe atrophy of the sphincter muscle.

25–11–71 implant rotated to vertical position using two needle knives.*

26–10–72 visual acuity 0.02. ECD and macular degeneration of the retina.

Case 298. Female, born 1923. Cataract of unknown origin OD.

9–11–67 intracapsular cataract extraction with horizontal iris clip lens implantation. Chymotrypsin and erysiphake used.

29– 6–70 macular oedema with pseudo-hole. Visual acuity 0.02.

16–11–71 incipient ECD nasally superiorly.

9–12–71 90° anti-clockwise rotation of the implant.

15–10–72 corrected visual acuity 1.0.

Case 329. Male, born 1905.

13– 6–68 intracapsular cataract extraction with iris clip lens implantation OD.

6– 8–68 corrected visual acuity 0.66.

12–12–68 corrected visual acuity 0.25. Macular oedema.

5–70 corrected visual acuity 0.66 (PEARCE, 1972).

* This was the first implant rotation BINKHORST performed.

Case 1014. Male, born 1917.

23– 8–68 intracapsular cataract extraction with horizontal iris clip lens implantation OD. Chymotrypsin used. Loop length $\frac{8.50}{8.50}$-mm.

8–11–68 corrected visual acuity 0.25. Macular oedema. Retrobulbar dexamethasone sodium phosphate (Decadron).

6– 6–69 corrected visual acuity 0.65. Some ECD peripherally at 12 o'clock.

16–11–71 fine bullae in the upper half of the cornea.

24– 2–72 rotation of implant since it was too mobile in the horizontal position.

9– 5–72 only a few bullae left near the limbus.

7–11–72 visual acuity 0.02. Macular degeneration of the retina (KROONENBERG).

Case 1038. Male, born 1903.

28– 2–69 intracapsular cataract extraction with horizontal iris clip lens implantation OS.

10– 3–60 herpes simplex keratitis. Débridement.

18– 3–69 relapse of herpes. Débridement.

6– 5–69 herpes cured. Flare +, cells ±. Retrobulbar dexamethasone sodium phosphate (Decadron).

8–69 corrected visual acuity 1.10 (JAPING).

11–10–69 visual acuity reduced relative to some weeks earlier, but improved with prednisone tablets (JAPING). Some star-shaped marking of the macula.

12– 2–71 corrected visual acuity 0.33.

29– 8–72 corrected visual acuity 0.45.

Case 432. Female, born 1890.

29–11–69 intracapsular cataract extraction with iris clip lens implantation OD. Chymotrypsin and erysiphake used. Post-operative macular oedema with pseudo-hole. Visual acuity not mentioned in records.

23– 9–70 corrected visual acuity 0.55.

11– 8–71 total posterior dislocation, non-operative repositioning.

11–12–71 total posterior dislocation.

13–12–71 repositioned with needle knife, implant rotated to vertical position, loop sutured to iris.

21– 8–72 death of patient.

7. *Decentration of the implant. Twenty-four cases (3.46%).*

Decentration occurred always within 6 months of the implant operation. It was due to either secondary cataract (6 cases), vitreous traction (4 cases), membranes (one case), iris incarceration after squeezing (one case), too tight a suture around the superior loops (one case), anterior synechia (7 cases), atropine (one case), paralytic pupil in (congenital?) syphilis (case 1021, see page 81) or no apparent cause (2 cases). In one case pupillary decentration was present before the operation. The direction of the decentration was upward (13), downward (3), nasally (5) or temporally (4) or in a combination of two directions.

Only an average amount of astigmatism was present in any of these cases. In 15 cases the decentration was slight and of no consequence to visual acuity. Thus, only large decentrations threatened visual acuity due to corneal contact, and required treatment, e.g. loop amputation.

In 4 earlier cases of secondary implantation, the lens implant had been recentred by anterior synechiolysis.

Surgical treatment was performed in 8 cases:

Case histories.
Cases 42, 69, 79, 95 showed recentration after anterior synechiolysis.

Case 198. Male, born 1878.
  7–10–65 intracapsular cataract extraction with iris clip lens implantation OS.
      Upward decentration caused by a fibrous membrane.
31– 3–66 needling of membranes, but centration not successful.
24– 4–66 corrected visual acuity 0.25.
24– 8–67 death of patient.

Case 335. See page 82. Amputation of nasal loop.

Case 484. Female, born 1907.
18–11–61 iridencleisis ODS (VAN DER DRIFT).
12–11–70 intracapsular cataract extraction with iris clip lens implantation OS. Chymotrypsin and erysiphake used.
      Posterior synechiolysis, coloboma sutured. The implant was decentred nasally. An attempt to centre it led to iridodialysis with haemorrhage.
  6– 5–71 needling of membranes.
  7– 6–71 corrected visual acuity 0.7.
  9– 4–73 corrected visual acuity 0.4, reason unknown. Intermittently raised IOP.

Case 485. Male, born 1896.
19–11–70 intracapsular cataract extraction with vertical iris clip lens implantation OD. The insertion at 6 o'clock was difficult, the implant sprang back temporosuperiorly, possibly due to vitreous interposition.
21– 5–71 amputation of temporal loop in view of its proximity to the cornea.
10– 1–72 corrected visual acuity 0.4.

8. *Dislocation of the implant.*

Dislocation of an iris clip lens is an awkward complication necessitating repositioning.

Dislocation occurred 73 times in 53 eyes (7.64%) belonging to 52 patients.

The interval between implantation date and dislocation date is shown in Fig. 27.

number of eyes	%	number of dislo- cations	♂	♀	aver- age age at opera- tion	interval between implantation date and dislocation date				aver- age in days	range in days
						frequency in groups					
						0–¼ year	¼–1 year	1–4 years	>4 years		
53	7.64	73	27	26	60.62	29	13	20	11	673	1–3043

Fig. 27

Interval between implantation date and dislocation date in 694 iris clip lens implantations performed by BINKHORST.

Sixteen patients had 20 dislocations from 1 to 4 years after implantation. Four of these patients had discontinued instilling pilocarpine and one patient was subject to a blunt trauma (case 153 on page 119).

Six patients had 11 dislocations more than 4 years after implantation. Three of these patients had discontinued instilling pilocarpine. Moreover, one had also been involved in a collision (case 26 on page 119).

The distribution of the directions of dislocation is shown in Fig. 28.

	anteriorly	posteriorly	total
nasal loop	16 times	5 times	21 times
temporal loop	4 times	3 times	7 times
superior loop	1 time	—	1 time
inferior loop	5 times	1 time	6 times
both loops	15 times	23 times	38 times
	41 times	32 times	73 times

Fig. 28

Distribution of the directions of iris clip lens dislocation.

In 20 out of 130 patients fitted bilaterally with iris clip lenses, dislocation occurred twice in both eyes at different times (cases 15/158 and 101/150), 15 times in the first eye only and 3 times in the second eye only. In 6 cases dislocation in the first eye suggested the use of a different surgical technique when operating on the second eye: 5 second eyes were operated on extracapsularly and one implant was sutured on the iris. After 1–1–1972 iridocapsular lenses were used routinely in second eyes when dislocation had occurred in the first.

Multiple dislocations in the same eye occurred in 15 eyes: in 11 cases twice, in one case 3 times, in one case 4 times, and in one case 5 times (see case 56 on page 98). Of the 11 cases with two dislocations, 8 had exactly the same type of dislocation each time.

Relationship to surgical procedure

Of these 53 cases with dislocation
16 out of 112 (14.29%) were secondary implantations,
37 out of 582 (6.36%) were primary implantations. Likewise,
45 out of 581 (7.75%) occurred after intracapsular extraction, and
 8 out of 113 (7.08%) occurred after extracapsular extraction.

Causes of dislocation

Dislocation has been caused by
1.   inadequate loop length (see Fig. 29).
In the first 96 implants the anterior loop length was about 7 mm. Henceforth and until no. 180 (3–6–65) it was about 8 mm.

Until 1969 the anterior and posterior loop lengths were 9 to 9.5 mm (to prevent dislocation). Since then it has been maximally 8 mm (to prevent ECD).

In the first 96 cases the posterior loop length was usually shorter than the anterior, for fear of the loops tangling. In later cases the posterior loop length was either 0.5 mm longer, or both loops were of the same length. This explains the overwhelming majority of anterior dislocations in the first group, and the preponderance of posterior dislocations in the later groups.

The fact that the percentage of dislocations of the first 8 mm group is larger than that of the 7 mm group (namely 23.81 against 15.62%) is paradoxical. However, it may be explained in part by the fact that 75.0% of the 7 mm group consisted of secondary implant operations where the behaviour of the pupil, a considerable time after the cataract extraction, was known, whereas 96.4% of the first 8 mm group consisted of primary implant operations where the post-operative behaviour of the pupil was a matter of speculation.

The main difference between the 8 mm groups is that
a) routine instillation of pilocarpine hydrochloride 2% eye drops twice daily was prescribed in the last group from the beginning.
b) both superior loops were sutured to each other (46 cases) or sutured loop to iris (13 cases) only in the last group.

94

	anterior and posterior loop length	number of eyes	number of eyes with dislocation	%	number of dislocations	%	number of anterior dislocations		number of posterior dislocations	
							eyes	dislocations	eyes	dislocations
11–8–58 until 3– 8–62	approx. 7 mm	96	15	15.62	25	26.04	15	24	1	1
9–8–62 until 3– 6–65	,, 8 mm	84	20	23.81	24	28.57	8	9	13	15
10–6–65 until 12–12–68	,, 9 mm	214	5	2.34	8	3.74	1	4	4	4
9–1–69 until 31–12–71	8 mm	300	13	4.33	16	5.33	3	4	10	12
11–8–58 until 31–12–71		694	53	7.64	73	10.52	27	41	28	32

Fig. 29. Incidence of dislocation relative to loop length period, in 694 iris clip lens implant operations performed by BINKHORST.

The importance of the loop length is clearly demonstrated in case 56/93 (for case 56 see page 98). In the first eye the $\dfrac{\text{anterior}}{\text{posterior}}$ loop length was $\dfrac{7.00}{7.00}$ mm, in the second eye it was $\dfrac{7.75}{8.75}$ mm. The patient persistently failed to instil pilocarpine drops. However, only the first eye was subject to 5 (!) anterior dislocations while the second had none.

The same applies to the patient of case 152/218 who, in error, had never been told to instil pilocarpine drops: with loop lengths $\dfrac{8.00}{9.00}$ and $\dfrac{9.00}{9.00}$ only the first implant dislocated into the vitreous. Similar cases are 112/226 ($\dfrac{8.00}{8.75}$ and $\dfrac{9.00}{9.00}$), with dislocation of the first implant into the vitreous, and 113/291 ($\dfrac{8.00}{8.75}$ and $\dfrac{9.00}{9.00}$) with two dislocations of the first implant, the patient having forgotten to instil pilocarpine drops in both eyes.

2.   Insufficient narrowing of the pupil.

Most important is the nocturnal pupillary diameter (darkness, coitus). In June 1965, after 176 implantations, it became clear that too wide a pupil was an important cause of dislocation. Pilocarpine drops twice daily have since been prescribed routinely. Patients originally operated upon before that date, have since been given the same instructions.

The application of atropine, apart from an early case (case 3 on page 99) where it was applied in error, resulted in 5 cases of dislocations (3, 28, 51, 106, 114).

3.   Blunt trauma to the eye. Three cases, see page 119.

The incidence of dislocations per hundred implantations is shown in Fig. 30. See also Fig. 37 on page 114.

It may be concluded from Figs. 29 and 30 that the incidence of dislocation decreased considerably after June 1965 due to pilocarpine drops instilled twice daily as well as to the loop length of $\dfrac{9.00}{9.00}$ mm. However, it increased slightly after 1–1–69 due to the re-introduction of a loop length of $\dfrac{8.00}{8.00}$ mm.

Prevention of dislocation

1.   Measurement of the anterior and posterior loop lengths before implantation is of the utmost importance. The surgeon remains responsible for any imperfections of the implant not noticed by the manufacturer.

2.   Instillation of pilocarpine hydrochloride 2% drops twice daily.

	implantation date no. 100, 200, etc.	dislocation of iris clip lens		
		number of eyes	number of dislocations	
			total	during first week only
1st hundred	20– 9–62	15	25	6
2nd hundred	7–10–65	20	24	3
3rd hundred	29–11–67	3	3	2
4th hundred	14– 2–69	2	5	—
5th hundred	26–11–69	6	6	5
6th hundred	15– 1–71	5	8	3
7th 94	9–12–71	2	2	—
total 694		53	73	19

Fig. 30

Incidence of dislocations per hundred iris clip lens implantations.

3. Suturing of either the superior loops to each other, or suturing the loop(s) to the iris (see page 56 ff.).

Treatment of dislocation

The technique used to reposition the implant is described on page 65. Non-operative repositioning was performed in 24 cases, with a blunt iris hook in 8 cases, with a needle knife in 21 cases, with an iris hook and a needle knife in 3 cases, with ZIEGLER's knife in two cases, and it was performed once with an iris repositor; for 9 cases the method was not recorded. A new implant was inserted in two cases (cases 11 and 28, below), the same implant was used in one case (case 17, below), one implant was extracted (case 353 on page 99), and one implant was left in the eye (case 204 on page 99).

A transcorneal loop iris suture was inserted in 5 cases (see page 118).

Case histories:
Case 11. Female, born 1888. (BINKHORST, 1962d).
30 -11–58 intracapsular cataract extraction OS.
19– 3–59 secondary horizontal iris clip lens implantation.
The $\dfrac{\text{anterior}}{\text{posterior}}$ loop length was $\dfrac{7.00}{6.50}$ mm (i.e. too short).
30– 8–65 anterior dislocation of temporal loop.
8– 9–65 exchanged for a new implant with loop length $\dfrac{9.00}{9.00}$ mm.
8–11–67 corrected visual acuity 0.55.
14– 5–69 death of patient.

Case 17. Female, born 1892. (BINKHORST, 1962bd).

18–12–58 intracapsular cataract extraction OD.

25– 6–59 secondary horizontal iris clip lens implantation.

23– 7–59 total dislocation into the anterior chamber due to the horizontal pupil width being too large in the dark.

Extraction of the implant and re-implantation in the vertical position (according to more up-to-date techniques the vertical re-insertion would have been carried out with only one or two needle knives).

29–11–60 corrected visual acuity 0.9.

14– 4–69 corrected visual acuity 0.5 caused by senile macular degeneration.

Case 28. Male, born 1909. Cataract of unknown origin OS (BINKHORST, 1962d).

15–10–59 extracapsular cataract extraction.

11– 2–60 secondary horizontal iris clip lens implantation.

Pilocarpine and atropine were instilled in view of difficulties with pupillary size during insertion.

12– 2–60 infero-temporal decentration of implant with pupil at its widest. Recentration by means of di-isopropylfluorphosphate (Diflupyl).

13– 2- 60 dislocation of implant into the vitreous (this was the only posterior dislocation amongst the first 96 cases).

Extraction of the implant with a blunt iris hook. Some loss of fluid vitreous.

15– 2–60 decentration of the pupil towards the wound.

14– 4-60 anterior synechiolysis.

19– 8–60 horizontal re-implantation of iris clip lens.

22– 8–60 anterior dislocation of nasal loop caused by temporal wound leakage (only one suture).

25– 8- 60 repositioned through nasal keratome incision.

26– 9-60 decentration caused by broad adhesion between iris and cornea.

28– 6–61 anterior synechiolysis. Recentration. Air injection.

10– 7–61 total ECD.

24– 1–69 visual acuity 0.02.

Case 56. Male, born 1902.

1– 6–61 intracapsular cataract extraction with iris clip lens implantation OD. Loop length $\frac{7.00}{7.00}$ mm.

21–10–68, 22–11–68, 27–1–69, 19–8–69 and 8–9–69: dislocation into the anterior chamber caused by irregular pilocarpine medication. Each time non-operative repositioning.

11– 9–69 both loops were sutured to the iris with perlon, through a transcorneal incision*.

5–70 corrected visual acuity 0.66 (PEARCE, 1972).

Case 124. Male, born 1902. His OS had been hit by his daughter's knee in 1952.

20– 6–63 intracapsular cataract extraction with iris clip lens implantation. Chymotrypsin used.

* This was the first transcorneal loop iris suture BINKHORST inserted.

98

22– 6–70 anterior dislocation of nasal loop caused by irregular pilocarpine medication. Non-operative repositioning under mydriasis, by manipulation of the patient's head. Miosis.

1– 2–71 anterior dislocation of nasal loop. Repositioning was unsuccessful.

4– 2–71 repositioned with needle knife.
The nasal loop was sutured to the iris with one perlon suture, through a small corneal incision.

11– 8–71 corrected visual acuity 0.7.

Case 204. Female, born 1887.

21–10–65 intracapsular cataract extraction with iris clip lens implantation OS.

30– 3–66 – 10.00 DS / – 1.00 DC × 80 gave 0.25 visual acuity. Low visual acuity due to myopic degeneration.

12– 8–71 implant dislocated to bottom of eye. Square pupil! No further complications.

Case 353. Female, born 1899. The left eye had been 'bad' since 1909.

31–10–68 intracapsular cataract extraction with iris clip lens implantation OS.

13– 1–69 dislocation into the vitreous. The patient was suddenly able to see the clock, indicating previous high myopia.

16– 1–69 extraction of implant with blunt iris hook through a temporal keratome incision.

10– 3–69 + 1.00 DS / + 4.50 × 80 gave a visual acuity of 0.6.

18– 5–71 visual acuity 0.5 (uncorrected).

Cases 204 and 353 are examples of spontaneous self-healing!

Consequences of dislocation

1. In 3 cases (0.43%) dislocation occurred twice and repositioning may have contributed to the development of ECD.

Case histories.

Case 3. Male, born 1903. Traumatic cataract OS due to being hit by a cow's tail in 1951 (BINKHORST, 1960c, 1962bd).

6– 2–58 intracapsular cataract extraction.

19–11–58 secondary horizontal iris clip lens implantation.
Local anaesthesia.

26–11–58 anterior dislocation of nasal loop due to atropine instillation and the shortness of the nasal loops.
Repositioned with blunt iris hook through a 1½ mm nasal keratome incision Miotics.

27–11–58 repeat dislocation, again due to atropine.

28–11–58 repositioned in the same manner. The nasal loops proved to be much shorter than the temporal loops.

12– 7–60 ECD in lower half of the cornea.

5– 4–62 total ECD.

14–11–69 visual acuity 0.02.

Case 28. See page 98. ECD after 7 operations.

Case 39. See page 83. ECD after 5 operations.

2. In two cases (0.29 %) anterior dislocation of respectively the nasal and the temporal loop caused local corneal oedema. This cleared after repositioning.

9. Endothelial corneal dystrophy (ECD.)

Incidence of ECD

Endothelial corneal dystrophy is the most insidious complication of iris clip lens implantations, because it frequently becomes manifest only a long or a very long time after the implant operation.

Cases with ECD may be divided into three groups:
1. total ECD: bullous keratopathy of the entire cornea.
2. partial ECD: local bullous keratopathy.
3. minimal ECD: local stromal and/or epithelial oedema.

The interval between implantation date and date of detection of incipient ECD relative to total, partial and minimal ECD, is shown in Fig. 31.

It appears from Fig. 31 that a post-operative interval of up to 8 years may exist before ECD becomes manifest and that there is no correlation between the duration of this interval and the severity of ECD that will ultimately develop.

Bilateral ECD was present in two patients. In 6 patients the implant in the fellow eye gave a good visual acuity without any ECD developing. The best advice is, of course, not to perform a second lens implant operation in cases where the first eye develops ECD.

Case histories.
Case 80/187. Male, born 1885. Syphilis.
24–11–61 intracapsular cataract extraction OD.
14– 2–62 secondary implantation of a biconvex iris clip lens. Loop length $\dfrac{8.00}{7.50}$ mm.
17– 6–65 intracapsular cataract extraction with iris clip lens implantation OS. Loop length $\dfrac{9.00}{9.00}$ mm.
8– 9–66 corneal ulcer OS.
16– 7–68 ECD in both eyes. Visual acuity ODS 0.02.
29–11–69 death of patient.

Case 195/203. See page 107. Loop length $\dfrac{9.00}{9.00}$ mm in both eyes.

	number	%	♂	♀	average age at operation	interval between implantation and the first detection of incipient ECD					
						frequency in groups				average in days	range in days
						0-¼ year	¼-1 year	1-4 years	>4 years		
total ECD	32	4.61	14	18	68.81	3	2	21	6	1088	0-2259
partial ECD	10	1.44	7	3	68.10	0	1	5	4	1346	287-2240
minimal ECD	22	3.17	7	15	64.50	2	6	7	7	1009	34-2830
total	64	9.22	28	36	67.22	5	9	33	17	1101	0-2830

Fig. 31. Interval between implantation date and date of detection of incipient ECD in 64 out of 694 iris clip lens implant operations performed by BINKHORST.

The frequency of ECD per 100 implantations in the whole series, is shown in Fig. 32 (see also Fig. 37 on page 114).

	implantation date, no. 100, 200, etc.	number of eyes with		
		total ECD	partial ECD	minimal ECD
1st hundred	20– 9–62	8	—	1
2nd hundred	7–10–65	7	4	3
3rd hundred	29–11–67	8	3	10
4th hundred	14– 2–69	6	2	2
5th hundred	26–11–69	3	1	2
6th hundred	15– 1–71	—	—	4
7th 94	9–12–71	—	—	—
total 694		32	10	22

Fig. 32

Incidence of ECD in 694 iris clip lens implantations performed by BINKHORST, for every 100 cases.

It may be concluded from Figs. 32 and 37 that the incidence of ECD decreased only after 1–1–1970 when the loop length was again reduced to $\frac{8.00}{8.00}$ mm (see page 28), and cases with a shallow anterior chamber or a small corneal diameter were fitted with iridocapsular lens implants. However, in view of the fact that the average interval between iris clip lens implantation and the appearance of the first signs of ECD is about three years, the possibility of ECD developing in patients of the last two groups cannot yet be totally excluded.

Relationship to surgical procedure

Of these 42 cases with total or partial ECD
 5 out of 112 (4.46%) were secondary implantations,
37 out of 582 (6.36%) were primary implantations. Likewise,
40 out of 581 (6.88%) occurred after intracapsular extraction, and
 2 out of 113 (1.77%) occurred after extracapsular extraction.

Factors promoting ECD

As we have seen on page 67 a variety of factors may be responsible for its occurrence. The distribution of these factors relative to the development of total, partial and minimal ECD, is shown in Fig. 33.

loop length	number of eyes	number of eyes with ECD	endothelial touch			pre-operative FUCHS' corneal dystrophy			serious operative and post-operative complications			reason unknown		
			total ECD	partial ECD	minimal ECD	total ECD	partial ECD	minimal ECD	total ECD	partial ECD	minimal ECD	total ECD	partial ECD	minimal ECD
approx. 7 mm	96	8	1	—	1	1	—	—	5	—	—	1	—	—
approx. 8 mm	84	6	—	1	1	—	—	—	—	—	2	2	—	—
approx. 9 mm	214	40	8	7	9	7	—	1	3	1	3	1	—	—
8 mm	300	10	—	—	5	3	—	1	—	—	—	—	1	—
total	694	64	9	8	15	11	—	2	8	1	5	4	1	—
grand total	694	64	32			13			14			5		
%	100	100	50.0			20.3			21.9			7.8		

Fig. 33. Factors promoting ECD, distributed over cases with total, partial and minimal ECD, and related to the loop length.

1. Endothelial touch.

Endothelial touch caused total, partial or minimal ECD in 32 cases (4.61 %), 24 of these occurring during the period where the loop length 9 mm was used. The relationship between ECD and loop length is shown in Fig. 34.

The importance of the loop length must be stressed once more. This became clear in Fig. 34 where the first 8 mm group shows a percentage of 7.14 ECD, the 9 mm group of 18.69 and the second 8 mm group of 3.33. The two 8 mm groups are chronologically separated by 6.5 years. One may assume that in another 6.5 years the 3.33 % will have increased to some extent, but improvements in design (loops bent back) and in evaluation before the operation (corneal diameter, anterior chamber depth) may prevent it from approaching the 7.14 % of the first group.

The total percentage of 3.17 in the second group is taken very liberally since it includes cases with even the slightest signs of ECD.

2. Pre-operative FUCHS' endothelial dystrophy.

Thirteen cases (1.87 %). This condition was present in 20 patients (3 ♂ and 17 ♀), of whom 24 eyes (3.46 %) were fitted with an iris clip lens, primarily after intra-capsular (and only one case of extracapsular) senile cataract extraction.

Of these 24 eyes, 13 (54.17 %) developed ECD with an average interval of 639 days (range 0–1453 days) after implantation, i.e. shorter than the average interval of 1219 days in the other 51 cases of ECD. The female cases developed total ECD (11), the male minimal ECD (2).

Of the remaining 11 cases, 3 patients died without ECD having been observed, and 8 eyes remained free from ECD during an average observation period of 1089 days (range 77–2855) after implantation.

Initially, BINKHORST considered FUCHS' dystrophy to be a contra-indication for iris clip lens implantation in view of case 63 (below). However, he changed his opinion later (BINKHORST, pers. comm. 11–4–1972) since
a) penetrating keratoplasty would be much safer;
b) the implant prevents vitreo-corneal contact;
c) an implant fitted in one eye only does not interfere with full stereopsis.

However, in view of the fact that ECD developed in 13 eyes (54.17%), 11 (45.83%) of which became subject to total ECD, and only some two years after implantation, the indication for iris clip lens implantation seems to be very doubtful in the presence of FUCHS' corneal dystrophy. On the other hand, the same may be true of cataract extraction without lens implantation, but pertinent statistical data could not be found in the literature.

anterior and posterior loop length		number of eyes	total ECD		partial ECD		minimal ECD		total %	eyes with implant dislocation
			no.	%	no.	%	no.	%	%	%
11-8-58 to 3- 8-62	approx. 7 mm	96	8	8.33	—	—	—	—	8.33	15.62
9-8-62 to 3- 6-65	approx. 8 mm	84	2	2.38	1	1.19	3	3.57	7.14	23.81
10-6-65 to 12-12-68	approx. 9 mm	214	19	8.88	8	3.74	13	6.07	18.69	2.34
9-1-69 to 31-12-71	8 mm	300	3	1.00	1	0.33	6	2.00	3.33	4.33
11-8-58 to 31-12-71		694	32	4.61	10	1.44	22	3.17	9.22	7.64

Fig. 34. Relationship between ECD and loop length in 694 iris clip lens implant operations performed by BINKHORST. The percentages of implant dislocations have been added for reasons of comparison.

105

Case history.

Case 63/186. Female, born 1888. Pre-operative FUCHS' corneal dystrophy.

22– 6–61 intracapsular cataract extraction with iris clip lens implantation OD. Loop

length $\dfrac{7.75}{7.25}$ mm.

19–10–61 needling of an opacity of unknown origin situated behind the implant.

8– 8–63 total ECD.

15–10–64 macular oedema and pseudo-hole.

17– 6–65 intracapsular cataract extraction with iris clip lens implantation OS.

Loop length $\dfrac{9.00}{9.00}$ mm.

5–70 shallow anterior chamber (PEARCE, 1972).

7– 7–70 visual acuity OD $1/\infty$, and OS 0.8.

14– 4–71 death of patient.

In the other 3 bilateral implant cases with pre-operative FUCHS' corneal dystrophy, an explanation of the unilateral development of ECD could not be found.

3. Serious operative and post-operative complications.

Fourteen cases (2.02%). Extra manipulations in the anterior chamber such as repositionings and re-implantations, may have contributed to the development of ECD.

Case histories.

Case 3. See page 99. ⎫
Case 28. See page 98. ⎬ these are the only 3 cases in which dislocation and reposition-
Case 39. See page 83. ⎭ ing of the implant was carried out twice, and seemed to have contributed to the development of total ECD (see page 99).

Case 12. Male, born 1892. (BINKHORST, 1961a, 1962d Fig. 1.; BINKHORST & LÉONARD, 1967e).

20– 1–58 intracapsular cataract extraction OS (KOK-VAN ALPHEN).

3– 2–59 anterior synechiolysis followed by the implantation of a DANNHEIM lens, modified after BARRAQUER (see page 19).

5– 2–59 extraction of the implant: loops too short.

21– 5–59 tertiary iris clip lens implantation.

25– 6–62 bullous keratopathy commencing supero-temporally. Visual acuity 0.1.

30– 9–64 total ECD. Visual acuity 0.02.

2– 4–67 death of patient.

Case 64. See page 49. According to BINKHORST, prolonged corneal oedema was due to the intracameral use of epinephrine.

Case 1004. See page 119. Severe ocular trauma.

106

4. Macular oedema was present prior to total or partial ECD in 7 cases (1.01 %).

All had been subject to intracapsular cataract extraction. If both conditions were completely independent, the chance of them occurring simultaneously, would be given by the product of their percent frequency, i.e. $3.31 \times 6.05 = 0.200\ 255\%$ or 1.4 eyes. According to the zero-independence hypothesis, the chance of this five-fold occurrence calculated on the basis of the FISHER test, is 0.000 23. Consequently, their occurrence is not completely independent. If the loops could touch the cornea easily, and the retina were under stress from small vitreo-retinal adhesions, a relatively large forward displacement of the vitreous in these intracapsular cases could very well be the explanation for both.

Prevention of ECD.

See page 67 as well as the next section.

Treatment of ECD.

Until 1st May 1972 ECD was treated in 17 cases.

In addition, a preventive intervention was performed in 5 cases of anticipated ECD, i.e. in cases in which the loops showed so much swinging motion during slitlamp examination that intermittent corneal contact could not be excluded. The results of treatment and prevention are shown in Fig. 35.

From this one may conclude that surgical correction of ECD can be successful only in incipient cases. Of late, however, good results have been reported about penetrating keratoplasty in cases of total ECD caused by contact between cornea and intraocular lens (KOK-VAN ALPHEN, pers. comm.).

Case histories of treatment of total ECD.
Case 182. Female, born 1895. Pre-operative FUCHS' corneal dystrophy.
10– 6–65 intracapsular cataract extraction with horizontal iris clip lens implantation OD. Loop length $\frac{9.00}{9.00}$ mm.
24– 6–65 nasal loop very close to the cornea.
2– 6–69 total ECD.
18–11–71 penetrating keratoplasty 7 mm.
7– 8–72 patient able to read newspapers with a loupe.
29– 5–73 ECD of corneal graft. Visual acuity 0.02.

Case 195/203. Male, born 1902.
9– 9–65 intracapsular cataract extraction with horizontal iris clip lens implantation OS. Chymotrypsin used. Loop length $\frac{9.00}{9.00}$ mm.

	total number	treated number	visual acuity results			
			penetrating kerato-plasty	corneal inlay design CHOYCE	loop amputation	implant rotation
total ECD	32	5	0.02, 0.35	0.02, 0.1, 0.02		
partial ECD	10	3				0.02 0.02 unknown
minimal ECD	22	9			0.5 0.55 0.6 0.7 0.9 clear cornea unknown	1.0 unknown
threatening ECD	5	5			0.4 0.5 0.6	clear cornea clear cornea

Fig. 35

Visual acuity in 17 treated ECD cases and 5 cases of prevention of ECD, ½ to 5 years after the intervention. The loop amputation applied in 5 cases to the nasal loop, in 4 cases to the temporal loop, and in one case to both loops. Rotation of the implant was always towards the vertical direction.

21–10–65 intracapsular cataract extraction with diagonal iris clip lens implantation OD. Loop length $\frac{9.00}{9.00}$ mm.

8– 7–68 ECD and occlusion of the central retinal artery OS.

6–10–69 corneal oedema OD, near the temporal loop.

19– 2–70 amputation of the temporal loop. No improvement.

24–10–70 penetrating keratoplasty OD 8 mm.

11– 8–71 incipient bullous keratopathy of the graft. Corrected visual acuity 0.35 (NORDLOHNE).

4– 6–72 penetrating keratoplasty OS 8 mm. Visual acuity at present unknown.

Case 39. See page 83. Loop length $\frac{8.00}{6.50}$ mm. Corneal inlay, design CHOYCE. Final corrected visual acuity 0.10.

Case 76. Male, born 1901. Experimental case!

18– 1–62 intracapsular cataract extraction with iris clip lens implantation OS. The implant had the shape of a meniscus (see page 29). Loop length $\frac{8.00}{8.50}$ mm. Acetazolamide (Diamox) was used for the first time. The vitreous did bulge, however.

26– 1–62 corrected visual acuity 0.5 (NORDLOHNE).

5– 8–65 total ECD.

24–10–68 corneal inlay, design CHOYCE.

9–12–68 the inlay had not taken, and was, therefore, removed.

24– 9–71 visual acuity 0.02.

13– 3–72 situation stationary.

Case 269. Female, born 1891. Pre-operative FUCHS' corneal dystrophy.

10– 5–67 intracapsular cataract extraction with iris clip lens implantation OS. Loop length $\frac{9.00}{9.00}$ mm.

10–11–67 total ECD.

11– 1–68 amputation of both anterior loops.

3–10–68 corneal inlay, design CHOYCE.

9– 4–73 visual acuity 0.02.

Case histories of treatment of partial ECD by implant rotation.

Case 121. Female, born 1898.

6– 6–63 intracapsular cataract extraction with horizontal iris clip lens implantation OD.

10–12–63 corrected visual acuity 0.5.

8– 4–66 intermittent corneal contact by the temporal loop.

15–11–71 partial ECD.

25–11–71 rotation of implant towards the vertical. Visual acuity at present unknown.

Case 216. See page 90. $\left.\vphantom{\begin{array}{c}a\\a\end{array}}\right\}$ these two cases showed temporary macular oedema as well.
Case 1014. See page 91.

Case histories of treatment of minimal or threatening ECD.

Case 193. Female, born 1898.

5– 8–65 intracapsular cataract extraction with horizontal iris clip lens implantation OS. Loop length $\frac{9.00}{9.00}$ mm.

5– 2–66 macular changes. Corrected visual acuity 0.35.

9– 3–68 temporal corneal oedema caused by swinging movements of the implant. Corrected visual acuity 0.5.

14–11–68 amputation of the temporal loop.

6–10–69 clear cornea.

13– 8–71 corrected visual acuity 0.7 (NORDLOHNE).

Case 224. Female, born 1887.

7– 7–66 intracapsular cataract extraction with horizontal iris clip lens implantation

OS. Loop length $\dfrac{9.00}{9.00}$ mm.

7– 1–67 the nasal loop nearly touching the cornea. Corrected visual acuity 0.66.

12– 1–67 amputation of the nasal loop*.

18– 8–71 cornea clear. Corrected visual acuity 0.8 (NORDLOHNE).

29– 2–72 corrected visual acuity 0.6.

Case 1010. Male, born 1904.

28– 6–68 intracapsular cryoextraction with iris clip lens implantation OD. Loop length

$\dfrac{9.00}{9.00}$ mm.

4– 3–69 temporal corneal thickening.

13– 6–69 amputation of the temporal loop.

23– 9–69 cornea clear.

16–11–71 cornea clear. Corrected visual acuity 0.55.

17– 3–72 condition stationary.

Case 335. See page 82. Amputation of nasal loop. Final corrected visual acuity 0.6.

Case 485. See page 92. Amputation of temporal loop. Final corrected visual acuity 0.4.

Case 405. Female, born 1894. Corneal diameter 10.00 mm.

28– 8–69 intracapsular cataract extraction with horizontal iris clip lens implantation

OD. Coloured implant, loop length $\dfrac{8.50}{8.50}$ mm (too long for this eye!)

6– 3–70 corrected visual acuity 0.9.

17– 8–71 the nasal loop nearly touching the cornea.

6– 9–71 macular changes. Visual acuity 0.02.

9–12–71 implant rotated.

The visual acuity at present is unknown.

Consequences of ECD.

In this series of 694 eyes, 38 (5.48 %) eyes with total (32) or partial (6) ECD failed to regain useful vision. However, four eyes with partial ECD had visual acuities of respectively 0.4, 0.5, 0.66 and 0.66.

10. *Retinal detachment. Thirteen cases (1.87%).*

The level of 1.87 % is a little lower than the 2 %, 1–4 % and 1–3 %, generally accepted for uneventful cataract surgery without implantation (DUKE-ELDER, 1969; URRETS-ZAVALIA jr. 1968; JAFFE, 1972b).

---

* This was the first secondary loop amputation that BINKHORST performed.

serial number	sex	L or R	cause of cataract	age at operation	operation date	surgical procedure of implant operation	retinal detachment date	interval in days	number of operations for retinal detachment	final visual acuity
99	♀	R	senile	59	13- 9-62	prim. intracaps. + chymotrypsin	20- 7-64	676	1 ×	1/∞ (recidive)
149	♂	L	senile	62	16- 4-64	prim. intracaps.	8- 3-65	326	3 ×	1.0
188	♀	L	senile	70	23- 6-65	prim. intracaps.	11-10-65	110	—	1/∞ (inoperable) See page 81.
196	♂	L	unknown	51	9- 9-65	prim. intracaps.	1-72	approx. 2313	3 ×	0.02 (recidive)
321	♀	L	senile	59	14- 3-68	prim. intracaps.	12- 9-68	182	1 ×	1/∞ (recidive and total ECD as well)
323	♂	R	senile	84	2- 5-68	prim. intracaps.	18-11-71	1295	—	0.02 (emboly central retinal artery)
347	♀	L	senile	67	10-10-68	prim. intracaps.	4- 4-69	178	1 ×	0.55
403	♂	R	senile	62	21- 8-69	prim. intracaps. + chymotrypsin	7-10-69	47	2 ×	0.40
412	♀	L	senile	75	2-10-69	prim. intracaps.	13- 2-70	134	2 ×	zero (recidive). Patient died 20-3-73.
428	♀	R	senile	59	26-11-69	prim. intracaps.	19-11-71	723	2 ×	0.02 (macular oedema)
451	♂	R	traumatic	30	23- 4-70	sec. extracaps.	20- 7-70	88	2 ×	1/∞ (retinal folds). See page 83.
452	♂	L	senile	69	14- 5-70	prim. intracaps. + chymotrypsin	3- 8-70	81	2 ×	0.15
550	♂	R	senile	60	16- 9-71	prim. intracaps. + chymotrypsin	7- 1-72	113	1 ×	0.66
IC 37	♂	R	traumatic	8	11- 1-68	sec. extracaps.	7-68	approx. 182	1 ×	0.55
IC 85	♂	R	traumatic	3	4-11-70	prim. extracaps.	1-71	approx. 61	—	? (patient abroad) See page 127.
IC 101	♂	L	traumatic	15	21- 5-71	sec. extracaps.	28-11-71	191	1 ×	0.02 (retinal damage) See page 130.

Fig. 36. Data and results of 16 cases with retinal detachment amongst 864 BINKHORST lens implant operations performed by BINKHORST.

Eight detachments appeared within six months after implantation, the others occurred after 11, 22, 24, 42 and 76 months.

Only one detachment occurred in the series of 113 extracapsular cataract extractions (0.88%), in a patient with a traumatic cataract.

The other 12 developed in the series of 581 intracapsular extractions(2.07%).

Treatment

The treatment of retinal detachment was not hampered in any of the patients by the narrow pupil inherent initially in eyes fitted with an iris clip lens implant. Good visibility of the peripheral fundus could always be obtained by careful mydriasis (BINKHORST pers. comm.). See also page 70. Data about and results of treatment are compiled in Fig. 36. The three cases of retinal detachment after *iridocapsular* lens implantation (1.76%) have been added.

It is interesting to note in Fig. 36 that four patients were operated on because of traumatic cataract, and that three of them were children comprised in the iridocapsular lens series (see also pages 70 and 161).

11. *Complications necessitating extraction of the implant.*

Four cases (0.58%). Extraction of the implant was necessary in four patients: in two cases of high myopia, because of the refraction, in one case due to infection and in another due to severe ocular trauma. The two cases of high myopia (a third where the lens had not been removed after dislocation into the vitreous, was case 204 on page 99), show the importance of determining the axial length where no earlier details of the case history are available.

Case histories.
Case 67. Male, born 1903.
18– 5–61 intracapsular cataract extraction OD.
20– 5–61 re-operation, because of iris incarceration.
 3– 8–61 secondary iris clip lens implantation.
17– 8–61 beginning of a severe infection with massive exudates. Intensive chemo-
        therapeutic and antibiotic treatment had no effect.
29– 8–61 temporal keratome incision. The iris was brought behind the posterior loop
        with a blunt iris hook. Extraction of implant and massive exudates.
        Sector iridectomy at 9 o'clock. Extraction of about ½ cc of vitreous.
        Irrigation with penicillin 20.000 units/cc.
15– 1–70 aphakic corrected visual acuity 0.9!

Case 181. Female, born 1893. The right eye had light perception only, since 1925.
10– 6–65 intracapsular cataract extraction with iris clip lens implantation OD.
17– 6–65 extraction of implant because the eye was very myopic. Small vitreous pro-

lapse. Extraction of about $^1/_2$ cc of vitreous, air injected, vitreous sweep. Vitreous haemorrhage.

5– 7–65 visual acuity 1/∞ due to extensive myopic degeneration. Projection good. Cornea clear; normal IOP.

22– 9–69 death of patient.

Case 1004. See page 119. Severe perforating trauma four weeks after implantation.

Case 353. See page 99. High myopia with dislocation of the implant.

12. *Complication necessitating enucleation.*

One case (0.14%).

In one case enucleation was unavoidable because of panophthalmitis following a perforating injury which occurred two years after implantation.

Case history.
Case 300. Female, born 1893.
29–11–67 intracapsular cataract extraction with iris clip lens implantation OD.
11– 7–68 corrected visual acuity 1.0.
15–12–69 patient fell on OD. Iris prolapse followed rapidly by panophthalmitis.
16–12–69 enucleation.
22–11–71 senile dementia.
26–11–72 death of patient.

SUMMARY

Complications, implant extractions and one enucleation in a series of 694 iris clip lens implantations were discussed in the approximate chronological order in which they may occur after implantation. Their frequency per 100 implantations in the whole series is shown in Fig. 37.

The improvement in the results in the course of time is mainly due to

1. a decrease of exogenous and endogenous infections thanks to the use of antibiotics and corticosteroids.

2. a reduction in the number of dislocations thanks to the use of miotics as well as the transient use of a loop length of $\frac{9.00}{9.00}$ mm, and finally, by suturing of both superior loops to each other, or suturing the loop(s) to the iris.

3. a decrease of ECD thanks to the use of a loop length of $\frac{8.00}{8.00}$ mm, and endothelium sparing surgery.

implantation date no. 100,200, etc.,	pupillary block	choroidal detachment	unintentional fistula	uveitis	macular damage	decentration	dislocation	total or partial ECD	retinal detachment	extraction of implant	enucleation
1st hundred 20– 9–62	2	1	7	6	5	6	15	8	1	1	—
2nd hundred 7–10–65	—	—	1	1	4	2	20	11	3	1	—
3rd hundred 29–11–67	—	—	2	3	4	3	3	11	—	—	1
4th hundred 14– 2–69	—	1	—	—	5	3	2	8	3	2	—
5th hundred 26–11–69	—	—	1	1	3	4	6	4	2	—	—
6th hundred 15– 1–71	—	—	—	—	2	5	5	—	3	—	—
7th 94 9–12–71	—	—	—	—	—	1	2	—	1	—	—
total	2	2	11	11	23	24	53	42	13	4	1
%	0.3	0.3	1.6	1.6	3.3	3.5	7.6	6.0	1.9	0.6	0.1

Fig. 37. Distribution of post-operative complications, implant extractions and one enucleation in 694 iris clip lens implant operations performed by BINKHORST, for every 100 cases.

Data and results of a group of special cases are shown in Fig. 38.

	number	%	average age at operation in years	average observation period in days	average visual acuity
diabetes mellitus:					
without retinopathy	42	6.05	69.48	667	0.59
with retinopathy	10	1.44	69.00	378	0.19
total	52	7.49	69.38	614	0.51
pre-operative glaucoma	29	4.18	70.72	753	0.50
mannitol	11	1.58	36.36	221	0.70
synechiolysis	37	5.33	53.11	659	0.63
chymotrypsin	121	17.43	58.99	707	0.65
erysiphake	18	2.59	58.05	532	0.74
cryoextraction	9	1.30	61.89	222	0.68
suturing of coloboma	19	2.77	62.58	192	0.54
suture around superior loops	46	6.63	64.74	193	0.73
loop suture WORST	13	1.87	70.77	161	0.67
transcorneal loop iris suture	5	0.72	58.80	1029	0.87
strabismus operations	7	1.01	29.57	553	0.63
ocular trauma upon implant	4	0.58	68.00	1790	0.38
needling intracapsular	9	1.30	63.22	1556	0.43
needling extracapsular	42	6.05	46.98	584	0.63

Fig. 38

Data and results of the group of special cases on which iris clip lens implant operations were performed by BINKHORST.

The group of special cases will likewise be discussed in the approximate chronological order in which they might occur in an individual case.

1. *Diabetes mellitus* was present in 39 patients (11 ♂ and 28 ♀) in whom 52 eyes (7.49%) were fitted with an implant. Five male and 8 female patients underwent a bilateral implant operation.

Three cases showed only a few micro-aneurysms in the macular area.

Ten eyes with diabetic retinopathy, had an average visual acuity of only 0.19 after an average observation period of 378 days. This was mainly due to the diabetic retinopathy. The other 42 eyes without diabetic retinopathy, had an average visual acuity of 0.59 after an average observation period of 667 days. In general, there were no more complications than one would normally expect. In two cases, however, the retinopathy grew worse during the post-operative period. Any relationship between retinopathy and the operation remains, of course, a matter of speculation.

From the results one may conclude that diabetes, with or without retinopathy, should not be a contra-indication for iris clip lens implantation (see also pages 166 and 193 ff.).

Case histories.
Case 542. Male, born 1907.
29– 9–68 intracapsular cataract extraction OD (REYNVAAN).
22– 7–71 secondary vertical iris clip lens implantation with an iris suture through holes in the optic portion.
 2– 8–71 corrected visual acuity 0.5.
18– 1–72 corrected visual acuity 0.1, caused by exacerbation of the diabetic retinopathy.
 8– 5–72 the perlon suture cut through the iris.

Case 1011. Female, born 1886.
28– 6–68 intracapsular cataract extraction with iris clip lens implantation OS.
10– 9–68 corrected visual acuity 0.45.
14– 7–70 corrected visual acuity 0.1, due to an increase in the diabetic retinopathy in addition to senile changes.
25– 9–71 death of patient.

2. *Pre-operative glaucoma* was present in 24 patients in whom 29 eyes (4.18 %) were dealt with. All 29 implants were fitted during primary and intracapsular operations.

Various glaucoma operations had been performed *prior* to implantation in 17 eyes of 16 patients, as follows: iridencleisis (7), ELLIOT trephining (5), sector iridectomy (2), unknown (2) and STALLARD (1). The corneal incision was made at 12 o'clock, except in the first of these cases where the incision was made at 6 o'clock (case 401).

Posterior synechiolysis was necessary in cases of iridencleisis (4), ELLIOT trephining (2) and unknown (2).

The coloboma was sutured with perlon in two cases of ELLIOT trephining (after radial iridotomy) and in all cases of iridencleisis and sector coloboma.

Chymotrypsin was always used to safeguard intracapsular extraction. An exception was a case with a sector iridectomy. With the exception of one eye, chymotrypsin was not used in any of the other 12 eyes of 8 patients who had not previously undergone an operation. On three eyes of two of these patients a cyclodialysis in the superior temporal quadrant was performed one year *after* implantation.

The intraocular pressure of these eyes was not significantly affected by the implantation.

From the above one may conclude that an unfavourable influence of the implant operation on the glaucoma could not be established. See also pages 166 and 229 ff.

3.   Since 10–10–1968 *mannitol* has been given intravenously to 11 patients (1.58 %). Seven of these were traumatic cataract cases on whom an extracapsular cataract extraction was made (with the exception of case 436, below) which was followed by a secondary implant operation. The remaining 4 cases were intracapsular extractions.

After 1–1–1972 BINKHORST's criteria for the use of mannitol have been: intracapsular cataract extraction, extracapsular extraction where the vitreous is in open communication with the anterior chamber, and when operating on children. Mannitol is given one hour before the operation; its dosage is 1 g per kg body weight, and it is only given with the consent of the physician.

4.   *Synechiolysis* was necessary 39 times in 37 cases (5.33 %): anteriorly 13 ×, posteriorly 24 ×, and twice both anteriorly and posteriorly. Among these were 14 traumatic cataract cases and 9 cases preceded by glaucoma surgery. The latter two groups were amongst the group of 28 cases in whom the synechiolysis was performed simultaneously with the implant operation. In 4 early cases anterior synechiolysis was necessary because of decentration (see page 92).

5.   *Chymotrypsin* was used in 121 cases (17.43 %). It was first used on 8–9–1959. None of these cases had wound leakage.

The reasons for its use have been (BINKHORST, pers. comm.):
a)   to lessen the risk of rupturing the capsule (97 cases);
b)   to facilitate intracapsular extraction in adults under 50 years of age (24 cases).

6.   *The erysiphake* was used in 18 cases (2.59 %). It was used for the first time on 3–10–1963. In 14 cases it was used in combination with chymotrypsin.

7.   *Cryoextraction* was performed in 9 cases (1.30 %). The first patient was an adolescent with a subluxated crystalline lens (case 436, see below); the others

were adults of 54 years and older who had a tense capsule (7), or a subluxated lens (1).

In all other cases capsular forceps were used for intracapsular extractions.

Case history.
Case 436. Male, born 1949.
    1– 1-60 fireworks hit OD. Upward dislocation of lens, iridodonesis, sphincter ruptures, vitreous prolapse.
    4–12-69 intravenous mannitol.
         Intracapsular (!) cryoextraction with iris clip lens implantation.
    12– 2-70 resection of internal rectus and recession of external rectus OD.
    23– 9-70 corrected visual acuity 0.66.

8. *Primary suturing of a coloboma* was performed in 19 cases (2.74%), the first having been done on 8-2-1968.

In 11 cases glaucoma surgery had been performed earlier: iridencleisis (7), ELLIOT trephining (2) and sector iridectomy (2). All of these underwent a primary iris clip lens implantation after intracapsular cataract extraction facilitated by chymotrypsin (one case of sector iridectomy was performed without the use of chymotrypsin, however).

In the other 8 cases, colobomata were present for other reasons: traumatic (3), optical iridectomy (2), radial iridotomy in view of a rigid sphincter (2), and sector iridectomy prior to cataract surgery (1).

9. *A primary suture around the superior loops* (technique described on page 58) was made in 46 cases (6.63%), from 6-3-1970 onwards. The general purpose was to prevent dislocation. Dislocation of the inferior loops occurred only once, and could easily be rectified.

10. Since 25-3-1971 a *primary loop suture after* WORST (technique described on page 57) was made in 13 cases (1.87%). In one case the suture cut into the iris, in another the upper rim of the implant was pressed against the iris. In a 14th case the preplaced suture had to be removed during the operation because it became entangled with the loops of the implant.

11. *Secondary transcorneal loop iris suture* (technique described on page 65) This was made in 5 cases (0.72%), starting on 11-9-1969 (case 56 on page 98). These 5 cases had dislocations 5, 4, 2, 2 and 2 times respectively. No further dislocations have occurred since.

12. *Strabismus operations* for divergent squints were performed 8 times in 7 cases (1.01%) of young adults, within six months of the implant operation. In these cases the interval between trauma and implantation was 2, 3, 10, 11, 17, 21 and 27 years. After 1-1-1972 strabismus operations were also performed in conjunction with implant operations.

13. Severe ocular trauma occurred in 4 cases (0.58%). It caused dislocation of the implant (3) and panophthalmitis (1).

Case histories.
Case 26. Male, born 1898.
11- 6–59 intracapsular cataract extraction OS.
31- 8–59 visual acuity with aphakic correction 0.9.
19-11-59 secondary horizontal iris clip lens implantation.
   3-68 anterior dislocation of the temporal loop due to a blow (when pilocarpine had not been instilled for a long time).
24- 6–68 repositioned with a needle knife. Instillation of pilocarpine resumed.
18- 8–71 corrected visual acuity 0.85 (NORDLOHNE).

Case 153. Male, born 1898.
 4- 6–64 intracapsular cataract extraction with iris clip lens implantation OD.
20- 9–67 clod of earth hit OD which caused a partial dislocation of a loop infero-temporally, with local corneal oedema.
 2-10-67 repositioned with needle knife.
 5-10-67 slight corneal oedema infero-temporally.
 9-12-67 clear cornea.
   5-70 corrected visual acuity 0.66 (PEARCE, 1972).

Case 300. See page 113. Panophthalmitis due to perforating trauma two years after implantation. Enucleation.

Case 1004. Male, born 1897.
15- 3–68 intracapsular cataract extraction with iris clip lens implantation OD.
30- 3–68 discharged.
12- 4–68 axe hit OD! Subconjunctival iris prolapse, iridodialysis inferiorly.
13- 4–68 extraction of implant, because it was displaced upwardly in a dangerous position by the iridodialysis.
17- 5–68 aphakic spectacle correction gave a visual acuity of 0.33.
   Incipient ECD adjacent to the incision (hyaloid keratopathy?).
11- 1–72 fully developed ECD.

14. Needling had to be carried out in 51 cases (7.35%). This was done in 4 extracapsular cases at some time prior to the secondary implant operation, and in 9 extracapsular cases before or after the implant operation. There were 9 post-operative needlings of thin condensed hyaloid membranes in 9 intracapsular cases (1.30%) at an interval of an average 411 (range 24 to 1704) days after implantation, and 46 post-operative needlings (twofold in 8 cases) in 38 extracapsular cases (5.47 %), at an average interval of 124 (range 0 to 937) days after implantation. The difference in these intervals is explained by the underlying cause: opacities of the anterior vitreous membrane develop much more slowly after intracapsular extraction than residual cataract after extracapsular extraction.

15. Simultaneous autokeratoplasty was performed in one aphakic case with central corneal degeneration. Notwithstanding, the visual acuity remained below 0.10 (case 573).

Simultaneous homokeratoplasty was performed on an 18 year old mongolian patient with bilateral aphakia and keratoconus, but the graft became opaque (case 343).

Introduction

Until 1–1–1972 BINKHORST inserted 170 iridocapsular lenses in 158 patients. The first operation took place on 16–9–1965*.

Initially, indication for the fitting of an iridocapsular lens was congenital or traumatic cataract in children, since the extracapsular cataract extraction necessary at that age, facilitated iridocapsular fixation (BINKHORST, 1967ac; BINKHORST & GOBIN, 1967d, 1970b, 1971b, 1972d). After 1970 MANSCHOT's histopathological findings (see Chapter VIII) and the desire to reduce dislocations and the development of ECD to a minimum induced BINKHORST to perform primary iridocapsular lens implant operations in cases with senile cataract as well. This explains the decrease in the fitting or iris clip lens implants in favor of iridocapsular lens implants (see Fig. 39). The distribution of the patients' ages in these 170 cases is, therefore, quite different from that of the 677 iris clip lens implant operations (see Fig. 40).

The technique of the iridocapsular lens implantation is described on page 59. Numerical data are shown in Fig. 41. Noteworthy in this table are the following points:

1. The average age at operation of 30.82 years which is very low compared with the 65.80 years for the iris clip lens series, may be explained by the relatively large number of children in this series (see Fig. 40).
2. The average observation period of 572 days is only 200 days fewer than the average observation period of 772 days for the iris clip lens series. However, the figure for senile cataract is only 416 days which is 356 days fewer, as shown in Fig. 43.
3. The average visual acuity of 0.62 is of the same order as that of the iris clip lens series (0.65).

Causes of cataract

The differences in the distribution of causes of cataract between the iridocapsular lens series and the iris clip lens series, are shown in Fig. 42.

The series of 51 iridocapsular lens implant operations in cases with senile cataract has been compared by the author with a series of 51 iris clip lens implant operations likewise performed in cases with senile cataract during the same period of time, and preferably with the same operation date. The average age at operation was 67.00 and 70.55 years respectively, the average observation period

---

* At present, 1-10-1974, the number of iridocapsular lens implant operations performed by BINKHORST totals 508.

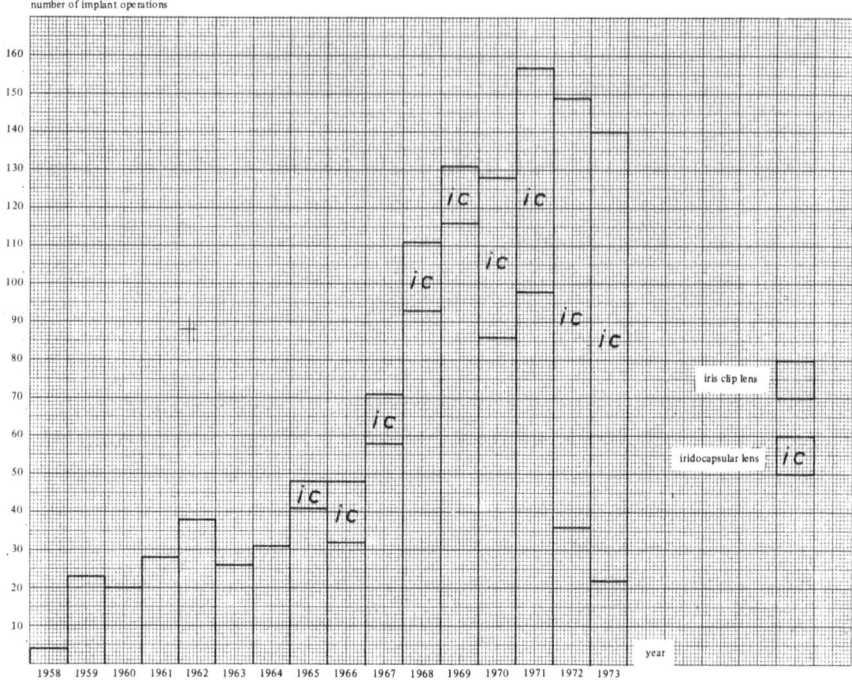

Fig. 39

Annual number of implant operations performed by BINKHORST.

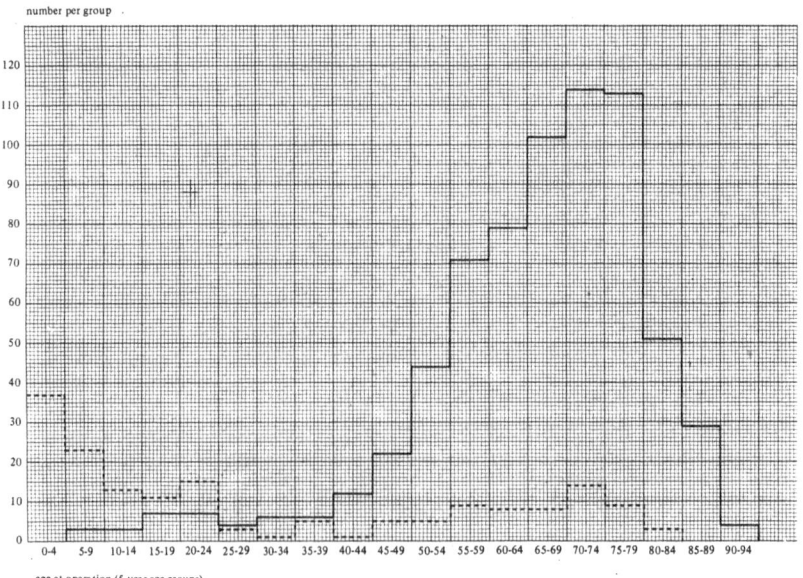

Fig. 40

Distribution of age at operation in 677 iris clip lens implant operations and 170 iridocapsular lens implant operations performed by BINKHORST.

	number	♂	♀	L	R	average age at operation in years	average observation period in days	average visual acuity
♂	106	106	—	55	51	28.70	566	0.60
♀	64	—	64	30	34	34.33	581	0.63
L	85	55	30	85	—	31.68	513	0.59
R	85	51	34	—	85	29.95	628	0.64
total	170	106	64	85	85	30.82	572	0.62
	(694)	(366)	(328	(329)	(365)	(65.80)	(772)	(0.65)

Fig. 41

Data and results of 170 iridocapsular lens implant operations performed by BINKHORST. The corresponding number of 694 iris clip lens implant operations is shown in brackets.

was 416 and 320 days respectively while the average visual acuity was 0.68 and 0.69 respectively. Thus, for senile cataract the short-term results of both series appear to be very similar.

Data and results of iridocapsular lens implant operations with respect to the cause of the cataract, are shown in Fig. 43.

1. *Congenital cataract*

The congenital cataractous lenses of 37 patients were replaced by 43 implants. They may be divided into unilateral and bilateral cataracts.

a) unilateral congenital cataract

Twenty-three eyes. All patients (except 7) underwent preliminary needling, on average 7 days (range 1 to 21 days) prior to the *primary* implantation. In one case a second preliminary needlig was necessary. Post-operative needling had to be performed very frequently in this group: once in 11 cases, twice in 4 cases, 3 times in 3 cases, 4 times in 1 case and even 5 times in another case.

A squint operation was performed in 3 cases. See also Fig. 44 on page 135. Post-operative surgical complications did not occur.

As is well-known this kind of cataract is often present together with other forms of congenital ocular pathology such as microphthalmia (7), slight microphthalmia (4), nystagmus (5), microcornea (1), persistent primary vitreous (1), retrolental membrane (1) or with mental retardation (1), or with a combination of these abnormalities (also: BINKHORST, 1943). Consequently, its prognosis is much worse than in binocular cataract: the three most successful cases of this

123

cause of cataract

	num-ber	average age at operation	senile	trauma-tic	un-known	compli-cated	hetero-chromic	thermic	radia-tion	conge-nital	juvenile	diabetic	average obser-vation period	average visual acuity
iris clip lens	694	65.80	567	52	51	14	4	2	1	1	1	1	772	0.65
iridocapsular lens	170	30.82	51	57	11	2	—	—	—	43	6	—	572	0.62
total	864	58.92	618	109	62	16	4	2	1	44	7	1	735	0.64
iris clip lens	694	65.80	81.7	7.5	7.3	2.0	0.6	0.3	0.1^5	0.1^5	0.1^5	0.1^5	772	0.65
iridocapsular lens	170	30.82	30.0	33.5	6.5	1.2	—	—	—	25.3	3.5	—	572	0.62
total	864	58.92	71.5	12.6	7.2	1.9	0.5	0.2	0.1	5.1	0.8	0.1	735	0.64

Fig. 42. Comparison of numbers (above) and percentages (below) of the data and results of 694 iris clip lens implant operations and 170 iridocapsular lens implant operations performed by BINKHORST.

cause of cataract		num-ber	♂	♀	L	R	average age at operation in years	average observa-tion period in days	average visual acuity
congenital	unilateral	23	11	12	11	12	2.74	680	0.10
	bilateral	20	15	5	10	10	5.95	444	0.49
traumatic at the age of									
0– 4 years		11	8	3	5	6	4.82	678	0 43
5– 9 years		14	10	4	8	6	10.93	892	0.57
10–14 years		13	10	3	8	5	17.69	808	0.66
15 years and over		19	16	3	8	11	28.42	581	0.74
complicated		2	1	1	1	1	4	?	0.55
juvenile		6	4	2	2	4	17.00	823	0.62
unknown		11	8	3	7	4	50.36	393	0.73
senile		51	23	28	25	26	67.00	416	0.68
total		170	106	64	85	85	30.82	572	0.62

Fig. 43

Data and results of 170 iridocapsular lens implant operations performed by BINKHORST, with respect to the cause of the cararact.

series obtained a visual acuity of 0.50, 0.20 and 0.10, but the average visual acuity attained was only 0.10.

The author agrees with BINKHORST that a lens implantation in cases of uni-lateral congenital cataract, is rarely called for.

In 5 cases a *secondary* implant operation was performed:
Case IC 26. Female, born 28–3–1965. Microphthalmia and cataract OD.
      Convergent squint OD.
   6–66 optical iridectomy (in Chile) with iridotomy at 6 o'clock.
12– 1–67 preliminary needling.
19– 1–67 lens extraction.
 9– 3–67 secondary iridocapsular lens implantation (secondary, because of prudence).
29– 2–72 pupil clear, downward decentration of implant, iris atrophy, slightly hazy fundus view (VERDONCK).

Case IC 35. Male, born 9–11–1966. Cataract OS with slight microphthalmia.
      Convergent squint with rotatory nystagmus.
 5–10–67 preliminary needling.
12–10–67 lens extraction during which the posterior capsule ruptured.
26–10–67 secondary iridocapsular lens implantation.
16–11-67 needling of lens remnants.
25– 4–69 no binocular vision. 10° convergent strabismus and rotatory nystagmus.

Case IC 45. Male, born 2-7-1966. Cataract with persistent primary vitreous OS.

18–10–67 needling (ZWIJSEN).

29–11–67 needling (ZWIJSEN).

26– 6–68 secondary iridocapsular lens implantation with sector iridectomy.

28–11–68 needling of lens remnants.

17– 1–72 visual acuity 1/∞. Vitreous opaque (ZWIJSEN).

Case IC 50. Female, born 4-1-1968. Microphthalmia and cataract OD.

19– 9–68 preliminary needling.

26– 9–68 extraction of lens remnants was very difficult, because they were extremely
  tough.

 6– 3–69 needling.

24– 4–69 needling.

28–11–69 extraction of after-cataract through the peripheral coloboma after secondary
  iridocapsular lens implantation (FEDOROV's method, see page 62).

 8–10–70 muscle operation for divergent squint.

 4– 9–71 visual acuity 0.02 (PRINS).

12– 3–73 visual acuity 0.08. Eccentric fixation.

Case IC 1005. Male, born 31-8-1957. Microphthalmia, cataract and convergent strabismus OD.

 8–11–68 preliminary needling.

15–11–68 lens extraction.

17– 1–69 secondary iridocapsular lens implantation.

14– 3–69 needling.

18– 3–69 corrected visual acuity 0.03.
  Convergent squint OD. No muscle surgery for fear of overcorrection.

 9– 8–69 corrected visual acuity 0.03. Eccentric fixation.

Some special cases:

Case IC 10. Male, born 23-5-65. Cataract with retrolental membrane OS.

 2– 2–66 preliminary needling.

 3– 2–66 primary iridocapsular lens implantation with excision of retrolental membranes after diathermic coagulation of retrolental bloodvessels.

17– 6–66 needling.

15– 9–66 needling.

  5–72 corrected visual acuity 0.01.

 9– 5–72 decentration due to a blow on the eye.

13– 6–72 corrected visual acuity 0.01.

Case IC 1018. Female, born 28-4-1967. Slight microphthalmia and cataract OS.

24– 4–70 preliminary needling.

31– 7–70 primary iridocapsular lens implantation. Capsulotomy.

14– 8–70 needling.

 2– 6–71 needling.

25– 4–72 visual acuity 0.04. Eccentric fixation, divergent squint, no binocular vision.

b) bilateral congenital cataract

Twenty eyes of 14 patients (10 ♂ and 4 ♀), with age varying from 1 to 17 years. Apart from one, all patients underwent a preliminary needling 7 days (range 1 to 21 days) prior to primary implantation. Post-operative needling was necessary once (9 cases), twice (3 cases) or three times (1 case). A squint operation was performed in one case. See also Fig. 44 on page 135.

Complications occurred neither during nor after surgery. The interval between the linked operations in the 6 bilateral cases varied from 0 to 441 days. Three of the patients who were mentally retarded, remained convergent. One of the patients operated on unilaterally, could not be examined orthoptically, because of mental retardation.

The average visual acuity attained was 0.49.

2. *Traumatic cataract*

Traumatic cataract was treated in 57 patients (44 ♂ and 13 ♀). There was no routine procedure for these cases since each case differed from another. In view of the fact that the functional result of the injured young eye is endangered by the development of amblyopia (BINKHORST, 1972e), results are discussed in 4 sections.

a) injury at the age of 0–4 years

Eleven cases (all of perforating traumata). The objects causing most injuries, were scissors (4). The interval between trauma and implantation varied from 0–7 years. Preliminary operations were performed 14 times in 7 cases, simultaneous anterior synechiolysis in 3 cases, post-operative needlings in 6 cases, 4 squint operations in 3 cases. See also Fig. 44 on page 135.

There were two cases of serious post-operative complications, viz. a case of retinal detachment (case IC 85, see below) and a case of infection where the implant had to be extracted (case IC 14, see below). Despite an average visual acuity of 0.43 and orthophoria in 8 of the 11 cases, orthoptic results lagged behind, partly because treatment was not always started immediately after trauma. See also Fig. 44 on page 135.

Important with respect to implant materials were two cases where a previously inserted DANNHEIM lens lost its supramide tips due to disintegration in the chamber angle.

Case histories.
Case IC 85. Male, born 29–1–1967. Scissors penetrated OD on 30–9–1970.
  2–11–70 preliminary needling.
  4–11–70 primary iridocapsular lens implantation with anterior synechiolysis.

14– 1–71 retinal detachment supero-nasally (ultrasonography GERNET).
Further details not available.

Case IC 14. Male, born 1–5–1957. An arrow perforated OS on 9–8–1960.
9– 8–60 iris prolapse. Conjunctival coverage (SATTLER). The lens opacified rapidly.
9–11–61 anterior synechiolysis, peripheral iridectomy at 12 o'clock, small needling
(BINKHORST).
20– 3–62 DANNHEIM lens implantation (BINKHORST).
4– 3–66 dislocation due to disintegration of the loop tips.
29– 8–66 extraction of DANNHEIM lens and implantation of iridocapsular lens.
9– 3–71 caustication of a corneal ulcer (DRAEGER).
30– 3–71 mixed injection, iridocapsular lens invisible due to exudates.
31– 3–71 extraction of the implant in view of ECD and infection (MÜLLER).

Case IC 77. Male, born 12–8–1960. Scissors injury to OD during October 1963.
29–11–63 extracapsular cataract extraction with peripheral iridectomy.
20– 2–64 DANNHEIM lens implantation with posterior capsulotomy.
17–12–64 needling.
28– 1–65 four muscle surgery, to correct a convergent squint.
7–70 dislocation due to disintegration of the loop tips.
30– 7–70 extraction of DANNHEIM lens and implantation of iridocapsular lens.
1– 3–71 corrected visual acuity 1.0. Simultaneous perception and fusion present.

b) injury at the age of 5–9 years

Fourteen cases (12 perforating). The majority of injuries were caused by scissors
(2) or arrows (5). The interval between trauma and implantation varied from 0
to 24 years. Preliminary operations were performed 11 times in 6 cases, simultaneous anterior and/or posterior synechiolysis in 7 cases, post-operative needling
9 times in 8 cases, excision of secondary membranes in one case, 10 squint
operations in 9 cases. See also Fig. 44 on page 135.

There were 4 cases with post-operative complications: dislocation occurred
in 3 cases, and retinal detachment in one. In one of the cases of dislocation the
iridocapsular lens was replaced by an iris clip lens.

Orthoptic results were far better here: 3 patients remained straight, 2 divergent squints became straight spontaneously after implantation, and 6 after muscle
surgery. Eight out of these 11 straight patients regained full binocular vision.
See also Fig. 44 on page 135. The average visual acuity attained was 0.57.

Case histories.
Case IC 6. Female, born 8–6–1956. A piece of wood perforated OD on 13–3–1962
(BINKHORST & GOBIN, 1967d; BINKHORST, GOBIN & LÉONARD, 1969d Fig. 7–4B,
1972e).
2–11–62 needling.
19–11–65 secondary iridocapsular lens implantation with posterior synechiolysis.

Posterior synechiae did not form: the implant became dislocated posteriorly 7 times!
21-11-68 implant replaced by an iris clip lens (see also case IC 130 on page 131).
7-12-71 corrected visual acuity 0.45.
Straight, with simultaneous macular perception and fusion (LÉONARD).

Case IC 30. Male, born 1947. Contusion OS in 1955 (BINKHORST, GOBIN & LÉONARD, 1969d Fig. 7-4G).
11- 5-67 primary iridocapsular lens implantation.
16- 5-67 dislocation behind the iris.
25- 5-67 repositioned spontaneously!
29- 6-67 needling. Muscle operation for divergent squint.
2- 2-68 corrected visual acuity 0.66. Straight, with simultaneous macular perception and fusion.

Case IC 55. Male, born 13-3-1964. Arrow in OS on 24-5-69 with extreme decentration and occlusion of the pupil (BINKHORST, KATS & LÉONARD, 1972e Fig. 18).
8- 9-69 formation of a pupil by means of iridotomy. The anterior chamber filled with vitreous.
23-10-69 secondary iridocapsular lens implantation in the artificial pupil, with anterior synechiolysis.
12-11-69 muscle surgery to correct a divergent squint.
27- 4-70 traumatic dislocation posteriorly after a punch on the eye. Attempt at non-operative repositioning was unsuccessful.
13- 5-70 repositioned with blunt iris hook while patient lay prone.
26- 1-71 corrected visual acuity 0.4.
Straight with simultaneous macular perception.

Case IC 37. Male, born 30-6-1960. Scissors in OD on 19-11-67 (BINKHORST, 1972e).
11-12-67 lens extraction.
11- 1-68 secondary iridocapsular lens implantation with anterior and posterior synechiolysis and peripheral iridectomy.
22- 5-68 needling.
7-68 retinal detachment (MACKENSEN).
9- 8-68 lamellar scleral resection with diathermy application (VAN BALEN).
30- 6-69 corrected visual acuity 0.55.
18- 5-71 straight with full binocular vision.

c) injury at the age of 10-14 years

Thirteen cases (9 perforating). Amongst the objects causing the injuries were scissors (2), arrows (4) and catapults (2).

The interval between trauma and implantation varied from 0-24 years.

Preliminary operations were performed 14 times in 11 cases, simultaneous anterior and/or posterior synechiolysis in 4 cases, post-operative needling 8 times in 6 cases, and 8 squint operations in 6 patients. See also Fig. 44 on page 135.

There was only one case with a serious post-operative complication, viz. a case of retinal detachment.

Orthoptic results were as good as in the previous group: 2 patients remained straight, four patients became straight spontaneously after implantation and three after muscle surgery. Eight out of these 9 straight patients regained full binocular vision. See also Fig. 44 on page 135.

The average visual acuity attained was 0.66.

Case history.
Case IC 101. Female, born 1956. Glass in OS on 15–8–1970. Aphakia with secondary cataract.
21– 5–71 secondary iridocapsular lens implantation OS with posterior synechiolysis.
26– 5–71 needling.
 9– 6–71 needling.
19– 7–71 corrected visual acuity 1.0.
19– 8–71 muscle operation to correct an exotropia.
28–11–71 retinal detachment.
30–11–71 encircling procedure with diathermy application (VAN BALEN).
13–11–72 visual acuity 0.02. Secondary cataract.
18–12–72 needling. Visual acuity remains 0.02 due to retinal damage (FALGER).

d) injury at the age of 15 years and over

Nineteen cases (14 perforating). The majority of injuries were caused by metal objects (7) and car accidents (5). The age at which the injury occurred varied from 15 to 47 years; the interval between injury and implantation varied from 52 days to 28 years.

Twenty preliminary operations were performed in 14 cases, simultaneous anterior and/or posterior synechiolysis in 6 cases, post-operative needlings 6 times in 5 cases, and 3 squint operations. See also Fig. 44 on page 135.

Two cases produced post-operative complications: in one case a decentration and in another a dislocation after which the iridocapsular lens was replaced by an iris clip lens.

Orthoptic results were good: 8 patients remained straight, 6 exotropias became straight spontaneously and 3 after muscle surgery. Seven out of these 17 straight patients regained full binocular vision. See also Fig. 44 on page 135.

The average visual acuity attained was 0.74.

Case histories.
Case IC 1. Male, born 1946. Traumatic cataract OD. (BINKHORST & GOBIN, 1967d).
25– 5–63 corneal perforation by iron wire at 5 o'clock. Small iris prolapse. Vitreous abcised; cornea sutured. Air injected. Antibiotics and atropine (WORST).

3– 1 64 needling with goniotomy needle and anterior synechiolysis (WORST). Lens material was washed out through a small incision in the opposing segment. Air injection.

7– 4–64 visual acuity was 0.75 with a contact lens.

23– 6–65 *Six contact lenses were lost. The patient was referred to* BINKHORST *for lens implantation.*

16– 9–65 secondary vertical iridocapsular lens implantation (BINKHORST). This iridocapsular lens was an iris clip lens of which the anterior loops had been removed.

7–12–65 corrected visual acuity 0.75.

The patient was licensed as a captain in the merchant navy.

28– 3–72 corrected visual acuity 1.0. Small exophoria. No fusion, no stereopsis.

Case IC 18. Male, born 1943. Iron fragment penetrated into (!) the lens OS on 9–6–1966 (BINKHORST, KATS & LÉONARD, 1972e Fig. 8; BINKHORST 1973 Fig. 14).

In the course of the following months the lens became opaque (NORDLOHNE).

3–11–66 irrigation and aspiration of lens material and the iron particle with primary iridocapsular lens implantation.

10–11–66 decentration was successfully rectified with a needle knife.

6–12–66 corrected visual acuity 1.0.

Case IC 130. Male, born 1949. Iron fragment penetrated the lens OD on 5–5–1971

27– 10–71 extracapsular cataract extraction including the iron particle with primary iridocapsular lens implantation.

8–11–71 anterior dislocation of inferior loop. Non-operative repositioning.

21– 2–72 iridocapsular adhesions did not form.

23– 2–72 implant replaced by an iris clip lens (see also case IC 6 on page 128). Corneal incision. Transiridectomy loop suture.

6– 3–73 corrected visual acuity was only 0.33 due to temporary corneal oedema.

14– 6–73 corrected visual acuity 1.20 (KIEWIET DE JONGE).

Special cases amongst the group of iridocapsular lens implant operations performed after traumatic cataract

1. In one case lens remnants were extracted through the peripheral iridectomy (FEDOROV's method, see page 62).

Case IC 51. Female, born 4–9–1959. Scissors injury OS on 21–12–66.

23– 3–67 needling (OUBORG).

9– 1–69 anterior synechiolysis, excision with extraction of secondary cataract through the peripheral iridectomy after secondary iridocapsular lens implantation (BINKHORST).

20– 3–69 needling.

6–11–69 muscle operation for exotropia.

27– 9–71 corrected visual acuity 0.25. Straight with full binocular vision.

2. The implant was fitted back to front in two cases where either a good iridocapsular cleft was absent or one could not be made. However, the reversed position had disadvantages, as follows:

a) the metal loops situated in front of the iris, glittered disagreeably.

b) needling became difficult.

Case histories.

Case IC 21. Male, born 1927. Iron fragment into OS on 1–10–48. (BINKHORST, KATS & LÉONARD, 1972e Fig. 17).

  1–10–48 conjunctival flap coverage of large corneal wounds (VAN DER VALK).

24– 3–66 anterior and posterior synechiolysis.

17–11–66 secondary implantation of an iridocapsular lens fitted back to front. The optic portion lay behind the capsular membrane, while the loops were bent in the opposite direction.

23– 1–67 corrected visual acuity 0.6.

 3– 3–67 divergent squint operatively corrected giving full binocular vision.

Case IC 91. Female, born 1950. Car accident on 13–9–69 with severe mutilation of the anterior segment OS: two large corneal ruptures, spontaneous vitreous loss, complete aniridia.

13– 9–69 corneal ruptures sutured (GEERTS) resulting in a dense corneal scar (BINK-HORST, 1972b Fig. 4d; BINKHORST, KATS & LÉONARD, 1972e Fig. 12).

14– 1–71 anterior synechiolysis.

28– 1–71 rotating corneal autograft, 7 mm, with secondary implantation of an iridocapsular lens, fitted back to front in a central capsular coloboma, using Mannitol infusion.

 8– 9–71 muscle operation for divergent squint.

 9–11–71 corrected visual acuity 0.20. Straight with full binocular vision.

3. *Complicated cataracts* were operated upon in 2 patients, both children, at the age of 4 years. See also Fig. 44 on page 135.

The ultimate results are not known at present since both children are still receiving orthoptic treatment.

4. *Juvenile cataracts* were operated upon in 5 patients. See also Fig. 44 on page 135.

In one case there was a slight brownish discolouration of the iris at 6 o'clock due to pressure of the optic portion.

All 5 patients became straight with full binocular vision.

The average visual acuity attained was 0.62.

5. *Cataracts of unknown origin* were operated upon in 11 patients. See also Fig. 44 on page 135.

In one case a transient air block, present on the first day after the operation, was eliminated by means of mydriasis. In the same patient the inferior loop caused some iris atrophy nasally, being visible through a kind of iris coloboma. The loops had not been adequately bent backwards.

Nine patients became straight with full binocular vision.

The average visual acuity attained was 0.73.

6. *Senile cataracts* were replaced by 51 implants in 46 patients. The age at operation ranged from 50 to 83 years. See also Fig. 44 on page 135.

Preliminary needling was performed in 7 cases of *immature* senile cataract, This was meant to make cataract extraction easier, but it turned out to be more difficult (BINKHORST, pers. comm.), because:
a) lens remnants were often sticky, and could not be washed out easily.
b) IOP was raised.
c) hyperaemia.

Post-operative needling was performed 28 times in 23 cases after a post-operative interval of 140 (range 13–1468) days. Half of these were performed within the first 3 months after the operation.

There were 6 cases with post-operative complications: 5 dislocations (all within the first 24 hours) and one macular oedema. ECD has not developed to date.

Orthoptic results were good: 4 patients remained exotropic, one of them was operated upon bilaterally but had an amblyopic eye (case IC 1017), and all other patients remained straight or became straight spontaneously with full binocular vision.

The average visual acuity attained was 0.68.

Case histories.
Case IC 17. Female, born 1895. PARKINSON's disease.
26–10–66 primary iridocapsular lens implantation OD under local anaesthesia.
27–10–66 total posterior dislocation.
28–10–66 non-operative repositioning.
 2–11–70 needling (after 1468 days!).
25– 8–71 corrected visual acuity 0.5 (NORDLOHNE).

Case IC 28. Female, born 1892. Diabetes mellitus since 1965.
11– 5–67 primary iridocapsular lens implantation OD.
12– 5–67 total posterior dislocation.
16– 5–67 spontaneous repositioning.
25– 8–71 corrected visual acuity 0.7 (NORDLOHNE).

Case IC 41/42. See page 223. Downward posterior dislocation of both implants on the 2nd day; repositioned under mydriasis with a needle knife.

Case IC 1008. Female ,born 1897. Diabetes mellitus since 1969.

13– 3–69 primary iridocapsular lens implantation OD.

14– 3–69 total posterior dislocation.

18– 3–69 repositioned under mydriasis.

26– 8–71 corrected visual acuity 1.10 (NORDLOHNE).

31– 3–73 spontaneous hyphaema.

23– 5–73 corrected visual acuity 0.66 due to senile macular changes.

Case IC 106. Female, born 1903.

3– 6–71 primary iridocapsular lens implantation OD.

23– 6–71 needling.

24– 1–72 macular oedema. Corrected visual acuity 0.25.

16– 4–73 corrected visual acuity 0.25.

Summary

Surgical data, results of orthoptic examinations and average visual acuity are summarised in Fig. 44.

Conclusions

1. it is still too early for a final evaluation of the results in the group with unilateral congenital cataract.

However, the initial orthoptic results and the low visual acuities obtained make the indication for a lens implantation under these circumstances look rather doubtful.

2. orthoptic results for the group of bilateral congenital cataracts were satisfactory in about half the cases (see Fig. 44).

3. patients with an injury at the age of 0 to 4 years produced the least satisfactory results because they often started to receive treatment too late with respect to their age so that binocular vision could not be regained any more.

4. patients subject to injury at a later age regained binocular vision fairly easily, even after muscle surgery in 18 out of 46 cases.

5. there was no relationship between the length of the interval between accident and implantation, and the re-establishment of binocular vision provided amblyopia had not developed.

6. patients with senile cataract produced short-term results that were very similar to those with iris clip lens implants. Early dislocation can be avoided by leaving sufficient lens material in the periphery in which the loops can be embedded (see also page 59). ECD has not developed to date.

Fig. 44. Surgical data, results of orthoptic examinations and average visual acuity in 170 iridocapsular lens implant operations performed by BINKHORST, relative to the cause of cataract.

	number of		before operation				preliminary operations			post-operative needlings		strabismus operations		average observation period in days	after operation				binocular vision						average visual acuity
	patients	eyes	straight	convergent	divergent	unknown	patients	number	simultaneous synechiolysis	patients	number	patients	number		straight	convergent	divergent	unknown	absent	simultaneous perception	fusion	stereopsis	unknown	mental retardation	
congenital																									
unilateral	23	23	?	?	?	23	21	31	—	20	37	3	3	680	4	11	5	3	4	—	—	1	17	1	0.10
bilateral	14	20	?	?	?	7	14	22	—	13	18	1	1	444	8	5	1	—	3	—	—	6	1	4	0.49
traumatic at the age of																									
0– 4 years	11	11	2	3	6	—	7	14	3	6	6	3	4	678	8	3	3	—	7	3	1	1	—	—	0.43
5– 9 years	14	14	3	6	5	—	6	11	7	8	9	9	10	892	11	1	1	1	1	2	3	8	—	—	0.57
10–14 years	13	13	2	1	9	—	11	14	4	6	8	6	8	808	9	—	1	3	1	3	1	8	—	—	0.66
15 years and over	19	19	10	—	9	—	14	20	6	5	6	3	3	581	17	—	—	2	—	1	—	7	11	—	0.74
complicated	2	2	2	—	—	—	1	2	—	2	2	1	1	?	1	1	—	—	—	—	—	2	—	—	0.55
juvenile	5	6	—	—	—	—	—	—	—	5	5	—	—	823	5	—	—	—	—	—	—	5	—	—	0.62
unknown	11	11	—	—	9	—	—	—	—	2	2	1	1	393	9	1	1	—	—	—	—	10	1	—	0.73
senile	46	51	—	—	—	—	7	8	—	23	28	—	—	416	42	—	4	1	1	—	—	45	—	—	0.68
total	158	170					81	122	20	90	121	27	31	572	114	22	13	11	17	9	5	91	32	5	0.62

This was only applied to two cases in which two-stage surgery was used.

Case histories.

Case F 1. Male, born 1948. Amblyopia with esotropia OD. The patient received iron
    particle in OS (!) on 19–11–63. This had not been noticed at the time.

19–12–63 incipient cataract with adhering leucoma at 1–2 o'clock. Uveal reaction.
    Metal foreign body detected by X-ray and foreign-body locator contact lens
    WORST.

23–12–63 sclerotomy and magnet extraction of a 5.5 mm long iron splinter at 5.30
    o'clock (SCHREUDER & NORDLOHNE).

29– 9–64 needling (SCHREUDER).

27– 7–65 visual acuity with aphakic correction 1.0.

*However, the patient preferred to use the amblyopic eye with only 0.25 visual acuity over
the aphakic eye with 1.0 visual acuity!* SCHREUDER *considered this to be an absolute
indication for an intraocular lens, and he referred the patient to* BINKHORST.

3–11–66 secondary implantation of FEDOROV's modification of the iris clip lens after
    posterior synechiolysis through the peripheral iridectomy (BINKHORST).
    The anterior loops lay vertically, the posterior loops horizontally.

17–11–66 needling of ELSCHNIG pearls.

1–11–68 corrected visual acuity 1.0 (NORDLOHNE).

Case F 2. Male, born 1914. Cataract of unknown origin OD.

26– 1–63 intracapsular cataract extraction (BIJNEN).
    Chymotrypsin used.

21– 2–63 visual acuity with aphakic correction 1.0.

The patient continually lost his contact lenses and was referred to BINKHORST *for lens
implantation.*

3–11–66 secondary implantation of FEDOROV's modification of the iris clip lens after
    posterior synechiolysis (BINKHORST).

16– 1–67 corrected visual acuity 0.66.

	number	pupillary block	choroidal detachment	unintentional corneo-scleral fistula	uveitis	macular damage	decentration	dislocation	total ECD	partial ECD	retinal detachment	extraction of implant	enucleation
secondary intracapsular	76	1	1	5	3	4	6	10	4	—	—	1	—
primary intracapsular	505	—	1	—	1	19	9	35	27	9	12	3	1
secondary extracapsular	36	—	—	1	1	—	4	6	1	—	1	—	—
primary extracapsular	77	1	—	5	6	—	5	2	—	1	—	—	—
total	694	2	2	11	11	23	24	53	32	10	13	4	1
%		0.3	0.3	1.6	1.6	3.3	3.5	7.6	4.6	1.4	1.9	0.6	0.1

Fig. 45

Distribution of post-operative complications, implant extractions and one enucleation in 694 iris clip lens implant operations performed by BINKHORST, relative to surgical procedure.

	number	pupillary block	choroidal detachment	unintentional corneo-scleral fistula	uveitis	macular damage	decentration	dislocation	total ECD	partial ECD	retinal detachment	extraction of implant	enucleation
congenital unilateral	23	—	—	—	—	—	—	—	—	—	—	—	—
congenital bilateral	20	—	—	—	—	—	—	—	—	—	—	—	—
traumatic at the age of													
0– 4 years	11	—	—	—	1	—	—	—	1	—	1	1	—
5– 9 years	14	—	—	—	—	—	—	3	—	—	1	1	—
10–14 years	13	—	—	—	—	—	—	—	—	—	1	—	—
15 years and over	19	—	—	—	—	—	1	1	—	—	—	1	—
complicated	2	—	—	—	—	—	—	—	—	—	—	—	—
juvenile	6	—	—	—	—	—	—	—	—	—	—	—	—
unknown	11	1	—	—	—	—	—	—	—	—	—	—	—
senile	51	—	—	—	—	1	—	5	—	—	—	—	—
total	170	1	—	—	1	1	1	9	1	—	3	3	—
%		0.6	—	—	0.6	0.6	0.6	5.3	0.6	—	1.8	1.8	—

Fig. 46

Distribution of post-operative complications and implant extractions in 170 iridocapsular lens implant operations performed by BINKHORST, relative to the cause of the cataract.

Until the middle of 1972 the number of cases with post-operative complications after iridocapsular lens implantation is about half that occurring after iris clip lens implantation; for corneal dystrophy it is only one-tenth (see Figs. 45 and 46).

A statistical comparison, however, cannot be made because the series are quite dissimilar in number, age and cause of cataract (see Figs. 40 and 42).

A comparison of senile cataract cases only (see page 121) shows that short-term results are similar.

The most remarkable advantages of the iridocapsular implant seem to be the marked decline in the incidence of ECD, decentration and macular damage. An average interval of 3 years after operation till the detection of ECD, as observed in iris clip lens implantations (see Fig. 31 on page 101) was reached by only 8.8% of the iridocapsular lens cases, as opposed to 64.0% of the iris clip lens cases. The principal factor promoting ECD, viz. the pair of anterior loops, is absent in the iridocapsular lens. It is, therefore, hoped that ECD too will remain absent. Only time will tell whether this expectation is justified.

CHAPTER V

RESULTS OBTAINED BY J. G. F. WORST

'I thought him a magician, but I did not
want to imitate him'.

Richard CHURCH, as cited by Karl KÖNIG
in: 'The Order of Birth in the Family
Constellation' (in the Chapter on the
Second Child).
The Cresset, Journal of the Camphill
Movement, Vol. IV 1957 and Vol. V 1958.

INTRODUCTION

This chapter deals with the results of BINKHORST lens implant operations
performed by J. G. F. WORST, the only surgeon apart from BINKHORST himself,
who performed more than 600 BINKHORST lens implant operations which have
been well documented.

Until 1st January 1972 WORST performed 665 BINKHORST lens implant operations: he inserted 485 iris clip lenses, 4 iridocapsular lenses, 3 iris clip lenses
modified after FEDOROV (see page 28) and 173 iris medallion lenses. He performed the first 15 operations at the University Eye Clinic of Groningen,
between 16-1-1967 and 12-12-1967, and the remaining 650 at the Refaja Hospital, Stadskanaal, 27 miles from Groningen. The annual number of operations
rose rapidly: 1967 (15), 1968 (4), 1969 (91), 1970 (237), 1971 (318), 1972 (353),
1973 (361). A small number of patients was operated on under local anaesthesia.
The implant was sutured to the iris in 420 eyes (63.16%). This was done for the
first time on 20th February 1969 (case 21). Suturing to the iris became a routine,
with some exceptions, from 2nd June 1970 (case 189) onwards.

Of the 665 cases, and excluding the deceased patients, it was possible to
trace all patients after 1st January 1970.

A general review of numerical data is given in Fig. 47 at back of book. They
are based on the data from WORST and his three associates, viz. LUDWIG,
MASSARO and MOSSELMAN, as well as from ophthalmologists who referred
patients, and the refractionists DE HAAN and VAN WELY. They have been classified by the author according to the cause of the cataract, sex of the patient,
L or R eye, binocular or monocular implantation, age at time of operation,

observation period in days between operation date and last refraction date, and the visual acuity at that date.

The group of binocular implant operations consists of 207 patients (78 ♂ and 129 ♀). Of these 207 patients, 84 (40.6%) left eyes and 115 (55.5%) right eyes were operated on first, and 8 pairs (3.9%) were dealt with during one session. The interval between implant operations in one patient ranged from 0 to 631 days, with an average of 43 days. This average interval was relatively short compared with the 515 days in the series of BINKHORST. The explanation becomes apparent when the comparative duration of the series is examined: 13½ years (BINKHORST) and 5 years (WORST) respectively. The chance of a long average interval is eo ipso greater in a series spread over many years.

Fig. 48 shows data and results of BINKHORST lens implant operations in binocular cases.

interval between implant operations in binocular cases	number of patients	average age at operation in years		average observation period in days		average visual acuity	
		1st eye	2nd eye	1st eye	2nd eye	1st eye	2nd eye
0– 7 days	137	74.81	74.81	162	161	0.57	0.57
8–14 days	33	75.36	75.36	261	261	0.37	0.46
>14 days	37	72.70	73.13	377	175	0.64	0.61
total	207	74.52	74.60	216	179	0.55	0.56

Fig. 48

Data and results of BINKHORST lens implant operations performed by WORST in binocular cases, relative to the interval between implantations.

The group of monocular implant operations consists of 251 patients (118 ♂ and 133 ♀). The number of 251 monocular cases as opposed to 207 binocular cases, is relatively low compared with BINKHORST (570 against 147), but this is in accordance with the fact that in the series of WORST senile cataract was present in 621 out of 665 eyes (93.4%), i.e. in a considerably higher percentage than in the series of BINKHORST (71.5%).

Implant operations were performed by WORST in all cases of cataract extraction, except in the presence of:

1. pre-operative axial myopia of more than 7 dioptres.
2. manifest diabetes with visible leakage of fluorescein from the iris.
3. FUCHS' corneal dystrophy.
4. severe macular degeneration.

TECHNIQUE (WORST, 1971d)

I. Preparation of the patient

a. mydriasis with phenylephrine 10% and cyclopentolate hydrochloride 0.5% (Cyclogyl).
b. general anaesthesia.
c. measures to lower the intraocular pressure (IOP):
    1. biochemically by means of acetazolamide (Diamox) pre-operatively (however, see page 43).
    2. mechanically by the elimination of external factors which might elevate the IOP:
        a. the use of a disposable self-adhering eyelid retractor of own design which is supposed to avoid pressure on the globe.
        b . the use of FLIERINGA's scleral supporting ring placed eccentrically upwards along the vertical meridian.

Prior to surgery the IOP is measured with a BARRAQUER surgical tonometer. This is an applanation tonometer with a fixed weight of 16 g and a second weight of 25 g.

d. sterility.
    1. a non-turbulent jet of filtered air (lamellar flow) is passed over the operation area*.
    2. milli-pore filters are used for all syringes during surgery.
    3. steridrape procedure: plastic covers glued to the skin of the eyelids and surrounding tissues, in small strips according to own modification.

II. Surgical technique (1st November 1971)

Moisture and transparency of the cornea are maintained by means of a dis-

---

* MUNKTELL sterile airflow AFH-11.

posable continuous drip system delivering about 2 drops per second, and a continuous suction procedure.

1. subconjunctival injection of saline at 12 o'clock, to facilitate proper cleavage of the subconjunctiva.
2. limbal-based conjunctival flap of 2–3 mm.
3. lamellar dissection of the cornea at 3 and 9 o'clock. This restricts bleeding since the actual corneo-scleral incision can be made less sclerally, i.e. in only slightly vascularised tissue.
4. half deep corneo-scleral incision made with a GILETTE blade held at an acute angle. The incision should start in scleral tissue and end in corneal tissue.
5. one virgin silk suture preplaced at two suture points (2 and 10 o'clock), i.e. in a U-shape. The needle is temporarily left bridging the half deep corneo-scleral incision at one of the sites so as to prevent inadvertent cutting of the suture when opening the anterior chamber.
6. opening of the anterior chamber with a GILETTE blade and widening of the incision with CASTROVIEJO scissors. For a smooth and atraumatic lens implant operation the section should extend over slightly more than 180°.
7. a 0.025 mm atraumatic perlon suture is passed twice through the iris, near the major collarette, with a horizontal interspace of 4 mm.
8. cryoextraction. Chymotrypsin is rarely used for fear of delaying the healing of the wound and because of its tendency to induce glaucoma. Moreover these complications are promoted by the corticosteroid drops given post-operatively.
9. lens implantation using irrigating forceps of own design (technique described on page 61). The preplaced suture is drawn through the axillae of the anterior loops (iris clip lens) or the holes (iris medallion lens), tied with three knots *behind* the implant and cut as short as possible. Miosis is obtained by means of acetylcholine irrigation.
10. one peripheral iridectomy.
11. the anterior chamber is restored with saline as early as possible.
12. wound closure. The two preplaced virgin silk sutures are temporarily closed, but are replaced later by 3 to 5 steel wire sutures. Having placed the steel wire sutures, a continuous perlon marline hitch suture is added. The conjunctiva is closed with another continuous perlon marline hitch suture or with interrupted sutures of virgin silk.

III. Post-operative care

Dexamethasone sodium phosphate (Decadron) and neomycin eye drops are administered 6 times daily. This medication is continued for two or three weeks.

An eye shield is fitted during one day and five nights. The average hospitalisation period is 5 days.

Causes of cataract

The differentiation of results with respect to the cause of the cataract is shown in Fig. 49.

cause of cataract	num-ber	♂	♀	L	R	average age at operation in years	average observa-tion period in days	average visual acuity
senile	621	249	372	297	324	73.06	203	0.57
traumatic (12 perf.)	20	12	8	10	10	30.55	310	0.61
unknown	15	9	6	7	8	46.40	242	0.57
complicated	5	–	5	3	2	68.20	213	0.25
heterochromic	2	2	–	2	–	23.00	112	0.55
congenital	2	2	–	–	2	2.50	453	0.08
total	665	274	391	319	346	70.78	208	0.57

Fig. 49

Data and results of 665 BINKHORST lens implant operations performed by WORST, with respect to the cause of the cataract.

Case histories.
1. *Senile cataract:* 621 cases.
2. *Traumatic cataract:* 20 patients.

Case 1. Male, born 1943. Perforating injury OS in 1964 led to cataract and divergent squint.
16– 1–67 needling, extraction and horizontal iris clip lens implantation.
23– 1–68 muscle operation for divergent squint (HAM).
    7–69 thumb in the eye. A membrane developed behind the implant due to reasons unknown. This required needling.
25– 2–71 corrected visual acuity 1.2.

Case 8. Male, born 1939. Intraocular foreign body OD on 7-6-67 resulted in a cataract.
 8– 6–67 extraction of foreign body.
20– 6–67 aspiration of lens material with a goniotomy needle.

143

10– 8–67 irrigation of the anterior chamber, to remove residual lens material, followed by iris clip lens implantation.

23– 4–68 corrected visual acuity 0.75.

Case 9. Female, born 1964. Perforating injury OD on 11–8–67 resulted in a cataract.

11– 8–67 aspiration of lens material, followed by iris clip lens implantation.

1– 9–67 needling of secondary cataract.

71 slight upward decentration. Precipitates on the anterior surface of the implant. Visual acuity 0.02.

In this case the mother did not co-operate with the orthoptist, and so the unfortunate child became amblyopic.

Case 10. Male, born 1930. Perforating injury OD on 16–8–67 resulted in a cataract.

22– 8–67 preliminary needling.

29– 8–67 irrigation of the anterior chamber, to remove residual lens material, followed by iris clip lens implantation.

23– 9–67 precipitates on anterior and posterior surface of the implant, due to the extracapsular extraction. Corrected visual acuity 0.3.

Case 460. Male, born 1947. Perforating injury OD in 1969, resulting in aphakia, vitreous loss and updrawn pupil.

9– 1–70 muscle operation for divergent squint.

26– 5–71 radial iridotomy at 6 o'clock. Inverted implantation of an iris medallion lens, i.e. with the holes at 6 o'clock, and a STRAMPELLI suture (see page 20) through each hole. A massive secondary cataract pushed the implant forward.

2–10–71 repositioning of subluxated implant.

Visual acuity 0.07. Needling necessary.

26– 1–72 repositioning of subluxated implant.

28– 5–72 incipient ECD due to corneal contact.

27– 9–72 extraction of implant was technically easy.

15–12–72 partial ECD.

3. *Cataract of unknown origin:* 15 cases.

4. *Complicated cataract:* 5 cases.

Case 137/146. Female, born 1903. Bilateral central corneal maculae resulting from scrophulosis. History of bilateral iridocyclitis. A sector iridectomy OS had been performed elsewhere.

5–11–69 intracapsular cataract extraction OS.

1– 4–70 secondary iris clip lens implantation. The lens was sutured on the iris, intentionally too high to avoid vision through the corneal maculae.

9– 4–70 intracapsular cataract extraction with iris clip lens implantation OD. The lens was not sutured on the iris.

20– 4–70 corrected visual acuity R 1.0 and L 0.8.

27– 8–70 corrected visual acuity R 0.5 and L 0.3. Macular degeneration ODS.
 5– 4–71 corrected visual acuity R 0.2 and L 0.2.

5. *Heterochromic cataract:* 2 cases.

Case 112. Male, born 1949.
21– 8–69 needling, and aspiration of lens material OS.
14– 1–70 iris clip lens implantation. The implant was not sutured on the iris.
 6– 3–70 posterior dislocation of temporal loop. Non-operative repositioning with
        strabismus hook under mydriasis.
 8– 9–70 muscle operation for divergent squint.
22– 2–71 corrected visual acuity 1.0. Diplopia still present.

Case 617. Male, born 1946.
 9–10–69 needling, and aspiration of lens material OS.
15–11–71 iris medallion lens implantation.
24– 1–72 corrected visual acuity 0.1. Cloudy vitreous.

6. *Congenital cataract:* 2 cases.

Case 94. Male, born 1968.
23– 5–69 preliminary needling OD.
27– 5–69 aspiration of lens material.
14–11–69 iris clip lens implantation, needling of secondary cataract.
27– 2–70 muscle operation for convergent squint.
21– 5–70 anterior dislocation of implant nasally inferiorly.
20– 8–70 progressive dislocation.
15–10–70 total dislocation.
23–10–70 extraction of implant.
17– 6–71 + 16.50 DS gave a visual acuity of 0.06.

Case 248. Male, born 1966.
 1– 5–70 needling, and aspiration of lens material OD.
12– 5–70 1st muscle operation for convergent squint.
16– 9–70 2nd muscle operation for convergent squint, iris clip lens implantation.
 9– 8–71 eccentric pupil: contact of the nasal loop caused some localised corneal
        clouding. Uncorrected visual acuity 0.16. Orthoptic treatment continued.

PRIMARY INTRACAPSULAR IMPLANTATION

Exclusion of cases

The majority (616) of the 665 implant operations was formed by the rather
homogeneous group of 447 primary iris clip lens and the 169 primary iris
medallion lens implant operations after intracapsular cataract extraction. Four

cases with a ruptured lens capsule which could be removed completely, were treated as intracapsular cases.

Forty-nine implant operations had to be excluded and were, for various reasons, dealt with as a separate group: iridocapsular lens (4), FEDOROV modification (3), secondary implantation (25), extracapsular extraction (22), extraction of implant (7), enucleation (1), incomplete data due to old age (10), or death (5) while many cases fell in more than one of these groups.

The numerical data of these 49 cases are shown in Fig. 47.

Notable are the low average age at operation, the high percentage of monocular cases, the long average observation period, and the low average visual acuity.

Data and results of remaining cases

The data and results of the remaining 616 primary intracapsular implant operations are:

a. the *age at operation* ranges from 38 to 92 years, with an average of 72.08 years. Fig. 50 shows the frequency curve. Its maximum is at 78 years. The relationship between age at operation and visual acuity is shown in Fig. 51. After the age of 70 results decline progressively for the average visual acuity obtained and for the percentage of eyes attaining a visual acuity of 1.0 and over when considered in age groups of 5 years. See also Fig. 40 on page 122 and Fig. 21 on page 76.

b. the *observation period* ranges from 8 to 1363 days with an average of 199 days. Fig. 52 shows the frequency curve. Its maximum is at 52 days. The relationship between observation period, age at operation and visual acuity is also represented in Fig. 52. The increase of average visual acuity is shown here over the first 50 days after the operation. See also Fig. 22 on page 77.

c. the *visual acuity* ranges from 0 to 1.20 with an average of 0.58. Fig. 53 shows its relationship with the age at operation. See also Fig. 25 on page 80. The main feature, the 80 cases (13.0%) of primary intracapsular BINKHORST lens implant operations having a visual acuity of 0.10 or less, is explained in the main by the 24 cases of senile macular degeneration, the 11 cases of ECD (see page 159), the 10 cases of retinal detachment (see page 161) and the 7 cases of cystoid macular degeneration (see page 156) in this group. Fifty-four out of these 80 cases attained a visual acuity of 0.05 or less.

Complications during operations

The operative complications in 665 BINKHORST lens implantations were
1. bulging vitreous, 3 cases (0.45%)

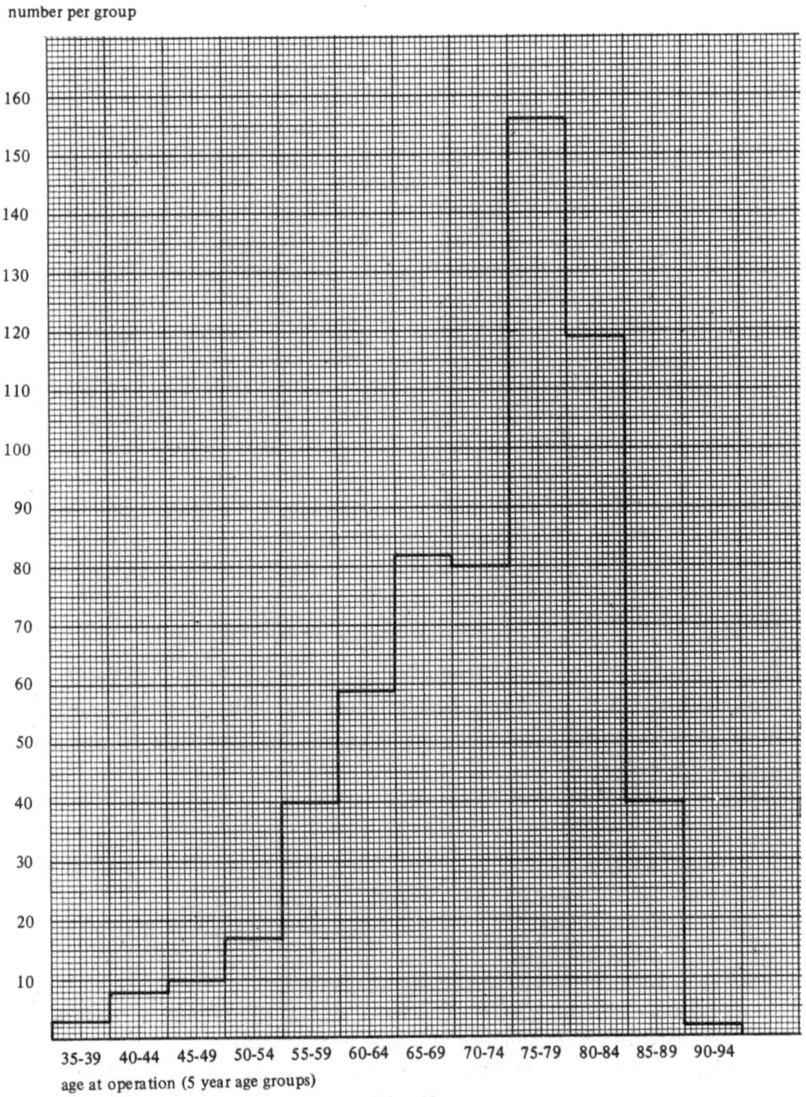

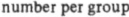

number per group

Fig. 50

Distribution of age at operation in 616 primary intracapsular BINKHORST lens implant operations performed by WORST.

2. vitreous in front of the implant, 7 cases (1.05%)
3. vitreous loss, 11 cases (1.65%)
4. minor accidents, 5 cases (0.75%)

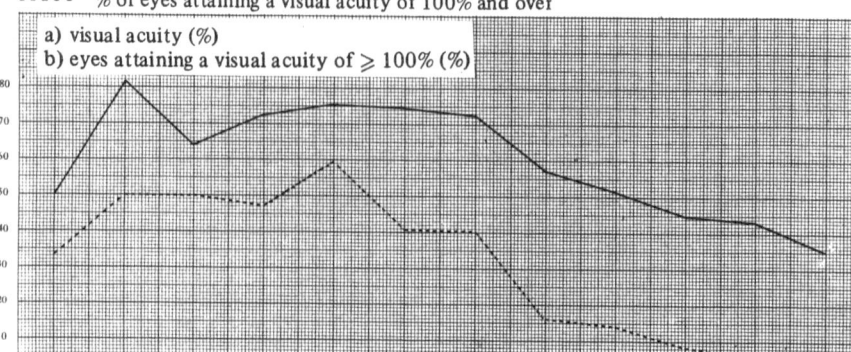

average visual acuity (%)

- - - - % of eyes attaining a visual acuity of 100% and over

a) visual acuity (%)
b) eyes attaining a visual acuity of ⩾ 100% (%)

age at operation (5 year age groups)

Fig. 51

Relationship between age at operation and visual acuity in 616 primary intracapsular BINKHORST lens implant operations performed by WORST.

re 1. *Bulging vitreous* was of no consequence to the final result.

re 2. *Vitreous in front of the implant* had no influence on the transparency of the cornea or the IOP. However, there was one case with upward decentration of the implant and another with retinal detachment one year after the operation (see also page 53).

Case histories.

Case 2. Female, born 1930.

1– 9–65 intracapsular cataract extraction OS (DONDERS).

24– 2–66 contact lens correction gave a visual acuity of 1.0. However, the contact lens could not be tolerated.

24– 5–67 secondary horizontal iris clip lens implantation.

25– 5–67 vitreous protruded in front of the implant, through the iridectomy which was too large, hence the implant was decentred upwards.

8– 9–70 repositioning of the implant, two STRAMPELLI sutures (see page 20) at 5 and 7 o'clock.

12–11–70 visual acuity 0.03 due to macular degeneration of the retina.

Case 534. Female, born 1895.

28– 7–71 intracapsular cataract extraction with iris clip lens implantation OS. Loop iris suture.

18– 8–71 small vitreous bubble in front of the implant.

30– 9–71 corrected visual acuity 0.15. Many precipitates on the implant. Vitreous opacities.

148

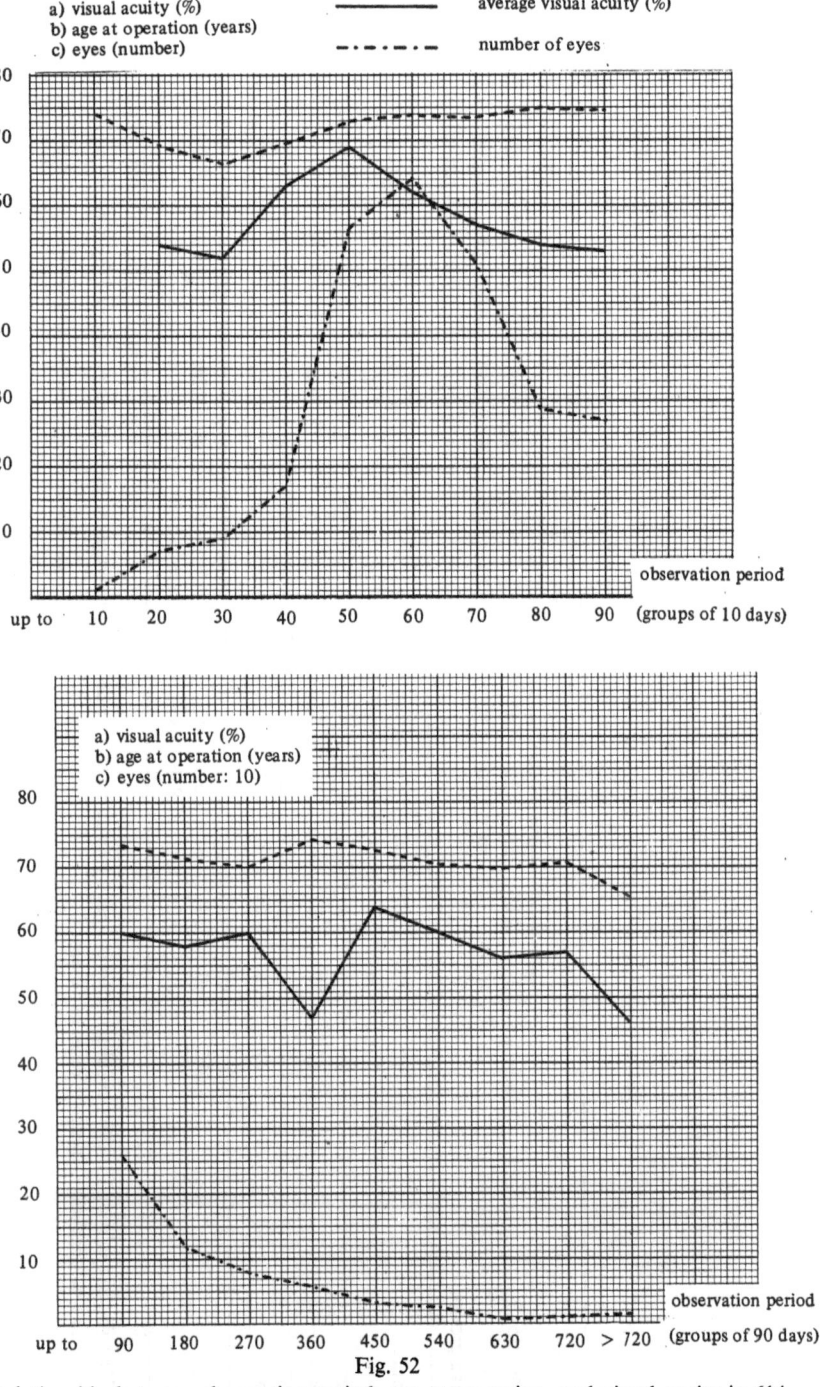

Fig. 52

Relationship between observation period, age at operation, and visual acuity in 614 BINKHORST lens implant operations performed by WORST.

In two cases the observation period was unknown.

The 261 cases with an observation period of up to 90 days are shown separately with a subdivision in groups of 10 days.

age at operation in 10 year age groups	number	percentage visual acuity												average visual acuity
		0–10	11–20	21–30	31–40	41–50	51–60	61–70	71–80	81–90	91–100	101–110	111–120	
35–44 years	11	1	—	—	1	1	1	—	2	—	5	—	—	0.73
45–54 years	27	4	1	1	3	—	1	2	2	—	11	—	2	0.69
55–64 years	99	5	4	5	3	6	9	3	22	1	37	—	4	0.75
65–74 years	162	17	6	6	14	12	25	2	31	3	42	—	4	0.65
75–84 years	275	47	19	26	25	28	57	4	37	—	31	—	1	0.49
85–94 years	42	6	4	6	6	5	9	—	3	1	2	—	—	0.43
total	616	80	34	44	52	52	102	11	97	5	128	—	11	0.58
%		13.0	5.5	7.1	8.4	8.4	16.6	1.8	15.8	0.8	20.8	—	1.8	

Fig. 53. Distribution of visual acuity results in 616 primary intracapsular BINKHORST lens implant operations performed by WORST, with respect to the age at operation, in age groups of 10 years.

1– 8–72 retinal detachment with a big tear at 11 o'clock.
14– 8–72 encircling procedure with a scleral pocket.
15– 9–72 visual acuity 1/∞. Relapse of the retinal detachment.

re 3.   *Vitreous loss* may be a contra-indication to implantation since vast experience is needed to solve the technical problems without taking undue risks although good results can be obtained when the appropriate technique is employed (see page 53).

However, if the surgeon is not extremely skilled, and does not take care about all the details described on page 53, he is likely to encounter a high incidence of complications typical of pseudophakia such as decentration and dislocation which entails the danger of ECD due to corneal contact. These complications may even occur to the very experienced surgeon as the following case histories may illustrate.

Case histories.
Case 188. Female, born 1962. Cornea and lens perforated OS.
30– 5–70 aspiration of lens material. Big vitreous loss. Iris clip lens implantation.
23– 9–71 upward decentration due to vitreous traction.
         Corrected visual acuity 0.3 due to vitreous opacities.

Case 384. Female, born 1907.
10– 2–71 intracapsular cataract extraction with horizontal iris clip lens implantation OD. Small vitreous loss.
23– 9–71 upward decentration due to vitreous traction, nearly caused corneal contact and produced diplopia with abnormal perspective. Corrected visual acuity 0.8.
 1– 5–73 extreme upward decentration of the implant, but no ECD.
         Corrected visual acuity 0.2.

Case 544. Male, born 1916. In 1961 the right eye was hit by a snowball which contained a stone.
 9– 8–71 intracapsular cataract extraction with iris clip lens implantation OD. Loop iris suture. Slight vitreous loss.
15– 9–71 corrected visual acuity 1.2.

Case 646. Female, born 1899.
 6–12–71 intracapsular cataract extraction with iris clip lens implantation OS. Loop iris suture. Some vitreous loss.
 8– 2–72 corrected visual acuity 1.0. Slight upward decentration due to vitreous traction.

re 4.   *Minor accidents.*
In a few isolated cases a posterior loop became distorted during the operation, one of the anterior loops broke, the point of a broken needle adhered to the iris, a piece of perlon suture remained behind the implant.

Data and results of post-operative complications, implant extractions and an enucleation are shown in Fig. 54.

	number	%	average age at operation in years	average observa- tion period in days	average visual acuity
pupillary block	3	0.45	60.67	359	0.30
choroidal detachment unintentional	3	0.45	73.67	166	0.72
corneo-scleral fistula	5	0.75	70.60	406	0.55
deposits on implant	10	1.50	60.00	462	0.23
uveitis (endogenous or exogenous)	15	2.26	67.27	465	0.37
cystoid macular oedema	23	3.46	66.83	712	0.29
decentration	7	1.05	50.43	188	0.59
dislocation	17	2.56	54.23	346	0.52
ECD	17	2.56	66.12	498	0.17
retinal detachment	12	1.80	64.33	504	0.08
extraction of implant	8	1.20	53.38	412	0.25
enucleation	1	0.15	86	322	0.00
cases with complications (total)	97	14.59	64.51	397	0.39
cases without complications (total)	568	85.41	71.85	175	0.60

Fig. 54

Data and results of post-operative complications, implant extraction and one enuclea- tion in 665 BINKHORST lens implant operations performed by WORST. The total number is 121, but the actual number of cases is 97 since some of the patients showed more than one complication. The total number of cases without complications has been added for comparison.

Post-operative complications and their sequelae will again be discussed in the approximate chronological order in which they may develop after the implant operation. For their distribution per 100 cases the reader is referred to Fig. 57 on page 164.

1. *Pupillary block*. Three cases (0.45%).

In two early cases (numbers 5 and 23) this complication was attributed to the air bubble in the anterior chamber. In both cases the air block was successfully dealt with by means of mydriasis. Nevertheless, WORST decided to abandon air insufflation. See also page 50. In case 20, pupillary block occurring 2 months after the operation was successfully treated by means of mydriasis too.

2. *Choroidal detachment.* Three cases (0.45%).

This complication which developed in two patients with glaucoma, owing to fistulising operations, was of no consequence: there was no shallow anterior chamber nor did corneal contact occur.

Case histories.
Case 413. Male, born 1896. Pre-operative ELLIOT trephining in both eyes (FLIERINGA).
12– 3–71 intracapsular cataract extraction with iris clip lens implantation and loop iris suture OD. Prolonged choroidal detachment.
26– 8–71 corrected visual acuity 0.6.

Case 415. Female, born 1883. Diabetes mellitus.
24– 3–71 intracapsular cataract extraction with iris clip lens implantation OS. Prolonged choroidal detachment.
31– 3–71 enucleation of the fellow-eye because of an intraocular tumour.
23– 9–71 corrected visual acuity 0.55.

Case 441. Male, born 1913. Glaucoma simplex.
26– 4–71 intracapsular cataract extraction with iris clip lens implantation and loop iris suture OS. Extremely bulging vitreous. Diathermy of the scleral wound edge between two corneo-scleral sutures to promote the development of a fistulising scar. Prolonged choroidal detachment.
21– 9–71 corrected visual acuity 1.0. Fistulising scar.

3. *Unintentional corneo-scleral fistula.* Five cases (0.75%).

In 3 cases the fistula was caused by a corneo-scleral virgin silk suture situated too deeply and left in place. In one case an unintentional corneo-scleral fistula caused prolonged flattening of the anterior chamber which resulted in ECD due to corneal contact. In the other cases, undesirable effects with respect to the final result were absent.

Case histories.
Case 7. Male, born 1906.
9– 8–67 intracapsular cataract extraction with iris clip lens implantation OD.
1– 9–67 flat anterior chamber due to wound leakage. Corneo-scleral wound resutured.
26– 6–69 visual acuity 0.05. Slight ECD.
4– 3–71 visual acuity through pinhole disc 0.2. Incipient ECD. Some precipitates on implant. Cloudy vitreous.

Case 68. Male, born 1888.

9–10–69 intracapsular cataract extraction with iris clip lens implantation OS.

24–10–69 corneo-scleral wound resutured because of wound leakage.

22–12–69 corrected visual acuity 0.4.

13– 8–70 death of patient.

Case 72. Female, born 1894.

12– 9–66 intracapsular cataract extraction OS (WORST).

16–10–69 secondary horizontal iris clip lens implantation.

29–10–69 resutured because of wound dehiscence temporally superiorly. Visual acuity not known owing to bad health.

1– 6–72 death of patient.

Case 601. Male, born 1891.

1–11–71 intracapsular cataract extraction with iris clip lens implantation OD. Loop iris suture.

16–11–71 corneo-scleral fistula. Not resutured. Spontaneous healing.

14–12–71 corrected visual acuity 1.0.

Case 663. Male, born 1912.

23–12–71 intracapsular cataract extraction with iris clip lens implantation OS. Loop iris suture.

18– 2–72 corrected visual acuity 0.6. Large bleb at 12 o'clock. Normal depth of anterior chamber.

4– 4–73 corneo-scleral wound resutured.

25– 5–73 corrected visual acuity 1.0.

4. *Deposits on implant.* Ten cases (1.50%).

These were of lenticular origin in 2 extracapsular cases, due to infection in 7 cases and of unknown origin in one case. Visual acuity in the infectious cases was impaired mainly due to the cloudy vitreous; not by the precipitates.

Case histories.

Case 3. Female, born 1894.

25– 5–67 intracapsular extraction of a hypermature cataract with iris clip lens implantation OD.

19– 1–71 corrected visual acuity 0.1.

Many precipitates on implant surfaces and vitreous membrane. Ophthalmoscopy impossible.

Case 7. See page 153. Cloudy vitreous and ECD.

Case 9. See page 144. ⎰ aspiration of lens material after perforating trauma.
Case 10. See page 144. ⎱

Case 12. Male, born 1907.

21– 9–67 intracapsular cataract extraction with iris clip lens implantation OS. A hypopyon which developed after the operation healed spontaneously.

154

22–12–67 uncorrected visual acuity 0.5. Some precipitates on implant.
23– 4–69 uncorrected visual acuity 0.8. Some precipitates on implant. Clear vitreous.
14– 1–71 status quo.

Case 119/127. Male, born 1889.
18– 2–70 intracapsular cataract extraction with iris clip lens implantation OD.
25– 2–70 ditto OS.
25– 5–70 corrected visual acuity R 0.6 and L 0.5. Precipitates on implant and cloudy
vitreous in both eyes.
16–12–70 corrected visual acuity R 0.15 and L 0.07.

Case 531. Female, born 1895.
23– 7–71 intracapsular cataract extraction with iris medallion lens implantation OD.
10–12–71 corrected visual acuity 0.3. Many precipitates on implant.

Case 534. See page 148. Many precipitates on implant.

Case 654. Male, born 1919. Cataract OS, cause unknown.
13–12–71 intracapsular cataract extraction with iris medallion lens implantation.
31– 1–72 many precipitates on implant.
Corrected visual acuity 0.3.

5. *Uveitis (endogenous or exogenous).* Fifteen cases (2.26%).

A low-grade iritis which must probably be considered to be a foreign-body
reaction, occurred in 12 cases. Post-operative infection developed in 3 cases
(numbers 14, 73 and 104). Recidives of pre-operative uveitis were not observed.
Visual acuity may be threatened by the development of membranes or by dislocation of the implant after atropine instillation, even in the presence of a loop
iris suture. However, with adequate treatment inflammation in the pseudophakic eye settled.

Case histories.
Case 3. See page 154. Precipitates on vitreous membrane.

Case 7. See page 153. Cloudy vitreous and ECD.

Case 12. See page 154. Hypopyon disappeared spontaneously.

Case 14. Male, born 1896.
4–12–67 intracapsular cataract extraction with iris clip lens implantation OS. A post-
operative purulent iritis caused by a virgin silk suture infection cured spontaneously after removal of the suture.
23– 4–69 corrected visual acuity 0.8.
22– 2–71 corrected visual acuity 1.2.

Case 73. Male, born 1901. Aphakia with secondary cataract OD.
17–10–69 secondary iridocapsular lens implantation.
27–10–69 violent iritis caused the development of membranes.

10–12–69 visual acuity 0.07.

5–12–72 visual acuity, determined through the pupil and a hole in the membranes, gave 0.8!

Case 104. Male, born 1888.

3–12–69 intracapsular cataract extraction with iris clip lens implantation OD. Loop iris suture.

16– 4–70 a foreign body on the cornea led to intensive intraocular inflammation resulting in iris bombé and a dense fibrinous exudate on the implant.

29– 4–71 visual acuity $1/\infty$. Pupil occluded by membranes.

Case 119/127. See page 155. Cloudy vitreous in both eyes.

Case 167. Male, born 1910.

8– 5–70 intracapsular cataract extraction with vertical iris clip lens implantation OS.

25–11–70 'vitritis'.

17–12–70 retinal detachment, not surgically treated because of its hopeless prospects.

22– 7–71 visual acuity 0.005.

3– 4–73 visual acuity 0.02.

Case 397/402. Female, born 1915.

22– 2–71 intracapsular cataract extraction with iris clip lens implantation OD.

26– 2–71 ditto OS. Loop iris suture in both eyes.

16– 3–71 uncorrected visual acuity R 0.5 and L 0.5.

21– 4–71 iritis ODS treated with atropine, dexamethasone sodium phosphate (Decadron) and subconjunctival hydrocortisone acetate suspended in water (Hydro-adresone).

27–10–71 corrected visual acuity R 0.5 and L 0.3.

Case 434. Female, born 1896.

19– 4–71 intracapsular cataract extraction with iris clip lens implantation OS. Loop iris suture.

28– 4–71 iritis, IOP = 40 mm Hg applanation. Same therapy as in case 397/402.

10– 6–71 dislocation due to atropine. Repositioned with needle knife.

29–10–71 corrected visual acuity 0.6.

Case 504. Male, born 1913.

30– 6–71 intracapsular cataract extraction with iris medallion lens implantation OD.

8–10–71 corrected visual acuity 1.0.

20–10–71 corrected visual acuity 0.5. Slight iritis.

Case 534. See page 148. Cloudy vitreous.

Case 654. See page 155. Implantation after extraction of a cataract of unknown origin. Many precipitates on the implant.

6. *Cystoid macular oedema.*

Twenty-three cases (3.46%), all operated intracapsularly, except one. It appeared unrelated to the development of ECD (see pages 89 and 107).

Case histories.

Case 13. Female, born 1906.

9–10–67 intracapsular cataract extraction with iris clip lens implantation OS. Sphincter muscle ruptured.

15–10–69 corrected visual acuity 0.3.
Cystoid macular oedema, treated with prednisone.

12–11–70 corrected visual acuity 1.2. Full binocular vision.

21–11–72 corrected visual acuity 1.0.

Case 209. Male, born 1889.

26– 6–70 intracapsular cataract extraction with iris clip lens implantation OD.

3–12–70 cystoid macular oedema, treated with prednisone.

16– 3–71 macular degeneration. Corrected visual acuity 0.05.

7. *Decentration of the implant.* Seven cases (1.05 %), all females.

Only upward decentration was observed. It was caused by either vitreous traction after vitreous loss (3), secondary cataract (1), a loop iris suture placed too high (1), or no apparent reason (2). One intentional decentration of the implant was mentioned on page 144 (case 137). In all cases only an average amount of astigmatism was present. Surgical treatment of unintentional decentration was required in two cases.

Case histories.

Case 9. See page 144. Secondary cataract caused slight upward decentration.

Case 170. Female, born 1920.

13– 5–70 intracapsular cataract extraction with vertical iris clip lens implantation OD.

26– 6–70 inferior loop sutured to iris because of upward decentration.

4– 2–71 corrected visual acuity 1.20.

Case 188. See page 151. Upward decentration due to vitreous traction.

Case 210. Female, born 1894.

29– 7–70 intracapsular cataract extraction with iris clip lens implantation OS. Loop iris suture.

27–11–70 corrected visual acuity 0.5.

23–12–71 STRAMPELLI suture (see page 20) at 6 o'clock in view of upward decentration.

24– 1–72 STRAMPELLI suture worked loose.

14– 2–72 new STRAMPELLI suture at 6 o'clock.

2– 3–72 visual acuity 0.05. Macular degeneration of the retina. Still corneal contact.

7– 5–73 total ECD.

Case 336. Female, born 1890.

7–12–70 intracapsular cataract extraction with iris clip lens implantation OS. The loop iris suture was preplaced too high.

20– 1–70 upward decentration. Corrected visual acuity 0.8.

Case 384. See page 151. Upward decentration due to vitreous traction.

Case 646. See page 151. Slight upward decentration due to vitreous traction.

8. *Dislocation of the implant.* Seventeen cases (2.56%).

Multiple dislocation in the same eye occurred in 1 case 3 times (see case 24 on page 64) and in 2 cases twice (see case 168 on this page and case 460 on page 144). All dislocations were partial, with the exception of case 94 (page 145). The average interval between operation date and dislocation date was 136 days, with a range of 2 to 454 days.

The distribution of the direction of the dislocation showed an anterior-posterior ratio of 5 : 11 (in 5 cases the direction had not been recorded). In 7 cases an inferior loop had become dislocated.

Out of 21 dislocations 15 cases occurred within 6 months after implantation. Two of them re-inserted spontaneously, the other cases were subject to operative (3) or non-operative (8) repositioning, one case was not treated and of one case no details were available.

The relationship between dislocation and the suturing of the implant to the iris is shown in Fig. 55.

		total number of cases	number of cases with dislocation	%	
not sutured implants	iridocapsular lens	4	1	25.00	3.67
	iris clip lens	241	8	3.32	
sutured implants	iris clip lens	247	5	2.02	1.90
	iris medallion lens	173	3	1.73	
total		665	17	2.56	

Fig. 55

Relationship between dislocation and suturing of the implant to the iris in 665 BINK-HORST lens implant operations performed by WORST. Three FEDOROV modifications (see page 28) are included in the group of 241 not sutured iris clip lenses.

It is to be noted in Fig. 55 that, after loop iris suturing, the dislocation percentage for the iris clip lens on its own decreased only from 3.32 to 2.02%. However, in case 168 (iris clip lens) the loop iris suture had been tightened too much, in case 387 (iris medallion lens) the iris suture was preplaced too far from the iris border. Without these two cases of technical imperfections, the dislocation percentage of the sutured iris clip lenses would have been decreased to 1.62%, and of all sutured implants to 1.43%.

Other causes of dislocation were not apparent, except the danger of an orgasm mentioned in case 24 (see page 64) or atropinisation in case 434 (see page 156).

Unfavourable results were related in this series to 2 cases of ECD. These ended with the extraction of the implant (cases 460 and 508).

Case histories.
Case 24. See page 64. Three dislocations after orgasm.

Case 94. See page 145. Dislocation→extraction→aphakia→amblyopia.

Case 112. See page 145. Posterior dislocation of the temporal loop.

Case 161. See page 163. Exchange of an iridocapsular lens for an iris clip lens because of dislocation.

Case 460. See page 144. Two dislocations of an iris medallion lens due to secondary cataract→incipient ECD→extraction.

Case 508. Male, born 1932. Perforating trauma OS in approximately 1942.
2– 7–71 intracapsular cataract extraction with iris medallion lens implantation OS.
30– 8–71 corrected visual acuity 0.5.
4– 1–72 dislocation of temporal loop.
6– 3–72 repositioned. Muscle operation for divergent squint.
17–10–72 corrected visual acuity 0.8.
25– 1–73 incipient ECD in a small superior segment due to intermittent touch.
1– 2–73 extraction of implant was technically easy.
27– 3–73 aphakic spectacle correction gave a visual acuity of 1.0. Clear cornea.

9. *Endothelial corneal dystrophy.* Seventeen cases (2.56%) until 1–2–1973.

The average interval between operation date and date of first detection of incipient ECD was 405 days, with a range of 0 to 1146 days, i.e. much shorter than in the BINKHORST series (see Fig. 31 on page 101). This can partly be explained by:
a. the rather short interval in the 4 cases of suture contact not present amongst the BINKHORST series,
b. the shorter average observation period in the WORST series compared with the BINKHORST series (208 days against 772 days).

The incidence of ECD in the 1st, 2nd, 3rd, etc. hundred implant operations, is shown in Fig. 57 on page 164.

The causes of ECD were: endothelial touch due to either the implant (7) or an iris suture (4), dislocation (2) and severe ocular trauma (1). In 3 cases the cause of the ECD was not clear. Suturing the implant to the iris did not prevent ECD (see page 168).

ECD was surgically treated in 8 cases: the implant was removed in 3 cases (numbers 201, 460 and 508), immobilised by means of loop iris sutures (numbers 163, 334) or a STRAMPELLI suture (no. 210), and the suture ends that touched the corneal endothelium were cut in 2 cases (numbers 132 and 602). Only case 132 regained a clear cornea and useful visual acuity after discharge.

Conclusion

In order to prevent ECD (see also page 67) careful attention should be paid to the
1. pre-operative evaluation: corneal diameter, condition of the corneal endothelium, condition of the iris, etc. (see page 42).
2. technique of wound suturing and implant suturing.

Case histories of cases treated by surgery:
Case 132. Female, born 1898.
27– 2–70 intracapsular cataract extraction with iris clip lens implantation OD. Loop iris suture.
30– 8–71 corneal oedema in the inferior half.
29– 9–71 the loose ends of the suture were cut in view of corneal contact.
21– 4–72 corrected visual acuity 0.8. Local ECD.

Case 163. Female, born 1889.
1– 5–70 intracapsular cataract extraction with horizontal iris clip lens implantation OD. Loop iris suture.
7– 7–70 corrected visual acuity 0.5.
31–10–72 ECD in superior half was due to contact between loops and cornea.
10–11–72 loop iris suture inferiorly.
20– 1–73 total ECD.

Case 201. Female, born 1893.
17– 6–70 extracapsular cataract extraction with iridocapsular lens implantation OD.
3– 7–70 corrected visual acuity 0.55.
30–10–70 the eye remained red.
14–12–70 eye was always tender.
4– 3–71 folds in DESCEMET's membrane, pericorneal injection, some cells and positive TYNDALL effect in the anterior chamber. Vascular ingrowth from the corneoscleral wound. Total ECD.
26– 3–71 implant extracted.

Case 210. See page 157. STRAMPELLI suture (see page 20) at 6 o'clock in view of upward decentration. Lasting corneal contact. Total ECD.

Case 334. Male, born 1907.
4–12–70 intracapsular cataract extraction with iris clip lens implantation OS.
7– 1–71 corrected visual acuity 0.8.
21– 9–72 incipient ECD caused by corneal contact of the nasal loop.
4–10–72 nasal loop sutured to the iris with perlon.
3–11–72 total ECD.

Case 460. See page 144. ⎰ partial and temporary ECD respectively, caused by endo-
Case 508. See page 159. ⎱ thelial touch which necessitated implant extraction.

Case 602. Female, born 1894.
1–11–71 intracapsular cataract extraction with iris medallion lens implantation OS.
22–12–71 corrected visual acuity 0.3.
23– 5–72 suture in contact with DESCEMET's membrane, local corneal oedema.
29– 5–72 suture removed.
14–11–72 total ECD.

10. *Retinal detachment.* Twelve cases (1.80%).

This percentage is a little lower than the generally accepted 2 to 3% after uneventful cataract surgery without implantation.

All detachments occurred after primary intracapsular implantation. In one case a small vitreous bubble was present in front of the implant (see case 534 on page 148).

Six detachments occurred within 6 months after the operation, the remaining six after 7, 8, 12, 13, 19 and 24 months.

It is a remarkable fact that no less than 10 out of 12 cases occurred in male patients. This is twice as frequently as one would expect from the ♂/♀ ratio of 41.2/58.8 in the 616 primary intracapsular implant operations. This distribution is at variance with the 6 out of 12 primary intracapsular implant operations in the BINKHORST series (see Fig. 36 on page 111). The author cannot offer an explanation for this discrepancy.

Treatment consisted of either an encircling procedure (9) or a scleral pocket (2). The data and results of the treatment are given in Fig. 56.

11. *Complications necessitating extraction of the implant.* Eight cases (1.20%).

Extraction was performed because of ECD (3), high myopia (1), dislocation (1), diabetes mellitus with rubeosis iridis (1) and severe ocular trauma (1). In one case the iridocapsular lens was exchanged for an iris clip lens because of dislocation of the former.

serial number	sex	L	R	cause of cataract	age at operation	operation date	surgical procedure of implant operation
16	♂		R	presenile	45	25–10–68	prim. intracaps.
70	♂		R	senile	81	14–10–69	prim. intracaps.
147	♂	L		senile	61	9– 4–70	prim. intracaps.
167	♂	L		senile	60	8– 5–70	prim. intracaps.
341	♂		R	senile	68	14–12–70	prim. intracaps.
407	♀		R	senile	72	3– 3–71	prim. intracaps.
410	♂	L		presenile	41	5– 3–71	prim. intracaps.
433	♂		R	senile	69	19– 4–71	prim. intracaps.
534	♀	L		senile	76	28– 7–71	prim. intracaps.
590	♂		R	senile	63	20–10–71	prim. intracaps.
613	♂	L		unknown	50	10–11–71	prim. intracaps.
664	♂	L		senile	86	23–12–71	prim. intracaps.

Fig. 56

Data and results of 12 cases with retinal detachment out of 665 BINKHORST lens implant operations peiformed by WORST. In the last 8 cases the implant was sutured to the iris. An iris medallion lens was inserted in cases 407, 590 and 664.

Case histories.

Case 94. See page 145. Extraction in view of intractable dislocation.

Case 136. Female, born 1901. Diabetes mellitus since 1965. Rubeosis iridis, diabetic
      retinopathy.
3– 3–70 intracapsular cataract extraction with iris clip lens implantation OD.
5– 6–70 iridectomy, the first being incomplete. Pilocarpine medication.
4– 8–70 IOP = 42 mm Hg. Corneal oedema. Acetazolamide (Diamox).
4– 9–70 extraction of the implant because of the intractable glaucoma.
9–10–70 partial rupture of the corneo-scleral wound.
6–12–71 IOP = 19 mm Hg. Shallow anterior chamber, cloudy cornea.
4– 6–73 IOP = 16 mm Hg. Stationary situation.

Case 201. See page 160. Extraction because of ECD and irritation.

Case 349. Female, born 1897. Details about earlier history not known.
21–12–70 intracapsular cataract extraction with iris clip lens implantation OS. Loop
      iris suture.
20– 1–71 the implant was extracted since the eye turned out to be myopic.
6– 3–72 + 3.00 DS / + 1.00 DC × 180 gave a visual acuity of 0.15.

Case 460. See page 144. Extraction because of ECD.

Case 508. See page 159. Extraction because of incipient ECD. Corneal transparency
      returned.

162

retinal detachment date	interval in days	number of operations for retinal detachment	final visual acuity	
7–11–70	743	1 ×	1/∞	(recidive)
22– 6–70	251	—	?	(death of patient on 13–8–1970)
31– 8–70	144	2 ×	0.25	
17–12–70	223	—	0.02	(inoperable, see page 156)
22– 2–71	70	2 ×	1/∞	(recidive)
10– 4–72	404	1 ×	0.60	
7– 8–71	155	spontaneous recovery	0.05	(vitreous opacities)
13–11–72	574	1 ×	zero	(massive vitreous traction)
1– 8–72	370	1 ×	1/∞	(recidive, see page 148 ff.)
13– 3–72	145	2 ×	0.03	(macular damage)
6– 4–72	148	1 ×	0.02	(recidive)
14– 3–72	82	—	0.003	(vitreous haemorrhage)

Case 554. Male, born 1887.

16– 8–71 intracapsular cataract extraction with iris clip lens implantation OS. Loop iris suture.

26– 9–71 patient fell, hitting the rim of the chamber pot with OS. The implant was forced through the ruptured corneo-scleral wound into the temporal superior subconjunctival space.

27– 9–71 extraction of implant. Sector iridectomy. Resutured. The present visual acuity is not known.

Case 161. Male, born 1910.

29– 4–70 extracapsular cataract extraction with vertical iridocapsular lens implantation OD.

4– 5–70 anterior dislocation of inferior loop.

2– 9–70 the iridocapsular lens was exchanged for a horizontal iris clip lens sutured to the iris.

27– 7–71 corrected visual acuity 1.0.

12. *Complication necessitating enucleation*. One case (0.15%).

In one case enucleation was unavoidable because of severe ocular trauma.

Case history.
Case 162. Female, born 1884.

1– 5-70 intracapsular cataract extraction with iris clip lens implantation OS. Loop iris suture.

27– 5-70 the demented patient fell and hit a key with OS. Iridodialysis, anterior chamber filled with blood, implant invisible.

23– 6-70 enucleation.

Summary and conclusions

Complications, implant extractions and one enucleation in a series of 665 BINKHORST lens implant operations are discussed in the approximate chronological order in which they may develop after implantation in the individual case. Their frequency per 100 implant operations in the whole series is shown in Fig. 57.

implantation date no. 100, 200, etc.	pupillary block	choroidal detachment	unintentional fistula	deposits on implant	uveitis (endogenous or exogenous)	cystoid macular oedema	decentration	dislocation	ECD	retinal detachment	extraction of implant	enucleation
1st hundred 21-11-69	3	–	3	5	5	2	1	3	2	2	1	–
2nd hundred 12- 6-70	–	–	–	2	4	6	2	8	3	2	1	1
3rd hundred 13-11-70	–	–	–	–	–	5	1	1	3	–	1	–
4th hundred 5- 3-71	–	–	–	–	2	3	2	1	5	2	1	–
5th hundred 30- 6-71	–	3	–	–	2	1	–	2	1	2	1	–
6th hundred 3-11-71	–	–	1	2	1	5	–	2	3	2	2	–
7th 65 23-12-71	–	–	1	1	1	1	1	–	–	2	–	–
total	3	3	5	10	15	23	7	17	17	12	7	1
%	0.5	0.5	0.8	1.5	2.3	3.5	1.1	2.6	2.6	1.8	1.1	0.2

Fig. 57

Distribution of post-operative complications, implant extractions and one enucleation in 665 BINKHORST lens implant operations performed by WORST, for every 100 cases.

Striking are the following features (see Fig. 57):

1. pupillary block occurred only in the early cases.
2. the decrease of endogenous and exogenous uveitis.
3. the decrease of dislocation after the suturing of the implant to the iris which

164

became routine procedure in June 1970. In view of Fig. 59 on page 168 the decrease seems somewhat flattered, however.

4. no effect of the suturing of the implant to the iris on ECD after June 1970 when it became standard practice.

SPECIAL CASES

Data and results of a group of special cases are shown in Fig. 58.

	number	%	average age at operation in years	average observation period in days	average visual acuity
diabetes mellitus					
without retinopathy	37	5.56	77.14	238	0.39
with retinopathy	10	1.50	74.60	79	0.09
total	47	7.07	76.60	204	0.33
pre-operative glaucoma	46	6.92	75.39	199	0.39
glaucoma with intentional					
corneo-scleral fistula	15	2.26	76.47	135	0.43
synechiolysis	8	1.20	62.25	120	0.53
chymotrypsin	5	0.75	52.40	156	0.90
suturing of coloboma	2	0.30	71.00	914	0.55
radial iridotomy	13	1.95	71.54	150	0.54
not sutured to iris	245	36.84	69.15	324	0.56
sutured to iris	420	63.16	71.73	142	0.58
iris clip lens	485	72.93	71.13	245	0.58
anterior loops cut	5	0.75	62.20	209	0.50
iridocapsular lens	4	0.60	43.00	398	0.09
FEDOROV modification	3	0.45	75.67	335	0.27
iris medallion lens	173	26.02	70.35	96	0.57
secondary implantation	25	3.76	34.68	393	0.44
STRAMPELLI suture	4	0.60	43.50	670	0.24
strabismus operations	9	1.35	34.22	409	0.55
trauma to implant	6	0.90	69.50	577	0.37

Fig. 58

Data and results of the group of special cases on which BINKHORST lens implant operations were performed by WORST.

The group of special cases will also be discussed in the approximate chronological order in which they might occur in an individual case.

1. *Diabetes mellitus* was present in 27 patients (8 ♂ and 19 ♀) with 47 eyes (7.07%). All male and 12 female patients were operated on bilaterally. Ten eyes had diabetic retinopathy, and an average visual acuity of 0.09 after an average observation period of 79 days. The low visual acuity was due mainly to their diabetic retinopathy. The other 37 eyes had an average visual acuity of 0.39 after an average observation period of 238 days. Moreover, six eyes of 4 patients were subject to pre-operative glaucoma simplex. Other pre-existing conditions in these 47 eyes were: amblyopia (1), branch thrombosis of the central retinal vein (1), vitreous opacities (2) that were often visible only after the cataract extraction, and corneal nebulae (2). In general, there were no more complications than usual: a single case of post-operative glaucoma (case 370/373 on page 167), of total ECD (case 214), of retinal detachment (case 407, see Fig. 56 on page 162 ff.) and of implant extraction (case 136 on page 162, rubeosis iridis!).

The author's conclusion is that apart from rubeosis iridis, diabetes with or without angiopathy is not a contra-indication for iris clip lens implantation (see also pages 115 and 193).

Case histories.
Case 280/291. Male, born 1905. Diabetes mellitus.
21–10–70 intracapsular cataract extraction with iris clip lens implantation OD. Loop iris suture.
 2–11–70 intracapsular cataract extraction with iris clip lens implantation OS. Loop iris suture.
26–11–70 corrected visual acuity ODS 1.2.
22– 7–71 corrected visual acuity OD 0.1 due to macular haemorrhages. Corrected visual acuity OS 1.2.
30– 5–72 corrected visual acuity OD 0.6. The macular haemorrhages have been absorbed.

2. *Pre-operative glaucoma* was present in 33 patients with 46 eyes (6.92%). All these patients had been treated for glaucoma for years, and some of them had visual field defects. All implant operations (except one) were primary and after intracapsular extraction.

Eight eyes of 7 patients had been operated on for glaucoma *prior* to the implant operation: ELLIOT trephining (4), iridencleisis (3), and trabeculotomy (1). The incision for cataract extraction in these cases was corneal in the first 2 and at 6 o'clock in the other 6, i.e. just the reverse of BINKHORST's development (see page 116). A radial iridotomy with preplaced suture(s) had to be performed in 7 cases. Chymotrypsin was not used. In 11 patients with 15 eyes an intentional corneo-scleral fistula was made during the same session (see cases 339 and 340 on page 169). This became routine after February 1971 for all non-operated glaucoma patients. In only one case, binocularly operated on, these fistulae closed again. In one case a cyclodialysis and later a fistulising operation was performed 7 months *after* the implant operation.

The conclusion is that, in general, an unfavourable influence of the implant operation on the glaucoma could not be demonstrated (see also pages 116 and 229 ff.).

Case histories.
Case 370/373. Female, born 1896. Diabetes mellitus.
22– 1–71 intracapsular cataract extraction with iris clip lens implantation OS. Loop iris suture.
27– 1–71 ditto OD.
26– 8–71 IOP = 80 mm Hg. Acetazolamide (Diamox) tablets 250 mg twice daily and pilocarpine hydrochloride 2% eye drops 4 times daily were prescribed.
27– 8–71 cyclodialysis OD.
24– 9–71 fistulising operation OD at 6 o'clock.
30– 9–71 fistulising operation OS with iridectomy ODS.
14–12–71 zero visual acuity ODS.
22– 3–72 death of patient.

3. *Synechiolysis* had to be performed prior to cataract extraction in 8 cases (1.20%): once anteriorly (perforating trauma) and 7 times posteriorly.

4. *Chymotrypsin* was only used in 5 cases (0.75%) that were all doing well having a visual acuity of between 0.7 and 1.0 (see also page 117). Indications for the use of chymotrypsin were traumatic cataract (2), cataract of unknown origin (2), and a previous operation for retinal detachment (1).

5. *Primary suturing of a coloboma* was performed in 2 cases (0.30%):

Case histories.
Case 15. Female, born 1902.
12–12–67 intracapsular cataract extraction with iris clip lens implantation OS. Sector coloboma sutured with perlon.
27– 3–68 corrected visual acuity 0.33.
5– 9–71 corrected visual acuity 0.6.

Case 108. Male, born 1892.
8– 8–68 iris prolapse OD as a result of a car accident. Sector iridectomy from 10 to 12 o'clock.
5–12–69 intracapsular cataract extraction with iris clip lens implantation and coloboma sutures. These sutures cut a little into the iris.
15– 3–71 corrected visual acuity 0.5.

6. *Radial iridotomy with preplaced suture(s)* was performed in 13 cases (1.95%). Four of these eyes were incised at 6 o'clock to avoid a previously made fistula at 12 o'clock. In the other cases iridotomy was necessitated by iris rigidity.

7. *The implant was sutured to the iris* in 420 cases (63.16%). The suturing was secondary in 2 cases of incipient ECD where it was carried out in order to immobilise the implant, however, without success (case 163 on page 160 and case 334 on page 161).

Fig. 59 shows the relationship between suturing of the implant and dislocation and ECD respectively.

	number			dislocation number of cases	%	ECD number of cases	%
iris clip lens	485	not sutured	238	8	3.36	4	1.68
		sutured	247	5	2.02	7	2.83
iris medallion lens	173	not sutured	–	–	–	–	–
		sutured	173	3	1.73	5	2.89
total		not sutured	238	8	3.36	4	1.68
		sutured	420	8	1.90	12	2.86

Fig. 59

Relationship between dislocation and ECD respectively, and the suturing of the iris clip lens or iris medallion lens to the iris, in 658 implant operations performed by WORST.

Notable features in Fig. 59 are
a. the small difference between the dislocation percentages for the not sutured and the sutured iris clip lens (3.36 and 2.02% respectively).
b. the inverse relationship between suturing and ECD (1.68 and 2.86% respectively) over the total number of 658 cases, even if the 4 cases where suture contacts occurred had been prevented (1.68 and 1.90% respectively).

The author's conclusion is that suturing of the implant to the iris may serve a purpose in that it decreases the percentage of dislocations slightly in cases where pilocarpine medication is not adhered to (iris clip lens), or in fixating the lens (iris medallion lens), but that it does *not* prevent ECD.

8. The *anterior loops were partially cut away* in 5 cases (0.75%). In 4 cases

the indication for this was a shallow anterior chamber, and in one case it was a mutilated anterior segment.

Case histories.
Case 339. Male, born 1888. Primary narrow-angle glaucoma.
9–12–70 intracapsular cataract extraction with iris clip lens implantation OD. Radial iridotomy with preplaced perlon iris suture. Both anterior loops were cut away. The posterior loops were sutured to the iris with the same suture. Intentional corneo-scleral fistula.
6– 1–72 corrected visual acuity 0.6.

Case 340. Female, born 1895. Primary narrow-angle glaucoma. Diabetes mellitus.
10–12–70 intracapsular cataract extraction with iris clip lens implantation OS. Radial iridotomy with preplaced perlon suture. Both anterior loops were cut away. The posterior loops were sutured to the iris with the same suture. Intentional corneo-scleral fistula.
11– 9–72 corrected visual acuity 0.8.

Case 354. Female, born 1896. Shallow anterior chamber.
6– 1–70 intracapsular cataract extraction with iris clip lens implantation OD. Both anterior loops were cut away. The implant was sutured to the iris.
25– 4–72 corrected visual acuity 0.55. A few vitreous opacities.

Case 391. Female, born 1897. Primary glaucoma. Diabetes mellitus.
17– 2–71 intracapsular cataract extraction with iris clip lens implantation OS. Both anterior loops were cut away. The implant was sutured to the iris.
25– 2–71 visual acuity: hand movements, due to diabetic retinopathy.

9. An *iridocapsular lens* was inserted in 4 cases (0.60%).

In a further case the iridocapsular lens was exchanged for an iris clip lens after dislocation (case 161 on page 163).

Case histories.
Case 17. Male, born 1950. Choroidal ruptures and aphakia with secondary cataract OS after an explosion.
3–12–68 secondary iridocapsular lens implantation.
19– 3–69 corrected visual acuity 0.3.

Case 73. See page 155. Complicated by a violent iritis which gave rise to membranes.

Case 201. See page 160. Extraction of implant because of ECD.

10. A FEDOROV *modification* (see page 28) was inserted in 3 cases (0.45%).

Case histories.
Case 27. Female, born 1901. Pre-operative glaucoma controlled by means of 1.66% di-ethyl-phosphoric acid-p-nitro-phenolester in pure sodium chloride (Mintacol).

1– 4–69 intracapsular cataract extraction with implantation of FEDOROV's modification of the iris clip lens OD.
5– 1–70 visual acuity 0.003. Macular degeneration.

Case 37. Male, born 1889.
23– 5–69 intracapsular cataract extraction with implantation of FEDOROV's modification of the iris clip lens OS.
19– 3–70 corrected visual acuity 0.2. Macular degeneration.

Case 38. Female, born 1890.
28– 5–69 intracapsular cataract extraction with implantation of FEDOROV's modification of the iris clip lens OS.
29– 7–70 corrected visual acuity 0.6.

11.   An *iris medallion lens* was inserted in 173 cases (26.02%), the first operation being performed on 18–12–1970. Four of these cases were preceded by extracapsular cataract extraction. A comparison with the iris clip lens is provided at the end of this chapter (see next page).

12.   *Secondary implant operations* were performed in 25 cases (3.76%) in which a primary implantation was not possible. It is a heterogeneous group, with many complications. That is the reason that 15 of these cases have already been mentioned in this chapter. In 2 of the remaining 10 cases the present visual acuity is not known; the other 8 cases are doing well having visual acuities between 0.5 and 1.0. Six of these patients are adults, one of whom had a traumatic cataract, two had contact lens troubles, and three underwent a secondary implant operation because the fellow-eye had been fitted with an implant primarily.

13.   A STRAMPELLI *suture* (see page 20) was used in 4 cases (0.60%).

Case histories.
Case 2.   See page 148. ⎫
Case 210. See page 157. ⎬ to prevent upward decentration.
Case 460. See page 144. ⎭

Case 401. Male, born 1934. Traumatic aphakia OS since 1962.
24– 2–71 secondary iris clip lens implantation, with STRAMPELLI sutures because of difficulties with centration.
    10–71 corrected visual acuity 0.8.

14.   A *strabismus operation* was required in 9 cases (1.35%), 2 taking place 16 and 4 months respectively prior to the implant operation, and 1 during the

same session. In the other 6 cases they were carried out 9, 2, 3, 3, 8 and 12 months respectively after the implant operation.

15. *Severe ocular trauma* in the post-operative period occurred in 6 cases (0.90%), resulting in membrane formation, iris prolapse, ECD, implant extraction or enucleation.

The wound ruptured in 4 out of 5 cases during the first 6 weeks after the operation.

This means that by wearing a protective eye-shield during the first six weeks after the operation the percentage of cases with complications would have been reduced by 0.75%, i.e. a reduction from 14.59 to 13.84%.

Case 1. See page 143. 2½ years after the implantation the eye was accidently hit by a thumb which caused the formation of membranes. These had to be needled.

Case 21. Blunt trauma on the 17th day led to wound rupture. Resutured.

Case 22. Blunt trauma on the 34th day led to wound rupture. Resutured. Total ECD.

Case 162. See page 163. Blunt trauma on the 26th day led to severe damage to the eye. Enucleated.

Case 554. See page 163. Blunt trauma on the 41st day led to wound rupture and dislocation of the implant into the subconjunctival space. Implant extracted.

Case 576. Rubbing of the eye on the 38th day produced an iris prolapse which had to be cut partly. Resutured.

Comparison of the results of iris clip lens implantations and iris medallion lens implantations

The distribution of visual acuity results for both types of implant is given in Fig. 60.

The conclusion must be that visual acuity results are about equal for both types of implant.

The distribution of post-operative complications, implant extractions and one enucleation for both types of implant is shown in Fig. 61.

It may be concluded that post-operative complications and their sequelae occur approximately equally frequently in both types of implant. ECD in 5 cases fitted with an iris medallion lens was due to suture contact (2), dislocation (2) and in one case the reason was obscure. They would have been avoided in some cases if the recently improved iris suturing technique had been applied (see page 142). However, the principal factor promoting ECD, viz. the pair of

	number	percentage visual acuity												average visual acuity
		0–10	11–20	21–30	31–40	41–50	51–60	61–70	71–80	81–90	91–100	101–110	111–120	
iris clip lens	473	65	30	34	40	37	69	6	75	6	100	—	11	0.58
iris medallion lens	166	23	7	12	12	16	34	6	26	—	29	—	1	0.57
%														
iris clip lens	100	13.7	6.3	7.2	8.5	7.8	14.6	1.3	15.9	1.3	21.1	—	2.3	
iris medallion lens	100	13.9	4.2	7.2	7.2	9.6	20.5	3.6	15.7	—	17.5	—	0.6	

Fig. 60. Distribution in numbers (above) and percentages (below) of visual acuity results in 473 iris clip lens implant operations and 166 iris medallion lens implant operations performed by WORST. In the remaining 19 cases the visual acuity was for various reasons unknown (see page 146).

	number	pupillary block	choroidal detachment	unintentional corneo-scleral fistula	deposits on implant	uveitis (endogenous or exogenous)	cystoid macular oedema	decentration	dislocation	ECD	retinal detachment	extraction of implant	enucleation
iris clip lens	485	3	3	4	8	10	17	7	13	11	9	4	1
iris medallion lens	173	–	–	1	2	2	6	–	3	5	3	2	–
	%												
iris clip lens	100	0.62	0.62	0.82	1.65	2.06	3.51	1.44	2.68	2.27	1.86	0.82	0.21
iris medallion lens	100	–	–	0.58	1.16	1.16	3.47	–	1.73	2.89	1.73	1.16	–

Fig. 61

Distribution in numbers (above) and percentages (below) of post-operative complications, implant extractions and one enucleation in 485 iris clip lens implant operations and 173 iris medallion lens implant operations performed by WORST.

anterior loops, is absent in the iris medallion lens, and consequently, it is hoped that ECD will not occur either. Only time will tell whether this expectation will come true.

CONCLUSION

Although the WORST series cannot strictly be compared with the BINKHORST series because of differences in the causes of cataract, surgical techniques e.g. suturing the implant on the iris and extracapsular extraction, observation period, and optotypes used for the determination of visual acuity, it may be said that visual acuity results and incidence of post-operative complications appear to be of the same order, especially if one considers only BINKHORST's last 400 iris clip lens implant operations (see Figs. 18, 37, 47 and 57).

CHAPTER VI

RESULTS OBTAINED BY THE AUTHOR

> After all, everybody takes pleasure
> in relating something about his own
> sphere of work and in talking about
> things which he knows thoroughly
> and from own experience.
>
> ERASMUS

INTRODUCTION

Initially, the author considered the technique of iris clip lens implantation to be beyond his surgical abilities. However, as ordinary cataract extractions continued to be successfully performed by him and successively produced good results, it was decided to attend operations performed by BINKHORST to evaluate the author's capabilities with respect to implant surgery. Having witnessed 20 of BINKHORST's implant operations in the course of six sessions the author came to the conclusion that iris clip lens implantation seemed technically feasible and, consequently, could be undertaken.

The first iris clip lens implant operation was performed on 19–1–1970, and the total number of implant operations up to 1-10-1974 was 144.

SELECTION OF CASES

Implant operations were performed only on patients over 50 years of age, since the author considered the technique of intracapsular cryoextraction to be less difficult than that of extracapsular extraction and because the risk of late complications was more acceptable in the older age groups. Therefore, until now patients under the age of 50 have been referred for implantation to BINK-HORST.

If the first eye of a patient was aphakic, an ordinary extraction without implantation was performed in the fellow-eye. There has been one exception only to this rule: in case 61 it was thought preferable to give an 84-year-old unilaterally aphakic patient who had a visual acuity of 0.35 and had not got used to her cataract lens, the benefit of the natural vision of her fellow-eye by means of an iris clip lens. This was fitted during a primary operation, and the result was a corrected visual acuity of 0.8.

All implants were fitted during primary operations.

TECHNIQUE

The author's technique was described on page 45.

General anaesthesia was used in all patients.

RESULTS

On.y the results of the first 72 implant operations will be evaluated in order to provide a sufficiently long period of post-operative observation. The primary operations were performed on 61 patients (21 ♂ and 40 ♀), 11 of which were binocular cases (6 ♂ and 5 ♀). Six patients (cases 2, 4, 6, 12, 20 and 40) were of Indonesian origin. Four patients (cases 4, 9, 19 and 64) were illiterates. The usual numerical data are given in Fig. 62.

	number	♂	♀	L	R	average age at operation in years	average observation period in days	average visual acuity
♂	27	27	—	15	12	70.37	429	0.67
♀	45	—	45	23	22	71.53	475	0.57
L	38	15	23	38	—	70.66	435	0.59
R	34	12	22	—	34	71.59	483	0.62
total	72	27	45	38	34	71.10	458	0.60

Fig. 62

Data and results of 72 iris clip lens implant operations performed by the author.

The patients were subjected to an extensive eye examination some time after implantation, preferably after more than six months. An account of this examination (except for gonioscopy) is given in Fig. 63 at back of book.

One patient (case 9) died before this examination could take place. Two other patients had to be excluded from this evaluation as well. In both of them there was vitreous loss, caused in one patient by the implant rupturing the vitreous membrane, and in the other patient the membrane was ruptured by a blunt iris hook used during implantation. The state of the anterior chamber after removal of the implant and having cut the vitreous, was no longer considered to be suitable for iris clip lens implantation in these two cases (see page 46).

Case histories of the above-mentioned patients:

1. Indonesian female, born 1914. Binocular cataract.
22–10–70 intracapsular cryoextraction OS. Vertical implantation was attempted notwithstanding the bulging vitreous. The implant jumped back when the special lens forceps were released, and the anterior vitreous membrane ruptured. This was likely to have been caused by contact with the implant. The implant together with a large amount of vitreous had to be removed. Twelve corneo-scleral perlon sutures were inserted. Vitreous sweep.
3–11–72 upward decentration of the horizontally elongated pupil. Visual acuity with aphakic correction was 0.85.
31– 8–73 corrected visual acuity 0.9.

2. Female, born 1896. Predominantly unilateral cataract OD.
10– 1–72 intracapsular cryoextraction OD. The zonules were extremely resistent. Vertical iris clip lens implantation. During the adjusting manoeuvre with the blunt iris hook (see page 49) the anterior vitreous membrane ruptured, and a large vitreous prolapse had to be cut off. The implant was removed for safety reasons. Fifteen corneo-scleral perlon sutures were inserted. Vitreous sweep.
14– 6–72 visual acuity with aphakic correction was 0.45. Updrawn pupil. The fellow-eye had a corrected visual acuity of 0.65, due to incipient cataract.

Discussion of Figs. 62 and 63.
1. Sex. The author's percentage of female cases (62.5 %) exceeds BINKHORST's (47.3 %) and WORST's (56.3 % or 273 out of 485 iris clip lens implant operations; see Fig. 79 on page 210) percentages. To some extent this difference in the iris clip lens cases is due to the amount of traumatic cases dealt with by each surgeon, namely zero, 52 (46 ♂ and 6 ♀) and 14 (10 ♂ and 4 ♀) respectively. Without these, BINKHORST's percentage of female cases would have been 50.2 and that of WORST would have been 57.1. The general percentage of about 55 % female cases (see Fig. 79 on page 210) is related to the fact that women tend to grow older than men.
2. The age at operation varied from 51 to 87 years, with an average of 71.10 years. This is higher than for BINKHORST's cases who had an average age of 65.80 years. This is due to the difference in indication for operation and the causes of cataract. It is similar to WORST's figure of an average of 71.13 years (see Fig. 58 on page 165).

3. Eye colour. This will be discussed in chapter IX (see page 229) in connection with IOP and tonography.

4. Cause of cataract. Senile cataract was present in as many as 67 cases (93.1 %). This percentage exceeds that of BINKHORST (81.7 %) and is similar to that of WORST (94.2 %, or 457 out of 485 iris clip lens implant operations). This is mainly due to the fact that BINKHORST, being the first to perform lens implant operations, operated on a relatively large group of patients with non-senile cataract referred to him.

5. Surgical procedure. This was intracapsular in 65 cases, and unintentionally extracapsular in the remaining 7 cases.

6. The average observation period of 450 days lies between that of BINKHORST (772 days) and WORST (245 days) since recently operated patients have been excluded (see above).

7. Visual acuity was determined with COLENBRANDER's optotypes (COLEN-BRANDER, 1955). The average visual acuity of 0.60 lies between that of BINK-HORST (0.64) and WORST (0.58) (see Fig. 79). The comparison, however, is only of limited value, because of differences in indication, observation period and the optotypes used for the determination of the visual acuity.

POST-OPERATIVE CHANGES IN VISUAL ACUITY

1. In 40 cases visual acuity reached its maximum after 6–8 weeks and changed only little afterwards.

2. In 16 uncomplicated cases visual acuity improved considerably after the 6–8 weeks period, increasing by 0.17 to 0.65 (average 0.32) above the initial level of visual acuity, and reached its maximum from 4 to 18 (!) months (average 12 months) post-operatively. This could be attributed to some extent to the decrease of corneal astigmatism (see Fig. 23 on page 78), but, the ocular media being clear, must have been due mainly to unknown retinal factors, possibly related to the Irvine Gass syndrome.

3. In 3 cases (17, 51 and 57; see pages 191 and 187) with uveitis, treated with decadron drops, optimum visual acuity of 0.65, 0.60 and 1.10 respectively, was not reached until 6, 4½ and 10 months post-operatively.

In one case (no. 62) the cornea remained slightly hazy for two months post-operatively. Dexamethasone sodium phosphate (Decadron) medication during 3 months produced an increase in visual acuity from 0.20 to 0.65 between the second and fifth month post-operatively.

4. In 4 cases (25, 32, 33 and 40) visual acuity deteriorated temporarily to 0.12, 0.02, 0.32 and 0.55 respectively, but returned to the initial level of 0.20, 0.50,

0.50 and 0.90 at respectively 14, 23, 8, and 13 months post-operatively having been treated with systemic and local corticosteroids. The reason for the deterioration was obscure, but in view of the clear media a maculopathy must be accepted as a cause: the pattern of decrease in visual acuity followed by a recovery is highly suggestive of the Irvine Gass syndrome.

5. In 3 cases the decrease in visual acuity was progressive, in one (case 15, see page 194) it was due to a diabetic retinopathy (decrease from 0.45→0.08), in another (case 36) to progressing macular degeneration of the retina (0.32→0.02) and in the third case (case 27) it was of an unknown nature (0.63→0.5→0.45→0.35).

6. In 5 cases deterioration of visual acuity to 0.02 was a consequence of ECD.

SPECIAL STUDIES

1. *Stereopsis*

The stereopsis of 60 patients was examined by means of the WIRT test*. See legend Fig. 63. In 4 patients it could not be determined because of old age (2) or for unknown reasons (2).

a. Stereopsis was fully present in 25 patients (41.7%).

b. Stereopsis was impaired in 6 patients (10.0%) due to a relative central scotoma in the operated eye (2), incipient cataract of the fellow-eye with visual acuity of 0.25, 0.30, 0.32 and 0.40 respectively (4).

c. Stereopsis was absent in 25 patients (41.7%) because of reduced vision of the

pseudophakic eye		*fellow-eye*		corrected visual acui-
due to		due to		ty 0.02 in 12 cases
ECD	5	cataract	15	and 0.10, 0.12, 0.16
amblyopia	1	aphakia without implant	1	in the remaining ca-
diabetic retinopathy	1	macular hole	1	ses
macular degeneration	1			
	8		17	

We may thus conclude that it is most likely that stereopsis, if present pre-operatively, returns after a successful lens implant operation. In view of its apparently strong relationship with the visual acuity of both eyes, one may

---

* Also known as the 'Housefly Test' or 'Stereo-Fly Test'. Made by Titmus Optical Co. Inc., Petersburg, Va., U.S.A.

expect that stereopsis will return after cataract extraction with lens implantation in the 19 (4+15) fellow-eyes mentioned above. This would increase the 41.7% of patients with full stereopsis to 73.3%.

These results compare well with those determined by the author in a series of 58 iris clip lens patients operated on by BINKHORST: stereopsis was fully present in 29 patients (50.0%), impaired in 10 patients (17.3%), absent in 18 patients (31.0%) and could not be assessed in one aphatic patient (1.7%).

2. *Direction of the implant*

Iris clip lens implant operations were performed
a. horizontally in 4 cases, because of a radial iridotomy at 12 o'clock (cases 17/52 and 26, see page 191) and for no particular reason in case 1 (see page 188).
b. *not* exactly vertically in 3 cases due to minimal surgical mishaps (see cases 21, 56 and 63, on page 183).
c. *exactly* vertically in all other 65 cases.

For the evaluation of the 'ultimate' position of the exactly vertically inserted iris clip lenses, 4 cases of repositioning after early (no. 19, 59 and 66) or late (no. 58) dislocation, one case of loop amputation (no. 14) and one case of early death (no. 9) had to be excluded. The distribution of the remaining 59 cases is shown in Fig. 64.

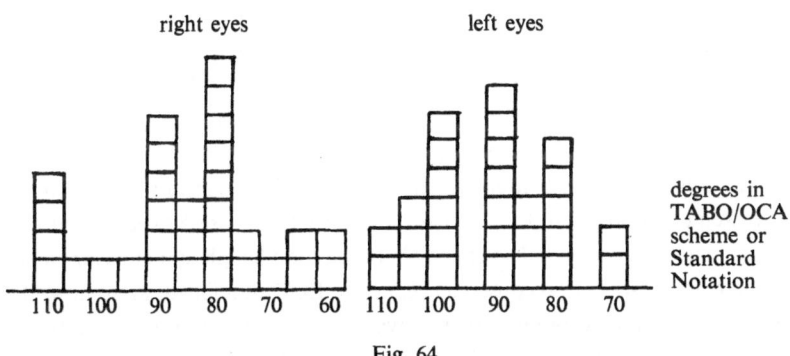

Fig. 64

31 right eyes with an average implant direction of 85° 19'
28 left eyes with an average implant direction of 91° 26'.

We may conclude that the 'ultimate' position of the exactly vertically inserted non-sutured iris clip lenses fluctuates around the vertical position; it may deviate up to 30°. Post-operative rotation is likely to explain this. The latter occurs only during a combination of eye movements and incomplete miosis, e.g. during the first days after the operation (see also JUNGSCHAFFER, 1972).

3. *Shape of the pupil*

Notwithstanding all patients were subject to pilocarpine medication, in 13 cases the pupil did not adopt a square shape. This was due to a sphincter lesion (2), sutured radial iridotomy (2), repositioning after dislocation (2), vitreous incarceration (1), large iris prolapse during operation (1) and a not fully successful blunt iris hook manoeuvre at 12 o'clock (5). It was of no consequence for the final visual acuity.

4. *Gonioscopic examination*

Gonioscopy was performed with a GOLDMANN two-mirror contact lens. In 3 cases (no. 1, 2 and 19) the chamber angle was invisible due to ECD.

1. A moderate amount of iris pigment in the lower chamber angle was present in nearly all cases, but not to a larger extent than was found to be normal by the author in a control group that had undergone an ordinary cataract extraction.

This means that pigmentation is caused mainly by surgical loss of pigment, and not by loop friction.

In 6 eyes (all with a blue iris!) larger pigment particles were observed. In case 55 the pigment was situated at the 4 – 5 o'clock position, probably due to the patient obstinately lying on his side after the operation.

2. A red film of encapsuled blood was present in the chamber angle of 6 eyes, even after 3 to 60 months. However, this did not provoke glaucoma although in 2 cases the nasal 180° was covered.

3. The anterior superior loop was in contact with DESCEMET's membrane at the extreme periphery in 3 cases: case 40 (page 182), case 59 (page 186) and case 63. This was due to a discrepancy between loop length and anterior chamber diameter. It was of no consequence, i.e. no ECD developed, up to now, the observation periods extending so far over 34, 21 and 3 months respectively. However, this is too short a period for proper evaluation.

4. The following technical failures were observed in the iridotomies (usually 3 iridotomies were made per eye):

a. not visible: in 2 patients, with 1 and 2 additional iridotomies respectively made to overcome a pupillary block (case 24 on page 185) and a vitreous incarceration of the 12 o'clock iridotomy (case 40 on page 182) respectively.

b. extremely small or closed opening: 19 iridotomies in 16 patients. Notwith-

standing the absence of any consequences it has to be stressed that, if iridotomies are made, it is preferable to produce at least 3. However, it is the author's
current opinion that it is safer to make one or two peripheral iridectomies.
5. The peripheral flap of 27 iridotomies (9 nasal, 9 central and 9 temporal) in
18 patients was attached to the wound (25) or to SCHWALBE's line (2) which did
not affect the aqueous dynamics of the eye.
6. Peripheral anterior synechiae over 5–30 degrees of the circumference of the
limbus, with the wound's edge (12) or SCHWALBE's line (7), were present in
19 eyes (26.4%). This is in good agreement with PEARCE's observations (1972)
who found some peripheral synechiae in 19% of 72 of BINKHORST's patients,
and in 35% of 115 of his own patients with an intracapsular cataract extraction.
However, the latter had been operated on without air having been insufflated
into the anterior chamber.

These 19 eyes with peripheral anterior synechiae had an average facility of
outflow of 0.10 as against 0.12 in 50 eyes without peripheral synechiae. Statistically speaking, this difference is not significant. The post-operative finding of a
shallow anterior chamber in case 14 (see page 189), and the pupillary block in
case 30 (see page 185), may act as a pointer to the development of peripheral
anterior synechiae, but in the other cases only the omission of iris repositionings
(see page 44) can be blamed.

The author was surprised to find that 10 out of 11 right eyes had temporal
synechiae, and 6 out of 8 left eyes had nasal synechiae. It seems, therefore, that
16 out of 19 synechiae amongst the author's cases are situated on the right-hand
side of the patient. This strongly suggests an asymmetrical trait in surgery,
probably in the incision or in the suturing.

OPERATION DIFFICULTIES AND COMPLICATIONS

A. Extraction

1. Cryoextraction occurred extracapsularly in 7 cases due to unintentional
rupturing of the lens capsule. The result was of no consequence with the exception of two cases where it was of minor importance: a slight downward
decentration due to a secondary cataract in case 37, and a slight upward decentration without a visible secondary cataract in case 67. Needling was not
necessary as thorough irrigation had removed all residual lens material. Thanks
to the clear ocular media obtained ultimately, visual acuity was not impaired
in any of these cases.
2. The cryoextractor inadvertently froze to the adjacent iris in 5 cases, and to
the cornea in one case. Lesions were not visible on slitlamp examination,

possibly because the probe was always immediately defrosted with saline of 37° C.

3. Vitreous loss occurred in 3 cases.

In 2 other cases an iris clip lens implantation had to be abandoned because of vitreous loss. These two cases were not included in this series. In both cases (see page 176) an upward decentration of the pupil developed, indicative of the danger an iris clip lens may pose for the corneal endothelium.

However, in 3 cases of vitreous loss where the author felt that the vitreous could be removed completely from the anterior chamber, an iris clip lens was implanted.

After observation periods of respectively 8, 6 and 17 months all three cases were considered to be successful.

Case histories.

Case 59. The vitreous adhered to the lens and had to be cut. On the fourth day a dislocation had to be treated by surgically repositioning it and making a loop iris suture. Anatomically, the result is 100% satisfactory. See page 186 and Fig. 65 opposite page 196.

Case 68. Liquefied vitreous appeared in the anterior chamber after the eye had been opened. It was rinsed out. Slight upward decentration. See page 191.

Case 70. The vitreous prolapsed at 12 o'clock after an unintentional extracapsular extraction, and it had to be cut. No ill-effects. Pupil central.

4. Between extraction and implantation the pupil remained unduly wide in 5 cases. In 4 of these cases the pupil proved to be square on the day after implantation, but in the case of an 84-year-old patient (case 32), the pupil remained wide after implantation, undoubtedly due to a sphincter lesion. However, visual acuity is good at present and no dislocation has occurred to date. Nevertheless, this case is an argument in favour of the narrow pupil method (see page 49).

B. *Implantation*

1. Bulging vitreous was present in 9 cases (12.5%). The anterior chamber regained its normal depth in all cases. After the introduction of curare by the anaesthetist (case 85), far less bulging vitreous was noticed. The application of the author's vertical implantation method described on page 52 was only required in 2 cases due to the amount of bulging vitreous.

Case history.
Case 40. Indonesian female, born 1896. Diabetes mellitus since 1969.

15- 2–71 intracapsular cryoextraction with iris clip lens implantation OS. Bulging vitreous with a tendency to iris prolapse. Author's method of vertical implantation (technique described on page 52). The vitreous presented itself nasally in the pupil as well as through the iridotomy at 12 o'clock.

For safety reasons the wound was first nearly completely sutured, and then two peripheral iridectomies were made at 3 and 9 o'clock. The air bubble filled up the anterior chamber in the usual way. Pupil central.

5- 5–71 visual acuity with – 2.75 DS / + 2.00 DC × 120 was 0.63.

Very many pigment nodules on the implant's surfaces. Square and central pupil. Position of the loops of the implant along the 70° meridian.

23- 3–72 visual acuity with – 1.50 DS was 0.90.

Gonioscopy: no iridotomies visible. The anterior superior loop was in contact with the corneal endothelium, and embedded in pigmented tissue of the iris.

Pilocarpine medication discontinued.

19- 3–74 visual acuity with – 1.50 DS was 0.80.

Despite the fact that the outcome of this case is good, the author is not satisfied with the position of the anterior superior loop. It would have been better if the implant had not been fitted.

2. Insertion of the loops was difficult:

a. at the 6 o'clock position in 3 cases,

b. at the 12 o'clock position in 7 cases, dependent on the degree of success of the blunt iris hook manoeuvre (see page 49).

Case histories.

re a)

Case 21. Failure at 6 o'clock; success at 5 o'clock. See page 184.

Case 24. Difficult, for no particular reason. See page 185.

Case 33. It was extremely difficult to place the loops astride the iris.

re b)

Case 11. The hook was caught up in some vitreous.

Case 54. Difficult, for no apparent reason.

Case 56. The hook inadvertently caught the superior loop, thus dislocating the inferior loops. Immediate repositioning. The only consequence was that the implant became located along the 60° meridian.

Case 63. Some vitreous appeared during the blunt iris hook manoeuvre.

Case 64. Incarceration of a vitreous bubble superotemporally. Later the pupil became square.

Case 65. The manoeuvre was successful only at the 4th attempt. See page 186.

Case 71. The manoeuvre was not completely successful due to incarceration of a vitreous bubble superotemporally. Consequently the pupil was not exactly square.

C. Early post-operative period

1. *Excessive vomiting.* Two cases (2.78 %).

The first 24 hours after the operation are very important because vomiting and restlessness of the patient while regaining consciousness may undo our achievements.

In case 55 excessive vomiting and walking during the first night after surgery did not upset the good result.

In case 2, however, excessive vomiting led to a shallow anterior chamber and the air bubble disappeared despite the fact that the corneo-scleral wound had been closed with 12 perlon sutures. Unfortunately, this led to the development of ECD (see page 189).

2. DESCEMET *folds* were present in 3 cases (4.17 %), but disappeared after a few days. Cases 2 and 19, however, where considerable intraocular manipulation had been necessary, ended in ECD (see page 189). This illustrates the danger of excessive manipulation, as mentioned on page 67 ff.

3. *Pupillary block* was observed in 5 cases (6.94 %). It was caused by iridotomies that were too small (case 24), iridotomies that had probably been blocked by blood (cases 1 and 30), iridectomies that had probably become blocked by blood, after a technically perfect operation (case 41), or for no apparent reason (case 21). Therefore, if the surgeon is not absolutely sure whether he has made good iridotomies, additional iridectomies should be made (see also page 180). It should be stressed that blood in the anterior chamber is a factor which promotes pupillary block by occluding the iridotomies or the iridectomies.

Case histories.

Case 1. See page 188. Pupillary block after re-implantation in a case where excessive bleeding occurred.

Case 21. Male, born 1909. Congenital downward decentration of both pupils (1.5 mm). Flocculi iridis.

24– 8-70 intracapsular cryoextraction with iris clip lens implantation OS. Implantation unsuccessful at 6 o'clock, but succeeded at 5 o'clock. Peripherally one iridectomy and two iridotomies.

27– 8-70 shallow anterior chamber with flattened remnant of the air bubble. Peripheral iridectomy at 2 o'clock after removal of the last temporal suture. Two new sutures. Air insufflation.

1–10–70 small subconjunctival haemorrhages after the lifting of heavy objects.

9–10–70 corrected visual acuity 0.45.

24– 6–71 corrected visual acuity 0.80.

2– 3–72 corrected visual acuity 1.00.

Gonioscopy: normal appearance of iridectomy and iridotomies.

To be on the safe side 3 iridectomies were made during the lens implantation in the patient's second eye (case 42).

Case 24. Female, born 1903. Diabetes mellitus since 1970. Myocardial insufficiency.

29– 9–70 intracapsular cryoextraction with iris clip lens implantation OD. The cryoextractor did not freeze at the tip. Besides, the instrument touched the iris temporally, and was immediately defrosted. Difficult implantation at 6 o'clock. Three iridotomies.

1–10–70 shallow anterior chamber with flattened remnant of air bubble.

Peripheral iridectomy between 10 and 11 o'clock, and air insufflation.

23–11–70 corrected visual acuity 0.8.

25– 6–71 corrected visual acuity 0.8.

Gonioscopy: no iridotomies visible! No goniosynechiae.

Case 30. Female, born 1907.

15–10–70 bilateral mature cataract. Visual acuity OD and OS 0.02. The patient had never visited an ophthalmologist. She was led into the room.

12–11–70 intracapsular cryoextraction with iris clip lens implantation OD. The zonular fibres were extremely strong. The cryoprobe was defrosted before the lens was completely born. Blood clot at 6 o'clock. Irrigation was necessary during implantation. three iridotomies, and much bleeding.

14–11–70 shallow anterior chamber with flattened remnant of air bubble. Patient laid on her side. Glaucosan eye drops.

15–11–70 normal anterior chamber. The pupil was not exactly square.

18– 1–71 corrected visual acuity 0.30. Myopia and astigmatism.

31– 3–71 corrected visual acuity 0.35.

6– 4–72 corrected visual acuity 0.50.

Gonioscopy: normal appearance of iridotomies, minimal peripheral anterior synechiae at 10 and 2 o'clock.

Case 41. Female, born 1892.

22– 2–71 intracapsular cryoextraction with iris clip lens implantation OS under general anaesthesia. After implantation the patient moved and as a result the implant with iris protruded half-way out of the eye. This produced the largest iris prolapse (180°) the author had ever seen; a horrible situation. Additional 2-bromo-2-chloro-1:1:1-trifluoroethane (Fluothane). Three corneo-scleral sutures were preplaced. The iris prolapse was repositioned with a flat spatula. The superior loop was re-inserted by means of an iris repositor and a blunt iris hook. Acetylcholine irrigation. Peripheral iridectomies at 9, 12 and 3 o'clock. Air insufflation. Wound closed. Blood remained in the anterior chamber.

26– 2–71 shallow anterior chamber with flattened residual air bubble. Additional peripheral iridectomies were made at 10 and 2 o'clock.

185

11– 5–71 the pupil was found to be elongated in the 12 o'clock direction. Corrected visual acuity 0.63.

28– 9–73 corrected visual acuity 0.65.

Gonioscopy: normal appearance.

4. *Wound leakage* giving rise to subconjunctival filtering blebs was not observed.

5. *Dislocation* occurred in 4 cases (5.55%): in two cases there was excessive bleeding during surgery, in the third case vitreous loss occurred and in the fourth there was vitreous incarceration. Instrumental repositioning had contributed to the development of ECD in the first two cases.

Case histories.

Case 1. See page 188. Surgery with excessive bleeding. Posterior dislocation of the temporal loop on the 4th day. Final result: ECD.

Case 19. See page 189. Surgery with excessive bleeding. Anterior dislocation of the inferior loop on the 5th day. Final result: ECD.

Case 59. Female, born 1902. Cataract of unknown origin OS since 1938.

6– 1–72 intracapsular cryoextraction with iris clip lens implantation OS. The vitreous adhered to the lens and had to be cut until it was entirely removed from the anterior chamber.

10– 1–72 posterior dislocation of the inferior loop.

Repositioning with a blunt iris hook was not successful. Five sutures around the 12 o'clock position were removed, and re-insertion was performed with non-toothed forceps. Resutured. The anterior chamber was filled with saline (and not with air for reasons of visibility). A perlon suture from the loop to the iris was passed through a tangential transcorneal keratome incision (technique described on page 65 ff.). Incision closed with 3 perlon sutures (see Fig. 65 opposite page 196). Air insufflated.

11– 1–72 air had nearly disappeared. The very shallow anterior chamber filled again after the patient had been put on her side.

29– 3–72 removal of the 3 intracorneal sutures. Anatomically perfect result.

18– 9–72 visual acuity 0.003 (amblyopia).

However, the patient was extremely happy with her 'new eye'. The dislocation was in this case probably due to vitreous threads pulling the posterior inferior loop up.

Case 65. Male, born 1910.

6– 3–72 intracapsular cryoextraction with iris clip lens implantation OS. The pupil remained wide after extraction, and was contracted by means of acetylcholine and by tapping on the eye. The manoeuvre with the blunt iris hook succeeded on the 4th attempt. Three corneo-scleral sutures were made followed by 2 peripheral iridectomies between the sutures, and one temporally. Air insufflation after 8 sutures. Once again acetylcholine irrigation. Complete wound closure.

10– 3–72 posterior dislocation of the inferior loop.
   Repositioned with a needle knife under general anaesthesia and maximal mydriasis. Acetylcholine in the anterior chamber produced an excellent miosis.
18– 9–72 pupil nearly square.
   Corrected visual acuity 0.60.
This dislocation was probably caused by a vitreous thread incarcerated at 6 o'clock, but freed after dislocation and mydriasis.

6. *Early developing uveitis* was present in 3 cases (4.17%). In one case with a complicated cataract a previous uveitis relapsed. In the other two patients no reason could be found. With corticosteroid therapy the final outcome was satisfactory in all cases.

Case histories.
Case 17. See page 191. Relapse of previous uveitis.

Case 51. Male, born 1897. Diabetes mellitus detected in 1955. Camp eyes.
2– 9–71 intracapsular cryoextraction of a hypermature lens with iris clip lens implantation OS.
   Continuous bleeding from the wound edges necessitated prolonged irrigation.
11–10–71 pain. Cell clumps on DESCEMET's membrane and in the anterior chamber. Dexamethasone sodium phosphate (Decadron) eye drops 3 times daily.
29–10–71 normal anterior segment. Corrected visual acuity 0.25.
19– 1–72 corrected visual acuity 0.60.
27–10–72 death of patient.

Case 57. Male, born 1912.
18–11–71 intracapsular cryoextraction with iris clip lens implantation OD.
21–12–71 slight pericorneal injection, cell clumps in the anterior chamber. Dexamethasone sodium phosphate (Decadron) eye drops 3 times daily.
10– 1–72 corrected visual acuity 0.85. Normal anterior segment.
18– 9–72 corrected visual acuity 1.10.

D. Late post-operative period

1. *Dislocation* was observed in one case (1.39%) only, and quite by chance during the extensive eye examination. After lens implantation the patient was told to instill pilocarpine drops immediately after waking up and before going to sleep. However, she used to go to sleep at irregular hours, which affected the miosis. Better advice would, therefore, be to instill the pilocarpine drops at a fixed time, e.g. 7 a.m. and 10 p.m. each day.

Until this time the rarity of late dislocation in the group using permanent pilocarpine medication was the reason for the author to suture an implant on the iris in special cases only (see page 191). This is supported by the only small difference in dislocation percentages in WORST's groups: 3.36% of not sutured iris clip lenses against 2.02% of sutured iris clip lenses (see Fig. 59 on page 168).

Case histoɪy.
Case 58. Female, born 1904.
25-11-71 intracapsular cryoextraction with iris clip lens implantation OD. Many blood clots.
18- 9-72 anterior dislocation of the superior loop.
19- 9-72 repositioned with a needle knife under general anaesthesia and maximal mydriasis.
12-10-72 square pupil. Direction of the loops along the 70° meridian. Corrected visual acuity 0.60.
3- 7-73 corrected visual acuity 1.0.

2. *Endothelial corneal dystrophy* (ECD) was present in 5 cases (6.94%). It was promoted by too many surgical manipulations (cases 1, 14 and 19), prolonged corneal contact (cases 1 and 2), intermittent corneal contact (case 14) and disposition to dystrophy, possibly FUCHS' corneal dystrophy (case 44). Greater surgical experience could have avoided ECD in some of these cases. *This is, of course, a strong argument for the optimal preparation of the ophthalmic surgeon who starts to perform implant surgery.*

The number of 5 cases of ECD lies between BINKHORST's 6 and WORST's 2 cases amongst their first 72 iris clip lens implantations, after an average observation period of 450, 1626 and 558 days respectively. Apart from the much longer observation period, it should, of course, be kept in mind that BINKHORST had to cope with all the difficulties encountered by any pioneer.

The first two cases of iris clip lens implantation that could also have been listed in the group of early complications, illustrate the importance of experience in the implantation technique for the final result. After these first two cases:
a. the 12 o'clock preplaced suture was omitted as it was felt to be too cumbersome.
b. vertical implantation was preferred as being technically easier.

Case histories.
Case 1. Male, born 1910. Familial cataract.
19- 1-70 intracapsular cryoextraction with horizontal iris clip lens implantation OS. Much bleeding and irrigation. Implantation fairly easy.
22- 1-70 posterior dislocation of the temporal loop.
Repositioning with blunt iris hook was only successful after the eye had been re-opened. Two extra iridotomies. Air insufflated.
26- 1-70 shallow anterior chamber with flattened residual air bubble.
1- 2-70 peripheral iridectomy at 3 o'clock.

16 - 2–70 DESCEMET folds and stromal cloudiness. Dexamethasone sodium phosphate (Decadron) eye drops 6 times daily.

2– 6–70 the lower segment of the cornea was clear.

5– 8–70 bullous keratopathy with band-shaped localisation.

18–10–72 the lower segment of the cornea continued to be clear. Visual acuity 0.02.

17–10–73 stationary situation.

In this case ECD developed exactly where the horizontal implant had been in contact with DESCEMET's membrane, because the anterior chamber was left shallow for too long. The extra peripheral iridectomy should have been made at once on 26–1–1970.

Case 2. Indonesian female, born 1908.

22– 1–70 intracapsular cryoextraction with horizontal iris clip lens implantation OS. After the first 3 corneo-scleral sutures, i.e. rather late, it became clear that both temporal loops were situated in front of the iris. Vertical re-insertion. No further difficulties. Excessive vomiting after the operation.

23– 1–70 shallow anterior chamber, the air bubble had almost disappeared. Corneal opacities.

7– 2–70 the corneal opacities were clearing up.

3– 3–70 pericorneal injection. Dexamethasone sodium phosphate (Decadron) eye drops 4 times daily.

25– 3–70 total ECD. Visual acuity 0.02.

19– 3–73 situation stationary.

In this case the anterior chamber should have been restored the day after implantation.

Case 14. Female, born 1893.

28– 4–70 intracapsular cryoextraction with iris clip lens implantation OD. No difficulties. Post-operative tendency for the anterior chamber to be shallow.

20– 5–70 corrected visual acuity 0.45.

15– 9–70 corrected visual acuity 0.60.

9–12–70 corrected visual acuity 0.80.

21– 8–72 excessive mobility of the inferior loop caused oedema in the lower half of the cornea.

28– 8–72 transcorneal amputation of the inferior loop with VANNAS scissors.

4–10–72 total ECD. Visual acuity 0.02.

In this case it would have been better for the loop amputation to have been carried out through a corneo-scleral incision. The trauma of the incision through the oedematous cornea proved to be too severe.

Case 19. Male, born 1900. Deaf-mute illiterate.

10– 8–70 intracapsular cryoextraction with iris clip lens implantation OS. Since the pupil was not wide enough, additional homatropine was instilled. The iris was extremely thick and, therefore, an iridectomy was made at 12 o'clock instead of an iridotomy. Much bleeding and irrigation. The anterior chamber could not be kept free of blood.

While waking up from the anaesthesia the patient fought with the unsterile nurse who tried in vain to keep him supine. There was no verbal contact at all.

14– 8–70 anterior dislocation of the inferior loop (during the fight?) became apparent. Repositioning with a blunt iris hook was not successful. The wound was completely re-opened, the implant was rotated clockwise through 90°, inserted nasally and both loops were sutured to the iris separately. During the last inspection the anterior loop was seen to be broken.

The sutures were cut again. During this difficult manoeuvre a hole developed in the iris temporally. Another iris clip lens was inserted horizontally. The new hole could be used for the suturing of the temporal loops to each other. The nasal loop was sutured to the iris. The implant was aligned with the 20° meridian.

15– 8–70 DESCEMET folds and stromal cloudiness.

2–12–70 the lower half of the cornea was clear.

16– 1–71 corrected visual acuity 0.20.

24– 6–71 partial ECD. The knots of the nasal loop iris suture had loosened. The slightly updrawn pupil was not exactly square.

13– 9–72 total ECD. Visual acuity 0.02.

In this case the preparation of the patient was insufficient. A handicap may form a contra-indication for implant surgery, and should be evaluated for each individual. The instillation of additional homatropine may have contributed to the dislocation.

Case 44. Female, born 1912. Diabetes mellitus since 1967.

4– 3–71 intracapsular cryoextraction with iris clip lens implantation OS. No difficulties.

29– 4–71 corrected visual acuity 0.16. Slight pericorneal injection. TYNDALL positive in the anterior chamber. Many pigment deposits on the surfaces of the implant impair ophthalmoscopy. Dexamethasone sodium phosphate (Decadron) eye drops 4 times daily.

5– 5–71 the eye's redness diminished. Anterior chamber clear. Corrected visual acuity 0.20.

16– 6–71 the pigment deposits had nearly disappeared.

14–12–71 pericorneal injection. Cell clumps in the anterior chamber. IOP = 13.4 mm Hg. Dexamethasone sodium phosphate (Decadron) eye drops 6 times daily.

21–12–71 slight corneal haziness in the periphery. Prednisone 3 × 10 mg daily.

17– 1–72 incipient ECD. Visual acuity 0.02. Prednisone discontinued.

13– 4–72 total ECD. The patient was referred to BINKHORST.

3–10–72 perforating keratoplasty 8 mm (BINKHORST).

13–11–72 corrected visual acuity 0.08. Thin condensed hyaloid membranes behind the implant.

26– 1–73 seclusio pupillae.

22– 2–73 needling of membranes.

1–11–73 corrected visual acuity 0.3. Full binocular vision (NORDLOHNE).

In this case the causative factor is not very obvious. According to BINKHORST FUCHS' endothelial dystrophy was present in the fellow-eye, but this diagnosis could not be confirmed by the author.

3. *Retinal detachment* was not observed.

4. *Late extraction of implant* has not been carried out.

5. *Enucleation* has not been carried out either.

1. *A loop iris suture* (see page 56) was made in 5 cases (6.94%), because of a radial iridotomy and, consequently, no sphincter action (cases 17 and 26), a restless patient (cases 19 and 68) and in order to prevent another dislocation (case 59).

Case histories.
Case 17. See page 191. For safety's sake, after a radial iridotomy.

Case 19. See page 189. For safety's sake, in a restless patient.

Case 26. See page 192. For safety's sake, after radial iridotomy.

Case 59. See page 186. To prevent another dislocation.

Case 68. Male, born 1896. Cataracta nigra.
17– 3–72 intracapsular cryoextraction with iris clip lens implantation OS. Liquefied vitreous appeared after the eye had been opened, and had to be rinsed out. The temporal loop was sutured to the iris, because it was known that the patient was somewhat mentally disturbed. During the post-operative period he wanted to go to his farm or to church, threw his eye-shield around the ward and had to be isolated. His mental condition improved when he was back at home.
19– 9–72 slight upward decentration (due to the suture?).
   Corrected visual acuity 0.55.

2. A *combination of synechiolysis, radial iridotomy and loop iris suture* had to be performed in 2 cases (2.78%) with a history of recurrent iridocyclitis. The author's technique is described on page 62.

Case 17/52. Male, born 1902. See Figs. 67 and 68 opposite page 196.
This patient had a history of recurrent iridocyclitis ODS since 1945. He had been treated in the Hochgebirg Augenklinik Guardaval in Davos during 1947–1948. The visual acuity of the right eye decreased to 0.15 in 1958 and 0.02 in 1961 as a result of a complicated cataract with nearly total seclusio pupillae (opening at 10 o'clock). The visual acuity of the left eye decreased to 0.25 in 1970, also as a result of complicated cataract, but this was only accompanied by a rigid pupil.
In spite of this pre-operative history it was decided to attempt an iris clip lens implant operation.

4– 6–70 intracapsular cataract extraction with horizontal iris clip lens implantation OD.

Posterior synechiolysis with the flat spatula through the opening at 10 o'clock. Radial iridotomy midway the iridic annulus, with two preplaced perlon sutures (see Fig. 69). Cryoextraction. Horizontal implantation. The preplaced sutures were knotted with three knots and cut extremely short. Because the pupil was still a little too wide temporally above, a secondary loop iris suture was added around the temporal loop. The operation was completed in the usual way.

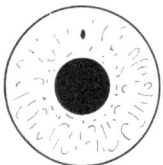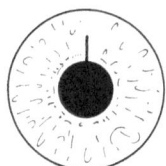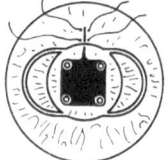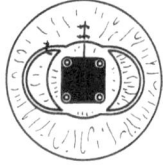

Fig. 69

Combination of radial iridotomy and loop iris suture.

a. a small hole is made in the middle of the iridic annulus.

b. radial iridotomy with DE WECKER scissors.

c. two preplaced perlon iris sutures, extraction, and horizontal implantation.

d. sutures tied and ends cut off as close to the knot as possible.

A secondary loop iris suture is placed and treated similarly.

13– 7–70 subjective decrease of visual acuity.

Clear anterior chamber, but greyish deposits on the implant were considered to be a sign that uveitis had recurred (see page 64). Dexamethasone sodium phosphate (Decadron) eye drops 3 times daily.

24– 7–70 subjective improvement of visual acuity.

Corrected visual acuity 0.35.

12–10–70 corrected visual acuity 0.60.

2–12–70 corrected visual acuity 0.65. Decadron discontinued.

28– 3–73 corrected visual acuity 0.55. Gonioscopy ODS: normal appearance.

This was the most gratifying case of this series.

This patient underwent an intracapsular cataract extraction with horizontal iris clip lens implantation of the left eye on 6–9–71 (case 52), but a radial iridotomy was omitted, the rigid sphincter was a little torn and the pupil remained wide, but not too wide. It became the patient's better eye having a corrected visual acuity of 0.65 on 28–3–1973. However, the case was less gratifying for the surgeon (see Fig. 68 opposite page 196).

Case 26. Female, born 1887.

This patient, too, had a history of recurrent iridocyclitis ODS since 1937, with complicated cataract ODS, extensive posterior synechiae ODS and visual acuity ODS reduced to 0.02 in 1962. The next visit to the ophthalmologist was on 4–9–1970.

15–10–70 intracapsular cataract extraction with horizontal iris clip lens implantation OS. The technique of synechiolysis, radial iridotomy and preplaced sutures, was the same as in the previous case. Because vitreous and iris were caving in (old eye!), implantation was only possible while simultaneous external pressure was applied by the sterile nurse.

Both loops were sutured to the iris, but the temporal loop was sutured too peripherally resulting in a local elongation of the pupil.

25– 6–71 corrected visual acuity 0.45.

3. *Overgrowth of an anterior loop by pigmented tissue of the iris* occurred in two Indonesian females (2.78%). Consequently, pilocarpine medication could be discontinued.

It seems that in the Malayan race the anterior layer of the iris tends to produce a proliferating reaction when a foreign body rests on it. The other 4 Indonesian patients, however, have not yet shown this phenomenon.

Case 20. Indonesian female, born 1910. See Fig. 66 opposite page 196.

18– 8–70 intracapsular cataract extraction with iris clip lens implantation OS. The zonules were very strong. The vertical implantation was rather difficult due to a mildly bulging vitreous.

9–12–70 corrected visual acuity 0.8.

24– 6–71 corrected visual acuity 1.0.

The entire nasal half of both anterior loops had become embedded in pigmented iris tissue. The rim of the optical portion was invisible between 8 and 12 o'clock. Pilocarpine medication discontinued.

29–11–71 corrected visual acuity 1.0.

The rim of the optical portion was not visible between 8 and 1 o'clock.

6–12–72 corrected visual acuity 1.0.

The rim of the optical portion was not visible between 7 and 1 o'clock.

17–12–73 corrected visual acuity 1.0. Status quo.

Case 40. See page 182. The overgrowth of the anterior superior loop can be observed only by means of gonioscopy. In view of the fact that this loop is in contact with the corneal endothelium the overgrowth, which improves stabilisation, has a beneficial side-effect.

4. *Diabetes mellitus* was present in 10 patients (2 ♂ and 8 ♀) with 12 eyes (16.67%). The data and results are shown in Fig. 70.

The average visual acuity in the 12 diabetic eyes (0.46) was clearly lower than in the 60 non-diabetic eyes (0.63).

When cases with diabetic retinopathy are excluded, the average visual acuity becomes 0.47. This figure lies between that of BINKHORST (0.59) and WORST (0.39), as does the average age at operation: 73.50 as compared with 69.48 and 77.14 years.

serial number	sex	diabetes detected at age (years)	age at operation (years)	cortex	nucleus	scattered	diabetic retinopathy	observation period in days	visual acuity	remarks
3	♀	75	76	+	—	+	—	1002	0.50	
36	♀	75	77	+	—	+	—	635	0.02	macular degeneration
12	♀	55	55	+	—	—	+	608	0.32	macular degeneration increased diabetic
15	♀	61	61	—	—	+	+	868	0.16	retinopathy
24	♀	67	67	—	—	+	—	787	0.80	pupillary block
40	♀	73	75	+	—	—	—	407	0.90	
44	♀	55	59	+	—	—	—	973	0.30	total ECD→penetrating keratoplasty
48	♂	56	77	—	—	+	—	492	0.63	
70	♂	56	78	—	—	+	—	204	0.63	vitreous loss
51	♂	58	74	+	+	—	—	210	0.60	
64	♀	80	83	—	+	—	—	207	0.25	
66	♀	78	79	—	+	—	—	193	0.40	
total	3 9	789	861	6	3	6	2	6586	5.49	
average		65.75	71.75					549	0.46	

Fig. 70

Data and results of iris clip lens implant operations performed by the author on 10 patients with diabetes mellitus.

Diabetic retinopathy progressed in one of the two cases.

Thus, diabetes with or without diabetic retinopathy, cannot be considered a contra-indication for BINKHORST lens implantation. See also pages 115 and 166.

Case 15. Female, born 1909. Diabetes mellitus was detected and treated by the physician in the pre-operative period.

1– 5–70 intracapsular cataract extraction with iris clip lens implantation OS.

10– 6–70 corrected visual acuity 0.45.

21– 8–70 corrected visual acuity 0.12.

The diabetic retinopathy had increased.

A stringent low fat diet was prescribed and maintained for one year.

20– 1–71 corrected visual acuity 0.08.

18- 1–72 corrected visual acuity 0.08.

15- 9–72 corrected visual acuity 0.16. The fellow-eye still had a corrected visual acuity of 1.0.

CONCLUSION

The results of this series of 72 iris clip lens implant operations performed by the author are in many respects comparable with those of the iris clip lens series of BINKHORST and WORST although it is much smaller and does not count amongst its number patients under 50 years of age or traumatic cases.

Fig. 65. Author's case 59

Cataract of unknown origin OS, present since 1938. See page 186. Vertical iris clip lens implantation after intracapsular cryoextraction with vitreous loss. A posterior dislocation of the inferior loop on the 4th day was treated by repositioning and a transcorneal loop iris suture. Visual acuity 0.003 (amblyopia).

Photographed by Dr. BINKHORST, on the 25th day after the operation.

Fig. 66. Author's case 20

Indonesian female with vertical iris clip lens implant OS after intracapsular cryoextraction. See page 193. The nasal half of both anterior loops is overgrown with pigmented iris tissue. Corrected visual acuity 1.0.

Photographed by L. H. LOONES, technical assistant to Dr. BINKHORST, 2½ years after the operation.

Fig. 67. Author's case 17.   Fig. 68. Author's case 52

Binocular case of a male patient with a history of recurrent iridocyclitis and complicated cataract. See page 191. Horizontal iris clip lens implantation after intracapsular cryoextraction, both eyes. Right eye with, and left eye without radial iridotomy and loop iris suture. Corrected visual acuity R 0.55 and L 0.63, after an observation period of 34 and 19 months respectively.

Photographed by Dr. BINKHORST, respectively 20 and 5 months after the operation.

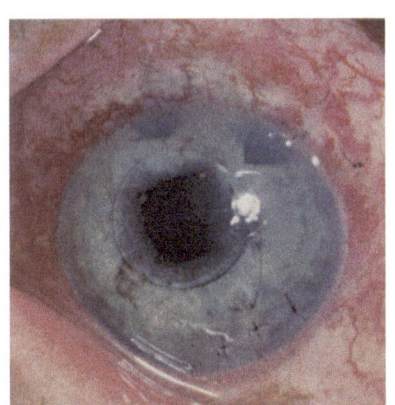

Fig. 65

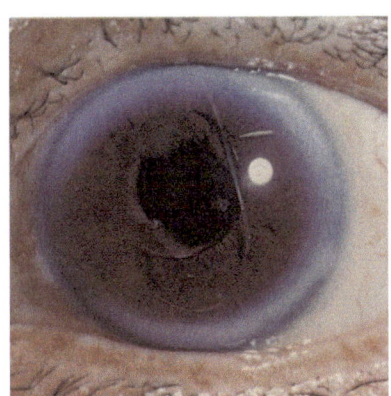

Fig. 66

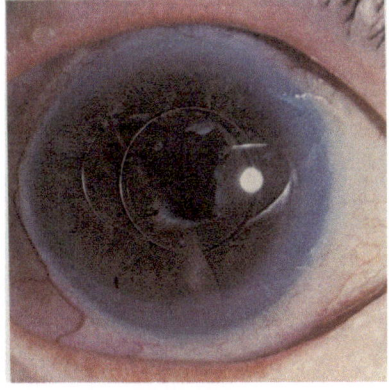

Fig. 67

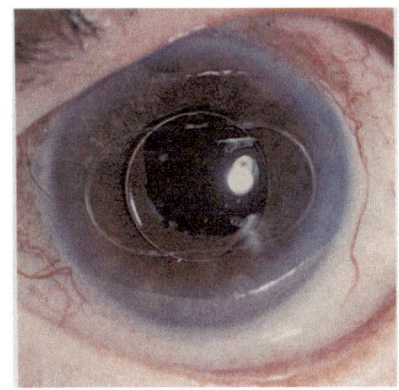

Fig. 68

CHAPTER VII

RESULTS OBTAINED IN THE NETHERLANDS WITH BINKHORST LENS IMPLANTS

This chapter deals with the experience of 26 Dutch ophthalmologists in fitting BINKHORST lens implants, as revealed by their replies to a questionnaire covering indications, techniques, complications, and post-operative visual acuity.

> Are we not drawn onward, we few, drawn onward to new era?
> English palindrome.

INTRODUCTION

A number of ophthalmologists in the Netherlands and abroad were inspired by C. D. BINKHORST's example to start fitting lens implants themselves. BINKHORST fitted the first iris clip lens on 11th August 1958 and the first iridocapsular lens on 16th September 1965. By 1st January 1972, at least 30 Dutch ophthalmologists had followed his example. Of these, 23 visited him in person in Sluiskil. Instructing surgeons included WORST (Groningen), JAPING (The Hague) and VAN BALEN (Rotterdam), each of whom had been personally instructed by BINKHORST. For many, the numerous films of operations by BINKHORST and WORST were also a stimulus (sometimes the only one) to start fitting BINKHORST lens implants. BINKHORST and his co-workers kept Dutch ophthalmologists regularly informed about results and new developments by means of lectures to the Dutch Ophthalmological Society. Foreign ophthalmologists were kept up-to-date by means of lectures abroad and by many publications in journals (see references.).

Many of the latter watched BINKHORST at work.

It took about 10 years before BINKHORST's many activities melted the initial distrust felt about lens implants in the Netherlands. Since that time, the number of ophthalmologists fitting implants has increased rapidly: 5 in 1969, 11 in 1970.

BINKHORST, *and others with· him, however, have always wondered whether* BINKHORST *lens implant operations can suitably be performed by any given ophthalmologist.*

Should this not be so:

a. a number of eyes would be subject unnecessarily to some loss of vision;
b. the BINKHORST lens would be discredited as a result of misuse.

To obtain a reply to this question, an investigation was held into the results

of implant operations for a total of approx. 2711 BINKHORST lenses fitted up to
1st January 1972 by 26 Dutch ophthalmologists.

INQUIRY

Interviews lasting from 1 to 4 hours with each of the 26 ophthalmologists who
had performed independently at least 8 BINKHORST lens implant operations before 1st January 1972, enabled the author to obtain an insight into motives,
preparations, indications, techniques, complications, and visual acuity obtained*.

A mainly written enquiry had to be resorted to in only 4 cases (ophthalmologists
H, L, M and Z). This applied also to the whole question of the ophthalmologists'
opinions on contra-indications arising out of their own experience.

The author found that all who contributed did their utmost to provide reliable
information. However, some were hindered by the absence of detailed records, which
meant that it was not possible to assemble absolutely all the data required (ophthalmologists B, D, L, M, R, V, W and Z).

The reliability of the data obtained is limited due to the following facts:
a.   the material is heterogeneous, especially as regards the cause of cataract and the
optotypes used.
b.   the investigation was retrospective.
c.   the author did not study all the case histories himself.

Fig. 71 (at back of book) gives a general review of the data obtained during
these interviews divided into general data, surgical technique, post-operative
complications and their sequelae, and opinions held on contra-indications based
in part on practical experience. The names of the ophthalmologists have been
replaced in chronological order by the letters A, B, C, etc.

The replies to the following questions could not be included in the table, or
only incompletely:

1.   *Question: Why did you start fitting* BINKHORST *lens implants?*

Answers:

a.   because the optical solution is much better than in the case of cataract
spectacles and contact lenses. Moreover, elderly people in particular have great
difficulty with these appliances and are consequently discontented (ophthalmologists A, F, I, K, N, T, X, Y, Z and the author).

---

* An additional 14 iris clip lenses and 6 iridocapsular lenses were fitted by 5 ophthalmologists. Their results are not included in this series since the number of implantations
performed by each was considered to be too small for evaluation.

b.   on account of unilateral cataract and traumatic cataract (A, B, G, H, P, S, V, W, Z).

c.   because BINKHORST's results were good (B, C, F, J, S, X) and, moreover, the experimental phase had been left behind (the author).

d.   because it is an important advance in ophthalmology (C, E, F, Z), one might even call it the apotheosis of cataract surgery (O, R, U).

e.   because patients ask for it (H, N, X, Z), and would otherwise consult other ophthalmologists (T, X).

f.   because the ophthalmologist himself considered it to be interesting (T) or even a challenge (U), and . . . because he would like to be able to join in the conversation (L).

2.   *Question: Why did you cease fitting* BINKHORST *lens implants?*

Answers:

a.   because of difficulties arising from the severe demands made on binocular vision during the operation (B).

b.   because it meant too much work and was too great a responsibility for such a small financial gain (L).

c.   because the results were unsatisfactory (V).

3.   *Question: How many* BINKHORST *lens implant operations did you watch before you attempted to perform the first yourself?*

The replies expressed in terms of 'sessions' and 'implantations' (one session may represent 1–4 implant operations) are shown in Fig. 72.

Four ophthalmologists (ISPX) had only watched films before they performed their first implant operation. One of these (I) went to watch BINKHORST after having performed 3 implant operations himself.

4.   *Question: Did you carry out your first implant operation on your own, or was there a surgeon experienced in implant operations at hand?*

Answers:

a.   on their own: 16 ophthalmologists.

b.   supervised:

1.   by BINKHORST: B F H J W

2.   by JAPING: K O T Y

3.   by VAN BALEN: M

ophthalmologists	number of sessions	ophthalmologists	number of implantations
author	6	F	120 (approx.)
E U	5	W	50
D N V Y	3	J	50
C T	1	H	tens
		Z	32 (approx.)
		B	25
		G	20
		K	18
		R	10 (assisted)
		T	8
		O	6
		M	several

Fig. 72

Number of sessions or implant operations attended by each of 21 Dutch ophthalmologists prior to starting fitting BINKHORST lens implants themselves.

5.   *Question: Is it your opinion that every ophthalmologist ought to be able to perform a* BINKHORST *lens implant operation?*

Answers:

a.   yes (G L O R), that is everybody could learn to perform it (N).

b.   no (the remaining 21 ophthalmologists):

1.   only ophthalmologists who are skilful, have a particular interest in surgery and specialise in it (S W X Z).

2.   only well-balanced and skilful ophthalmologists who also maintain sterility, and not everybody falls into this category (C).

3.   a fairly high degree of surgical training and manual dexterity is essential, and not everybody possesses these requirements (E).

4.   in a number of practices the opportunities for maintaining surgical skill are limited (J).

5.   only ophthalmologists who are sufficiently skilled and have performed a large number of uncomplicated cataract extractions. Moreover, they should have an above-average reputation as regards complications and post-operative astigmatism (F G K and the author).

6.   only ophthalmologists who feel confident in anterior chamber surgery, and who have mastered the whole technique of cataract extraction. Ophthalmologists who perform cataract extraction with VON GRAEFE'S knife followed by one suture are unsuitable as implant surgeons (D).

7. there is a danger of it becoming a status symbol (B).

8. if all ophthalmologists start performing these operations, many accidents will occur (T U).

9. only ophthalmologists who are enthusiastic about lens implantation (V).

10. ophthalmologist F points out the importance of the mentality of the implant surgeon, in particular his preparedness to allow free access to the operating theatre and patients' records.

The question whether every ophthalmologist should be able to perform a BINKHORST implant operation is associated with the question of the desirability of dividing ophthalmological training in the Netherlands into intraocular and non-intraocular eye surgery. Seven ophthalmologists (A E J P S X and the author) are in favour of such a division into ophthalmic surgeons and ophthalmic medical practitioners.

Ophthalmologist A suggested that a special endorsement should be granted for ophthalmic surgery, ophthalmologist J suggested a 5-year training course which would include surgery, and a 3-year course without it; two ophthalmologists suggested that the future ophthalmic surgeon take an examination (T), or a test which would be judged by experienced ophthalmic surgeons. This could be done post-graduate (P).

Three ophthalmologists (A I P) advocated establishing centres for eye surgery in the Netherlands, while ophthalmologist H stressed the desirability of one member of any team of two or more ophthalmologists being competent to perform lens implant operations.

Four ophthalmologists stressed the necessity of having well-trained operating theatre staff and adequate nursing facilities (A D S Z). A hospital prepared to provide perfect nursing facilities for ophthalmic patients is a sine qua non, assistance by ophthalmic nurses is imperative (A D).

6. *Question: How should the future implant surgeon prepare himself?*

The answers may be summarised as follows:

a. by studying literature and films (A B J X).

It is considered advisable that there should be a booklet providing a good description of a standard technique (Y).

b. in addition, by acting as assistant to an experienced implant surgeon. Training at this level should include:

1. attending lens implant operations (A B C D E F G H I J K M O R T U V W X Z and the author).

2. assisting with lens implant operations (C D H M R W X).

3. being assisted with lens implant operations (C I J M Z and the author).

c. if necessary, changing one's technique of cataract extraction in order to fulfil the following conditions of lens implantation:

1. non-traumatic, endothelium-sparing technique (A J).
2. watertight closure of the corneo-scleral wound (A J).

Ophthalmologists N and X were strong advocates of the use of the operating microscope. However, ophthalmologist A and the author are of the opinion that the operating microscope is not necessary for the implantation technique, and that it has disadvantages as well, e.g. the reduced manoeuvrability of the ophthalmologist which makes it difficult to observe details from every angle, the reduction of the field of view, and the fact that the perlon suture may be blown against the microscope (see page 46). It is of interest to note that the ophthalmologists with the greatest experience, namely BINKHORST and WORST, do not use the operating microscope.

Finally, it was recommended starting on one's own with the bad risk cases (R), the iridocapsular lens (B), LÉONARD's modification (F; see page 28) or the iris clip lens in unilateral cataract in elderly people (the author).

7. *Question: Which technique did you use for the cataract extraction with* BINKHORST *lens implantation?*

The answers to this question are tabulated in Fig. 71 at back of book.
    The great variation is due to:

a. the stage reached in the development of the technique when the ophthalmologist started to perform this operation.

b. the technique used by the surgeon who instructed the ophthalmologist, his standpoint with respect to the FLIERINGA ring, BEAVER knife no. 66, and air insufflation.

c. personal preference.

8. *Question: What difficulties did you encounter during the operation?*

Answers:

a. bulging vitreous was considered by 20 ophthalmologists to be the most important problem to be dealt with immediately prior to implantation. Three of the remaining six ophthalmologists had not encountered bulging vitreous, partly because they had fitted exclusively iridocapsular lenses (P S), or because of hypotensive general anaesthesia (Z). Two ophthalmologists (B X) massaged the globe just before the operation, but this was not a success in every case.

Only six (K M N T V X) of the 20 ophthalmologists considered bulging vitreous to be a contra-indication for BINKHORST lens implantation, the remaining 14 would continue the implant operation (technique described on page 52). This vitreous problem is the main reason for warning the patient in advance that a new lens can only be implanted provided no technical problems crop up during the operation (T).

b. visibility problems during the insertion of the loops caused by blood or increasing corneal opacity due to DESCEMET folds, for example (E F G J and the author).

Problems encountered less frequently were:

c. pupil too small before the implantation, or remaining too large after the implantation (E F O).

d. iris caved in (I and author).

e. air behind the iris (E, case 4).

9. *Question: Which post-operative complications did you encounter?*

The answers to this question are summarised in the table of Fig. 71. The incidence of the most important post-operative complications and of their sequelae is shown separately for the iris clip lens and the iridocapsular lens in Fig. 73 in which ophthalmologists A (BINKHORST), E (WORST), W and Z (data incomplete) have been excluded.

The data obtained for another important complication, viz. uveitis (endogenous or exogenous), do not lend themselves to reliable evaluation. This is because it is a complication which cannot very well be expressed numerically in view of the many gradations between slight cellular reaction and panophthalmitis. Many ophthalmologists will not have recorded the lower degrees such as slight cellular reaction. Post-operative uveitis subsided under local corticosteroid treatment in 18 out of at least 28 cases. However, in 8 out of 10 cases considered by the Dutch ophthalmologists to be exogenous infections, the final result was bad: 2 of the 4 iris clip lenses, and all 6 iridocapsular lenses, had to be removed.

1. Dislocation occurred in 39 cases (3.20%), i.e. in 30 iris clip lens cases 2.97%) and 9 iridocapsular cases (4.33%). Fourteen of the 39 cases occurred during the first week, and 2 during the second week after implantation. Repositioning was performed in 34 cases. Two cases were not treated: the first (under ophthalmologist T) because it was only a partial, posterior dislocation of one loop in a 91-year-old patient (after rubbing the eye), and the second (under ophthalmologist G) because it was considered to be too dangerous. However, ECD developed in the latter case, and eventually the implant had to be extracted. In 3 other cases (under ophthalmologists L, T and V) extraction of the implant was also considered necessary.

2. ECD developed in 28 cases (2.30%), i.e. in 27 iris clip lens cases (2.67%)

ophthalmologist	iris clip lens						iridocapsular lens						total					
	number	dislocation	ECD	retinal detachment	extraction of implant	enucleation	number	dislocation	ECD	retinal detachment	extraction of implant	enucleation	number	dislocation	ECD	retinal detachment	extraction of implant	enucleation
B	20 approx.	—	1	—	—	—	25 approx.	—	—	—	—	—	45 approx.	—	1	—	—	—
C	300 approx.	1	3	2	—	—	1	—	—	—	—	—	301 approx.	1	3	2	—	—
D	3	1	—	—	—	—	3	1	—	—	—	—	6	2	—	—	—	—
F	30	—	—	—	—	—	30	4	—	—	—	—	60	4	—	—	—	—
G	5	2	3	—	2	—	1	—	—	—	—	—	6	2	3	—	2	—
H	157	9	3	3	2	—	87	—	—	2	3	1	244	9	3	5	5	
I	23	1	—	—	—	—	6	2	—	—	—	—	29	3	—	—	—	—
J	24	1	—	—	—	—	9	—	—	—	—	—	33	1	—	—	—	—
K	24	—	3	—	2	—	2	—	—	—	1	—	26	—	3	—	3	—
L	10	1	—	—	1	—	3	—	—	—	1	—	13	1	—	—	2	—
M	5	—	—	—	—	—	4	—	—	—	—	—	9	—	—	—	—	—
N	38	—	—	1	1	—	—	—	—	—	—	—	38	—	—	1	1	—
O	48	1	1	1	—	—	—	—	—	—	—	—	48	1	1	1	—	—
P	—	—	—	—	—	—	12	1	—	—	1	—	12	1	—	—	1	—
Q	72	5	5	—	—	—	—	—	—	—	—	—	72	5	5	—	—	—
R	90 approx.	2	—	—	1	—	—	—	—	—	—	—	90 approx.	2	—	—	1	—
S	—	—	—	—	—	—	9	1	—	—	—	—	9	1	—	—	—	—
T	15	2	—	—	1	—	1	—	—	—	—	—	16	2	—	—	1	—
U	34	1	1	—	1	—	4	—	1	—	1	—	38	1	2	—	2	—
V	9	2	4	—	1	—	4	—	—	—	—	—	13	2	4	—	1	—
X	79	1	1	—	—	—	7	—	—	—	—	—	86	1	1	—	—	—
Y	25	—	2	—	—	—	—	—	—	—	—	—	25	—	2	—	—	—
tot.	1011 approx.	30	27	7	12	—	208 approx.	9	1	2	7	1	1219 approx.	39	28	9	19	
%		2.97	2.67	0.69	1.19			4.33	0.48	0.96	3.37	0.48		3.20	2.30	0.74	1.56	0

Fig. 73

Incidence of dislocation, ECD, retinal detachment, implant extraction and enucleation in approx. 1219 BINKHORST lens implant operations performed by 22 Dutch ophthalmologists. Iris clip lens implants and iridocapsular lens implants are shown separately and combined.

Ophthalmologists A (BINKHORST; see chapter IV), E (WORST; see chapter V), W and Z (data not available) have been excluded.

and one iridocapsular lens case (0.48 %). In 7 cases the cause was endothelial touch, in 2, pre-operative FUCHS' corneal dystrophy. In 10 cases serious operational and post-operative complications were responsible: chlorhexidine gluconate 0.5 % (Hibitane) on the cornea (1), too much manipulation (2), flat anterior chamber (2), and dislocations (5). In 9 cases there was no detectable reason. Treatment consisted of repositioning the dislocated implant (2), loop amputation (2), extraction of the implant (7) and penetrating keratoplasty (2). The final outcome of these 28 cases, as regards the condition of the cornea and the visual function, was generally bad whether they had been treated or not.

3.   Retinal detachment occurred in 9 cases (0.74%), i.e. 7 iris clip lens cases (0.69%) and 2 iridocapsular lens cases (0.96%). An encircling procedure performed in all these cases, had some success in 4 as regards re-appositioning of the retina. The final visual acuities in the latter cases were 0.1, 0.2, 0.4 and 1.0.

4.   Extraction of the implant was performed in 19 cases (1.56%), i.e. 12 iris clip lens cases (1.19%) and 7 iridocapsular lens cases (3.37%). Motivation included ECD (6 iris clip lens cases and one iridocapsular lens case), severe reaction of the anterior segment (2 iris clip lens cases and 6 iridocapsular lens cases), dislocation (3 iris clip lens cases) and vitreous incarceration with decentration (one iris clip lens case).

5.   Enucleation was necessary in one iridocapsular lens case (0.08%) with a purulent endophthalmitis ending in phthisis bulbi (see case history page 220 ff.).

Fig. 74 gives a comparison of some complications experienced by 13 ophthalmologists who performed their first BINKHORST lens implant operation on their own and those encountered by 9 ophthalmologists who performed their first BINKHORST lens implant operation under the supervision of a surgeon experienced in implant operations.

A comparison of the results of BINKHORST and WORST and those obtained by the other 22 Dutch ophthalmologists is shown in Fig. 75.

10.   *Question: What is the visual acuity obtained in your patients?*

The answers to this question have been summarised, together with some other details, in the table in Fig. 76, for all BINKHORST lenses. Fig. 77 shows the details for the iris clip lenses. With the exception of the cases of ophthalmologist H, they are all based on detailed information about each patient.

A comparison of BINKHORST, WORST, and 16 other Dutch ophthalmologists is given in Figs. 78, 79 and 80.

	number	disloca-tion	ECD	retinal detach-ment	extrac-tion of the implant	enuclea-tion
13 ophthalmologists operating from the first alone	713 approx.	22	18	3	10	—
9 ophthalmologists operating first under supervision	506 approx.	17	10	6	9	1
13 ophthalmologists operating from the first alone		3.09	2.52	0.42	1.40	—
9 ophthalmologists operating first under supervision		3.36	1.98	1.19	1.78	0.20

Fig. 74

Comparison of numbers (above) and percentages (below) for dislocation, ECD, retinal detachment, extraction of the implant, and enucleation, as encountered by 13 ophthalmologists who performed their first BINKHORST lens implant operation on their own and 9 ophthalmologists who performed their first BINKHORST lens implant operation under the supervision of a surgeon experienced in implant operations.

Numbers

	iris clip lens (including FEDOROV modification (11) and iris medallion lens (178))							iridocapsular lens							total						
	number of implantations	average observation period in days	dislocation	ECD (total or partial)	retinal detachment	extraction of implant	enucleation	number of implantations	average observation period in days	dislocation	ECD	retinal detachment	extraction of implant	enucleation	number of implantations	average observation period in days	dislocation	ECD (total or partial)	retinal detachment	extraction of implant	enucleation
BINKHORST	696	771	53	42	13	4	1	170	572	9	1	3	3	1	866	735	62	43	16	7	1
WORST	661	206	16	16	12	6	1	4	398	1	1	—	2	1	665	208	17	17	12	8	1
22 Dutch ophthalmologists	1022	314	30	27	7	12	—	208	314	9	1	2	7	—	1230	314	39	28	9	19	1
total	2379 approx.	418 approx.	99	85	32	22	2	382 approx.	430 approx.	19	3	5	12	2	2761 approx.	421 approx.	118	88	37	34	3

Percentages

	iris clip lens					iridocapsular lens					total				
	dislocation	ECD	retinal detachment	extraction of implant	enucleation	dislocation	ECD	retinal detachment	extraction of implant	enucleation	dislocation	ECD	retinal detachment	extraction of implant	enucleation
BINKHORST	7.61	6.03	1.87	0.57	0.14	5.29	0.59	1.76	1.76	—	7.16	4.97	1.85	0.81	0.12
WORST	2.42	2.42	1.82	0.91	0.15						2.56	2.56	1.80	1.20	0.15
22 Dutch ophthalmologists	2.94	2.64	0.68	1.17	—	4.33	0.48	0.96	3.37	0.48	3.17	2.28	0.73	1.54	0.08
total	4.16	3.57	1.35	0.92	0.08	4.97	0.79	1.31	3.14	0.26	4.27	3.19	1.34	1.23	0.11

Fig. 75. Comparison in numbers (above) and percentages (below) of dislocation, ECD, retinal detachment, extraction of implant, and enucleation in approx. 2761 BINKHORST lens implant operations performed by BINKHORST, WORST and 22 other Dutch ophthalmologists. Iris clip lens implants (including FEDOROV modification and iris medallion lens implants) and iridocapsular lens implants are shown separately and combined.

ophthalmologist	number of implantations	♂	♀	L	R	binocular implant	monocular implant	average age at operation in years	average observation period in days	average visual acuity
C	222	66	156	104	118	90	132	73.74	217	0.99
F	22	17	5	13	9	—	22	38.36	558	0.78
G	9	4	5	4	5	—	9	58.89	1073	0.52
H	179					18	161	65.95	401	0.72
I	29	11	18	14	15	12	17	64.24	230	0.81
J	33	16	17	14	19	4	29	70.97	61	0.72
K	26	9	17	16	10	12	14	71.38	504	0.69
N	38	16	22	15	23	2	36	72.84	205	0.62
O	19	7	12	10	9	10	9	76.79	389	0.47
P	12	10	2	8	4	—	12	5.92	367	0.47
Q	72	27	45	38	34	22	50	71.10	450	0.60
S	9	6	3	2	7	2	7	7.11	755	0.46
T	16	4	12	5	11	6	10	71.31	115	0.81
U	38	14	24	17	21	10	28	63.95	343	0.60
X	86	33	53	39	47	30	56	68.67	140	0.82
Y	10	3	7	8	2	—	10	74.80	74	0.67
total	820	243	398	307	334	218	602	67.46	314	0.78
%		37.9	62.1	47.9	52.1	26.6	73.4			

Fig. 76

Data and results of 820 BINKHORST lens implant operations performed by 16 Dutch ophthalmologists.

Detailed information from ophthalmologists B, D, L, M, R, V, W, and Z relating to approx. 208 BINKHORST lens implant operations performed up to 1st January 1972, was not available. Details about the work of ophthalmologist H were available in part only.

ophthalmologist	number of implantations	♂	♀	L	R	binocular implant	monocular implant	average age at operation in years	average observation period in days	average visual acuity
C	179	54	125	82	97	78	101	73.64	270	0.99
F	9	7	2	6	3	—	9	54.56	503	0.83
G	5	3	2	3	2	—	5	65.00	1187	0.24
H	157					16	141	68.49	401	0.72
I	23	7	16	12	11	12	11	73.78	177	0.83
J	24	12	12	9	15	2	22	74.17	61	0.72
K	24	7	17	15	9	12	12	73.29	527	0.68
N	38	16	22	15	23	2	36	72.84	205	0.62
O	19	7	12	10	9	10	9	76.79	389	0.47
P	—	—	—	—	—	—	—	—	—	—
Q	72	27	45	38	34	22	50	71.10	450	0.60
S	—	—	—	—	—	—	—	—	—	—
T	15	3	12	5	10	6	9	74.73	84	0.80
U	34	10	24	14	20	10	24	70.88	317	0.67
X	79	28	51	35	44	30	49	73.14	141	0.82
Y	10	3	7	8	2	—	10	74.80	74	0.67
total	688	184	347	252	279	200	488	71.78	314	0.78
%		34.7	65.3	47.5	52.5	29.1	70.9			

Fig. 77

Data and results of 688 iris clip lens implant operations performed by 14 Dutch ophthalmologists.

Detailed information from ophthalmologists B, D, L, M, R, V, W and Z, relating to approx. 168 iris clip lens implant operations performed up to 1st January 1972, was not available. Details about the work of ophthalmologist H were available in part only. Ophthalmologists P and S had fitted iridocapsular lenses only.

	number of implantations	♂	♀	L	R	binocular implant	monocular implant	average age at operation in years	average observation period in days	average visual acuity
BINKHORST	866	474	392	415	451	294	572	58.87	735	0.64
WORST	665	274	391	319	346	414	251	70.78	208	0.57
16 Dutch ophthalmologists	820	243	398	307	334	218	602	67.46	314	0.78
total	2351	991	1181	1041	1131	926	1425	65.23	441	0.67
%		45.6	54.4	47.9	52.1	39.4	60.6			

Fig. 78. Data and results of 2351 BINKHORST lens implant operations performed by BINKHORST, WORST and 16 other Dutch ophthalmologists.

	number of implantations	♂	♀	L	R	binocular implant	monocular implant	average age at operation in years	average observation period in days	average visual acuity
BINKHORST	694	366	328	329	365	265	429	65.80	772	0.65
WORST	485	212	273	237	248	297	188	71.13	245	0.58
14 Dutch ophthalmologists	688	184	347	252	279	200	488	71.78	314	0.78
total	1867	762	948	818	892	762	1105	69.39	472	0.68
%		44.6	55.4	47.8	52.2	40.8	59.2			

Fig. 79. Data and results of 1867 iris clip lens implant operations performed by BINKHORST, WORST and 14 other Dutch ophthalmologists.

percentage visual acuity

	number	0–10	11–20	21–30	31–40	41–50	51–60	61–70	71–80	81–90	91–100	101–110	111–120	121–130	131–140	141–150	151–160	161–170	171–180	181–190	191–200	average visual acuity
BINKHORST	489	58	22	20	40	35	29	93	22	41	110	3	6	10	—	—	—	—	—	—	—	0.63
WORST	473	65	30	34	40	37	69	6	75	6	100	—	11	—	—	—	—	—	—	—	—	0.58
13 Dutch ophthal-mologists	526	46	10	9	26	37	30	41	70	29	128	14	69	5	2	4	1	—	—	—	5	0.79
total	1488	169	62	63	106	109	128	140	167	76	338	17	86	15	2	4	1	—	—	—	5	0.67
BINKHORST	489	11.9	4.5	4.1	8.2	7.2	5.9	19.0	4.5	8.4	22.5	0.6	1.2	2.0	—	—	—	—	—	—	—	0.63
WORST	473	13.7	6.3	7.2	8.5	7.8	14.6	1.3	15.9	1.3	21.1	—	2.3	—	—	—	—	—	—	—	—	0.58
13 Dutch ophthal-mologists	526	8.7	1.9	1.7	4.9	7.0	5.7	7.8	13.3	5.5	24.3	2.7	13.1	1.0	0.4	0.8	0.2	—	—	—	1.0	0.79
total	1488	11.4	4.2	4.2	7.1	7.3	8.6	9.4	11.2	5.1	22.7	1.1	5.8	1.0	0.2	0.3	0.1	—	—	—	0.3	0.67

Fig. 80. Comparison in numbers (above) and percentages (below) of the distribution of visual acuity results in 1488 iris clip lens implant operations performed by BINKHORST, WORST and 13 other Dutch ophthalmologists. The visual acuity of 5 cases treated by members of the group of Dutch ophthalmologists was unknown.

An inquiry amongst 26 Dutch ophthalmologists produced the following information:

1. BINKHORST lens implant operations were attempted for very diverse reasons, but mainly because of the better optical correction of aphakia, the restoration of binocular vision in unilateral senile or traumatic cataract, and because BINKHORST's results continued good after the experimental phase had been passed.

2. BINKHORST lens implant operations were discontinued by 3 ophthalmologists in view of difficulties of various kinds.

3. In general, preparation for the first independently-performed implant operation was good.

4. The first implant operation by 16 of the 26 ophthalmologists (61.5%) was carried out without the assistance of an experienced implant surgeon. The author maintains that this is not the correct procedure: beginners should be assisted by an experienced ophthalmologist for some time because, especially in the beginning, technical difficulties often have to be overcome.

5. Only 5 ophthalmologists (19.2%) are of the opinion that every ophthalmologist should be able to perform a BINKHORST lens implant operation.

The remaining 21 (80.8%) do not agree, holding that it should only be performed by ophthalmologists skilled in surgery, assisted by well-trained ophthalmic nurses, in very well equipped operating theatres.

The author agrees with COLENBRANDER (1971) who said that 'the risk of this operation is only acceptable at the hands of a very experienced surgeon'.

Three ophthalmologists therefore advocate the establishment in the Netherlands of centres for ophthalmic surgery. According to the author, such centres already exist, namely the University Eye Clinics and the Ophthalmic Hospital of The Hague apart from the more peripheral centres of BINKHORST and WORST.

6. The author agrees with the general opinion about the best way of training future implant surgeons: study of the literature and films followed by an assistantship with an experienced implant surgeon. This should involve observing, then assisting, and finally being assisted. The surgical technique used up to now for the extraction of cataracts may have to be modified in order to fulfil the conditions required for implantation. On the basis of his own experience the author feels that being assisted during the first implant operation(s) is most important. He would recommend starting independently with vertical iris clip lens implant operations in unilateral cataract in elderly people, since these are less difficult and carry the least risk. He is opposed to starting with bad risks since these eyes require the utmost care. If the results were unsatisfactory,

the ophthalmologist might become too disillusioned to continue his implant surgery.

The prospective implant surgeon will, of course, have to form his own opinion, based on the experience of others, about the contra-indications for BINKHORST lens implantations (see also page 217 and Fig. 71 at back of book).
7. The operating technique used was usually that of the instructing ophthalmologist, with numerous personal variations. Striking features were the preference for keratome incision and cryoextraction, the gradual change from horizontal to vertical implantation, the preference for peripheral iridectomy over iridotomy, and the progressive change from virgin silk to perlon corneo-scleral sutures.

The fact that the large variety of surgical techniques employed by the Dutch ophthalmologists did produce acceptable short-term results, is, according to the author, an indication that the most important point about surgical technique is that it should fulfil the conditions required for implantation (see page 46).
8. Twenty ophthalmologists (76.9%) considered bulging vitreous to be the prime problem prior to implantation.

In the author's opinion, this shows how important it is to have a very good anaesthetist for lens implant surgery. He must be familiar with the demands that eye surgery imposes on anaesthesia, in particular the promotion of a good hypotony of the eye. For instance, the author noticed a reduction in the bulging of the vitreous after the introduction of curare by the anaesthetist (see page 182). Massaging the globe just before the operation could help to reduce the volume of the vitreous.
9. Figs. 74 and 75 reveal the following noteworthy facts about the most important post-operative complications and their sequelae:
a. the percentage of *dislocations* is lower in the iris clip lens group than in the iridocapsular lens group (2.94 against 4.33). This, too, is the case with the last 494 cases of BINKHORST's iris clip lens series (see Fig. 30 on page 97), in which there were 18 eyes with dislocation(s) (3.64), as opposed to his iridocapsular lens series (5.29). This shows that the fixation of the iridocapsular lens poses more problems than that of the iris clip lens. This applies mainly to the early post-operative period: taking all the Dutch ophthalmologists together, i.e. including BINKHORST and WORST, 13 of the 19 iridocapsular lens dislocations occurred during the first two weeks after the implant operation.

The extraction of no less than 3 dislocated iris clip lenses, and a fourth because of dislocation *and* ECD, is in striking contrast with the results of BINKHORST and WORST, each of whom extracted only one dislocated lens. Moreover, it emphasizes the value of continuing instruction.

b.   the percentage of *ECD* cases, both total and partial, is much higher in the group of iris clip lens cases than in the group of iridocapsular lens cases (2.64 against 0.48). This, too, is the case with BINKHORST's series (6.03 against 0.59), even for the last 494 cases of his iris clip lens series where there were 23 cases of total or partial ECD (4.66). This goes to show the importance of the omission of the anterior loop for the prevention of ECD.

The percentage of ECD cases may decrease as the implant surgeon becomes more experienced, especially as far as the group of iris clip lens cases is concerned. But it may also increase during an observation period longer than the present average of about 314 days: in the BINKHORST series of 694 iris clip lens implantations, the first signs of total or partial ECD were detected within the first year in only 6 cases, whereas an additional 26 cases (3.75%) of total or partial ECD developed in the following three years (see Fig. 31 on page 101).

The fact that after nearly one year ECD had developed in 2.64% of the cases of the 22 Dutch ophthalmologists, as opposed to 0.86% after one year in BINKHORST's series, seems to be serious. However, these percentages cannot really be compared, since one year in the case of the 22 Dutch ophthalmologists indicates an *average* observation period and in BINKHORST's series it represents a *fixed* period of observation. Future evaluation of the long-term results must bring clarity in this very important matter.

c.   BINKHORST's percentages for dislocation and ECD are high (7.16 and 4.97). This is a result of his pioneering problems. For the 5th hundred iris clip lens implantations these percentages had dropped to 6 and 4, for the 6th hundred to 5 and zero, and for the last 94 cases it had dropped to 2.13 and zero (see Fig. 37 on page 114) after an average observation period of 383, 281 and 151 days respectively.

d.   the percentage of cases with retinal detachment (0.73) in the group of cases of the 22 Dutch ophthalmologists is low compared with BINKHORST's (1.85) and WORST's (1.80) figures. The author has no explanation for this discrepancy.

e.   the percentage of implant extractions in the iris clip lens series is lower than in the iridocapsular lens series (1.17 against 3.37), also in BINKHORST's series (0.57 against 1.76). This may be explained by the difference in frequency, known for BINKHORST's series (see Fig. 42 on page 124), in the use of iris clip lenses and iridocapsular lenses in cases that tend to produce complications. The latter applies to cases with congenital cataract (0.15 and 25.3) and traumatic cataract (7.5 and 33.5). The total percentage (1.54) is higher than in either BINKHORST's series (0.81) or WORST's series (1.20). This may be due to a vain hope that the extraction of an implant would exert a favourable influence on ECD, or to inexperience in repositioning dislocated implants.

214

f. As for post-operative uveitis (endogenous or exogenous), the incidence of at least 28 cases out of approx. 1230 cases (2.28 %) exceeds BINKHORST's 12 out of 866 cases (1.39 %) and is equal to WORST's 15 out of 665 cases (2.26 %). However, the number of cases considered to be exogenous infections (10) is relatively higher than in BINKHORST's series (3). The same holds good for the extraction of implants considered necessary in these cases: 8, 2, and zero, respectively. Surgical difficulties resulting in infection, and lack of experience in the treatment of the infection, may account for the difference. The explanation does *not* lie in the fact that the 22 Dutch ophthalmologists had not made a pre-operative conjunctival culture (see Fig. 71 at back of book), for BINKHORST and WORST had not done this either!

g. Ophthalmologists who performed their first BINKHORST lens implant operation alone, show slightly lower percentages for the most important post-operative complications and their sequelae than those who first operated under the supervision of a surgeon experienced in implant operations. It is precisely ECD, however, that is the exception.

10. The visual acuities obtained are very good, compared with those of BINKHORST and WORST. The percentage of iris clip lens implants with a visual acuity of 0.10 or less (8.7) is also lower than that of either BINKHORST (11.9) or WORST (13.7). The 46 cases with a visual acuity of 0.10 or less (see Fig. 80 on page 211) are explained for the greater part by 16 cases of total ECD and 9 cases of macular degeneration. Thirty-five of these 46 cases attained a visual acuity of 0.05 or less.

However, the difference in the kind of optotypes used to determine visual acuity seems to play an important part. Variations in results may, to some extent, be explained by this difference. Without the exceptional 0.99 average visual acuity obtained by ophthalmologist C, which was clearly overrated for patients with an average age of nearly 74, the average visual acuity of the Dutch ophthalmologists' patients would have been 0.70 instead of 0.78. This more nearly approaches the results of BINKHORST and WORST. It is the author's opinion that the fact that this series is based on non-homogeneous material affects the results.

Generally speaking, however, these good visual acuity results indicate that the Dutch ophthalmologists have profited by the experiences of BINKHORST and WORST, and are doing quite well.

11. The Dutch ophthalmologists' opinions on contra-indications for BINKHORST lens implant operations, formed partly as a result of their own experience, is expressed in order of votes in Fig. 71 at back of book. Noticeable is the high number of votes for *severe* diabetes mellitus as a contra-indication.

According to the author (ophthalmologist Q; see Fig. 71 at back of book)

FUCHS' corneal dystrophy should not be considered a contra-indication for BINKHORST lens implantation, because he believes that the risk to the corneal endothelium after cataract extraction *with* implantation of a BINKHORST lens, preferably without the anterior loops, is no greater than *without* implantation (see also page 104). Nor does he consider a history of uveitis a contra-indication, for the same reasons and in view of his own good results in case 17/52 on page 191 and case 26 on page 192.

12.   Besides BINKHORST and WORST, the 24 Dutch ophthalmologists are also a positively selected group from the viewpoint of their common interest in surgery. This is obvious from their results which prove that with good preparation technically skilled ophthalmologists can achieve good short-term results. Unfortunately, a large series of long-term results is not yet available.

PROSPECTS FOR THE FUTURE

BINKHORST lens implantation was initiated by some very skilled ophthalmologists (first group). Their results improved in the course of time thanks to improvements in implant design, indication and surgical technique.

They were later joined by a number of ophthalmologists with a special interest in surgery (second group), whose initial results were better than those of the first group. Obviously, however, all the experience of the first group could not be conveyed to the second group so that they had to learn again in part from the same mistakes. Examples of this are insufficient sparing of the corneal endothelium, little experience in repositioning dislocated lenses and the treatment of uveitis.

At present the second group is increasing all the time and soon a new group may form (third group) which will include almost all the remaining ophthalmologists. Whether or not this third group will actually develop probably depends on whether or not the second group's long-term results are acceptable. Unfortunately, these long-term results are not yet available.

Evaluation of the acceptability of the long-term results will naturally depend on individual standards. Whereas one ophthalmologist will be willing to tolerate 3 % ECD in view of the important optical advantages of the other 97 %, another ophthalmologist will find even one case of ECD unacceptable. Clearly a happy medium must be found.

Taking into consideration the initial problems that had to be solved, the author holds that the long-term results of the first group represented by BINKHORST and, in part, by WORST, are acceptable. The author also considers the short-term results of the second group, represented by the other 22 to 24

Dutch ophthalmologists, acceptable. Despite the fact that the study of their material is of limited value as the material is heterogeneous and the investigation retrospective, it seems justifiable to say that these acceptable short-term results do not exclude the possibility of the long-term results turning out to be acceptable too. However, since this remains to be seen, no definite answer can be given to the question posed on page 197, namely whether BINKHORST lens implant operations could suitably be performed by any ophthalmologist.

It is the author's firm conviction that an ophthalmologist who does not possess avowed surgical skill and interest should not start performing BINKHORST lens implant operations *at this moment*. It may even be that he should never start at all if the long-term results of the second group turn out to be unacceptable. An increase in the number of implants fitted would definitely be irresponsible under such circumstances. This implies that lens implant operations should not form part of the course of ophthalmological training *at this moment*.

It is possible, according to the author, that the long-term results will reveal a clear distinction between the first and second group of ophthalmologists, or between the second and third group. In the first case lens implant operations should be limited to a few very skilled ophthalmologists; in the second case they should be limited to ophthalmologists with a special interest in surgery. The latter possibility which the author feels to be a probability, would mean a division into ophthalmologists who do, and who do not perform implant operations.

Surgical results would improve as a result of such a division, because

1. it would produce a positive selection of ophthalmic *surgeons*.

2. these ophthalmic surgeons would gain experience more rapidly in the ophthalmic surgery centres and group practices, and the transfer of experience would be better, because a large part of the time spent working as a team would be devoted to ophthalmic surgery.

3. the technical facilities of these centres could be raised to a higher level than would be economically possible for the ophthalmic surgeon working on his own.

However, as long as all this has not been realised the author would suggest that only ophthalmologists with an interest in surgery should start to perform BINKHORST lens implant operations, and that in accordance with the guidelines set out on page 212 and in that particular order (see also page 201), after they have formed an opinion about the contra-indications as mentioned on pages 33, 53, 82, 123 and in Fig. 71 at back of book.

In the future, the long-term results of the second group will show whether the number of ophthalmologists performing implant operations can justifiably be increased.

In addition, the author would not exclude the possibility that in future the intraocular lens may yield ground in some areas to an improved contact lens. However, this would only apply in the case of patients young enough to learn to insert and remove the contact lens and also only in the case of binocular aphakics because of the degree of aniseikonia in unilateral aphakic contact lens wearers.

APPENDIX

BINKHORST lens implantation has not remained confined to the Netherlands. BINKHORST lenses have been fitted in about 20 countries from 1963 onwards (LÉONARD, 1973).

Detailed reports by an Australian, an English and an American ophthalmic surgeon are discussed below.

1. MAXWELL STUBBS (1967) fitted his first iris clip lens in October 1963 and reported in 1967 on 15 iris clip lens cases and 4 EPSTEIN lens cases. Complications mentioned include: threatened corneo-scleral iris prolapse due to the use of an insufficient number of sutures (1), epithelial oedema (3) which led in one patient to ECD, stromal oedema due to excessive manipulation during implantation (1), iritis (1), vitreous loss (1), retinal detachment (1), epithelial downgrowth (1), late corneal clouding or ECD (6) which was caused in 4 cases by increased IOP.

However, the most embarrassing complication was the formation of a membrane posterior (usually) or anterior to the implant (7) which necessitated needling (3). This was not associated with cellular intraocular reaction (MAXWELL STUBBS, 1967). MAXWELL STUBBS himself is convinced that the membrane was produced by iris epithelium growing over the surface of the lens. His conviction is based on the observation that no membranes were encountered when pilocarpine was prescribed for the night only instead of immobilising the iris completely by means of 4 instillations of pilocarpine per day (pers. comm. 25-10-1973).

The surgical facts mentioned such as the excessive manipulation of the lens during implantation resulting in endothelial damage and ECD, the vitreous loss resulting in upward decentration and ECD, and in addition the positioning of the superior loops in front of the iris (3) which resulted in upward decentration and incipient ECD (1), may have contributed towards the threshold of the maximum amount of tolerable endothelial trauma being passed, even when this did not become apparent immediately after the operation. It seems, therefore, that technical and surgical imperfections are responsible for the failure rate of about 30 % amongst the first 19 cases, not the implant itself.

2. FEDOROV inserted iris clip lenses in 8 patients after 1963. Since 1964 he has fitted 243 patients with his first modification (see page 28), and 876 patients with another modification (see Fig. 7 on page 30) since 1968. Also, since 1965 he has fitted 21 patients with an iridocapsular lens.

'The results of intraocular lens implantation gradually improved as the lens was further perfected, its weight reduced and advances made in surgical techniques. The best results were obtained with the last modification of the iris clip lens (three loops and three pintles): no ECD was detected in 876 implantations. The percentage of retinal detachments is insignificant, being smaller after the lens implant operations than after ordinary intracapsular cataract extraction. There were 9 cases of endophthalmitis.' (FEDOROV, pers. comm. 31-10-1973).

3. DALLAS (1970) fitted his first iris clip lens in January 1966, and reported in 1970 on 92 primary iris clip lens implantations (60 ♂ and 32 ♀, varying in age from 44 to 89 years) after zonulolytic intracapsular cryoextraction of cataracts of varying origin. He started with strictly unilateral cataract in adult patients, but later extended the indication to almost all types of cataract.

Complications mentioned include: vitreous loss (2) resulting in poor centration (1) and glaucoma (1), iris prolapse with delayed healing which ended in gross infection and evisceration (1), shallow anterior chamber (4), marked striate keratitis (3, of which 2 were persistent), uveitis (15, all cured), updrawn pupil (7), glaucoma (2), ECD (4), dislocation (3) necessitating extraction of the implant (1). The implant was extracted in another 5 cases because of: displacements (3), one of which necessitated evisceration, loss of the anterior chamber after removal of the suture (1), and persistent keratitis with pain ending in glaucoma (1). One case of gross corneal opacification required corneal grafting. Two cases of decentration required amputation of a temporal loop.

The favourable influence of growing experience is clearly demonstrated by the rising number of good results:

	first 48 eyes	last 44 eyes
successful operations	34 (70.8%)	40 (90.9%)
unsuccessful operations	6 (12.5%)	2 (4.55%)
unsatisfactory operations	8 (16.7%)	2 (4.55%)

4. HIRSCHMAN (1971) reported in 1971 on 150 implantations of either an iris clip lens or its FEDOROV modification. The first operation was performed in December 1967. He, too, initially selected only unilateral cases, but later on fitted other cases without contra-indications. Contra-indications were previous uveitis, severe diabetes mellitus, glaucoma requiring a filtering procedure later, cornea guttata or early dystrophy, narrow angles and extensive synechiae.

Complications mentioned include:

a. implant extraction (6) due to corneal touch resulting in ECD (1), chronic irritation after two retinal detachment operations (1) or after three dislocations (1), threatened corneal touch (2) and dislocation (1).

b. dislocation (17), treated by surgical manipulation (6, of which 5 occurred in the first 50 cases), by eye drops (10) or implant extraction (1).

c. retinal detachment (4) of which 3 were successfully treated with the lens left in place.

Difficulties arose more frequently amongst the first 50 cases than amongst the last fifty.

In 96% of cases the eye tolerated the lens without any reaction. Approximately 90% of the cases achieved a corrected visual acuity of 0.5 or better, whilst this level was reached by 33% without a correction.

CHAPTER VIII

HISTOPATHOLOGY

MANSCHOT is the only person who has performed extensive histopathological studies of eyes fitted with an iris clip lens or an iridocapsular lens (MANSCHOT, 1972, 1974). He has been kind enough to provide the author with additional information concerning his histological findings in 9 cases:

post-mortem: 6 eyes fitted with an iris clip lens.

2 eyes fitted with an iridocapsular lens.

post-operative: 1 eye fitted with an iridocapsular lens.

Case histories.

1.   Female, born 1906. Diabetes mellitus with bilateral diabetic retinopathy. BINK-HORST, case 143/171.

5– 3–64 intracapsular cataract extraction with iris clip lens implantation OD.

9– 2–65 ditto OS.

8–10–65 corrected visual acuity OS 0.55 (small aneurysm near the fovea centralis).

12– 4–67 posterior dislocation of implant OD.

15– 4–67 non-operative repositioning by tapping the eye under maximal mydriasis and with the patient in TRENDELENBURG position.

22– 4–67 uncorrected visual acuity OD 0.65.

30– 6–69 death of patient.

Histopathology. MANSCHOT, lab. no. O.482 R/L.

a)   The pupillary margin of both eyes showed severe pressure atrophy at the site of the four posterior loop attachments. These had made deep grooves, and an interruption of the sphincter muscle was observed (Figs. 81 and 82).

b)   These were the only two eyes in this series showing a remarkable lymphocytic infiltration of the iris stroma adjacent to the sphincter muscle accompanied by proliferation of stromal cells (Fig. 83). The latter finding might be an argument in favour of the view that it was probably mechanical irritation, not a toxic influence from the acrylic implant that was of predominant aetiological importance.

The disappearance of iris pigment epithelium in large areas must have been due to mechanical pressure and friction by the supramid wire loops.

c)   In both eyes the site of pigment epithelium loss had been partly covered by a thin layer of hyalin tissue.

2.   Male, born 1946. Rotterdam Eye Clinic case.

25–12–57 blunt air-gun accident OS which gave rise to a cloudy cortical cataract. A corneal perforation could not be found, and an X-ray examination revealed no intraocular foreign body.

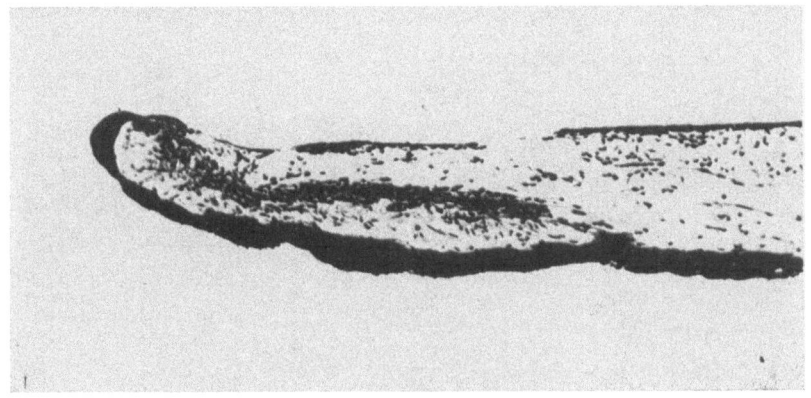

Fig. 81

Case no. 1, left eye. Pupillary margin between two posterior loop attachments. No pressure atrophy. Small ectropion uveae.

O.482 L, c. 120; H.E., ×225. Neg. 3036 (Courtesy W. A. MANSCHOT, M.D.).

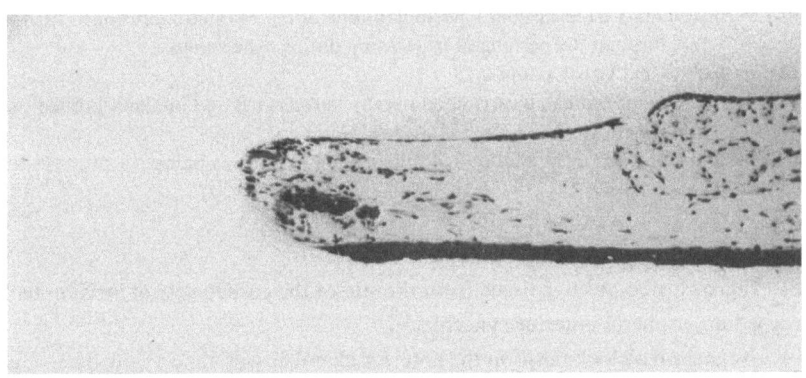

Fig. 82

Case no. 1, left eye. Pupillary margin at the site of a posterior loop attachment. Severe pressure atrophy; the sphincter muscle has almost disappeared.

O.482 L, c. 70; H.E., ×225. Neg. 3067 (Courtesy W. A. MANSCHOT, M.D.).

2– 7–58 preliminary needling (WAGENAAR).
7– 7–58 aspiration of lens material (WAGENAAR).
7– 8–62 needling of secondary cataract (WAGENAAR).
   Visual acuity with aphakic correction 1.0.
8– 4–65 diplopia. A contact lens was not tolerated.

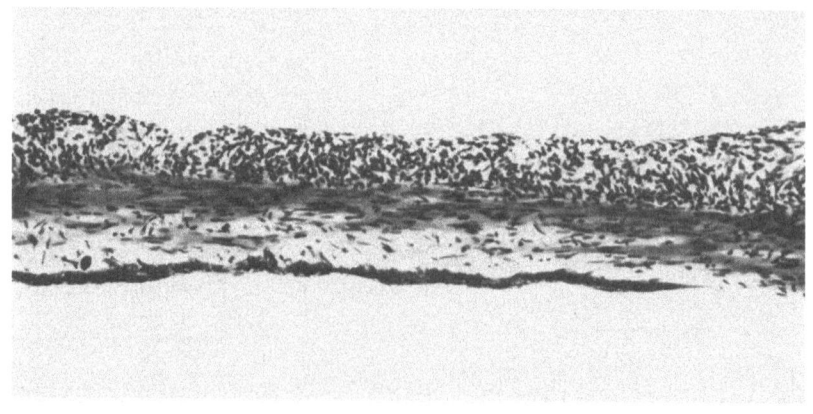

Fig. 83

Case no. 1, right eye. Hypercellularity anterior to the sphincter muscle due to infiltration by lymphocytes and proliferation of stromal cells.

O.482 R, c. 40; H. E., ×140. Neg. 22815 (Courtesy W. A. MANSCHOT, M.D.).

7– 1–70 secondary iridocapsular lens implant operation. Mannitol infusion. Vitreous loss through the peripheral iridectomy during synechiolysis.

14– 1–70 corrected visual acuity 0.75.

16– 1–70 a vitreous bubble, incarcerated nasally between iris and implant, pushed the implant forward.

18– 1–70 incipient purulent endophthalmitis ending in phthisis bulbi.

25– 2–70 enucleation.

Histopathology. MANSCHOT, lab. no. O. 517.

a) Ingrowing connective tissue from the site of the corneo-scleral incision had caused a peripheral anterior synechia.

b) Near the 6 o'clock position the anterior chamber was abnormally deep, due to shrinkage of a thick layer of connective tissue which occupied the pupillary area and had formed a cyclitic membrane. A ring-shaped SOEMMERING cataract adhered to the latter (see Fig. 84). This fibrous membrane was severely infiltrated by inflammatory cells; its shrinkage had also caused detachment of the ciliary body and of the peripheral parts of the retina and choroid.

c) The lower anterior part of the vitreous housed an abscess.

3. Female, born 1895. BINKHORST, case 214.

20– 1–66 unintentional extracapsular cataract extraction with iris clip lens implantation OD. Chymotrypsin used.

14– 7–69 uncorrected visual acuity 0.7.

7– 5–70 death of patient.

222

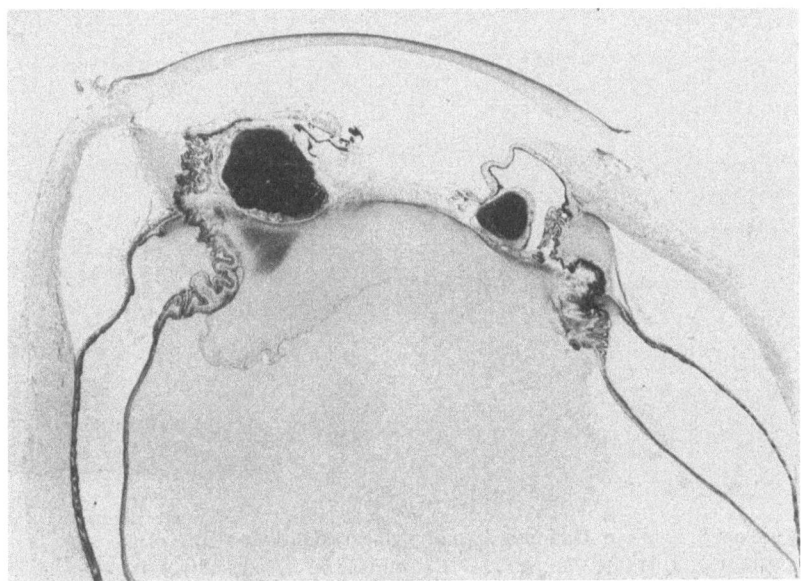

Fig. 84

Case no. 2, left eye. SOEMMERING cataract; layer of connective tissue in pupillary area. Abscess in anterior vitreous.

O.517 L, c. 12; H.E., ×6. Neg. 26717 (Courtesy W. A. MANSCHOT, M.D.).

Histopathology. MANSCHOT, lab. no. O.532.

a)   Pressure on the pupillary margin by the posterior loop attachments had caused complete local disappearance of the pupillary part of the iris and of the sphincter muscle.

b)   Local atrophy or disappearance of the pigment epithelium (see Fig. 85).

c)   Minor hyaline degeneration of the pupillary part of the stroma between sphincter muscle and pigment epithelium.

d)   No lymphocytic infiltration.

4.   Male, born 1892. Tuberculosis of lungs and vocal chords. BINKHORST, case IC 41/ IC 42.

1– 2–68 extracapsular cataract extraction with iridocapsular lens implant operations ODS.

2– 2–68 dislocation of both implants behind the iris due to the extremely posterior position of the capsular membrane.

5– 2–68 repositioned under mydriasis, with a needle knife. Pilocarpine hydrochloride 2% eye drops, twice daily, were prescribed.

18– 5–68 corrected visual acuity of each eye was 0.35.

1– 6–70 death of patient.

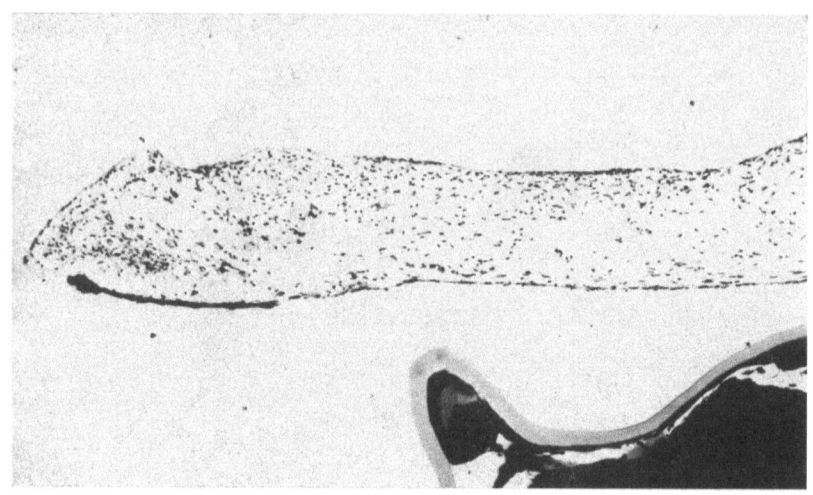

Fig. 85

Case no. 3, right eye. Disappearance of pigment epithelium.
O.532 R, c. 4; H.E., ×70. Neg. 26736 (Courtesy w. a. manschot, m.d.).

Histopathology. manschot, lab. no. O.533 R/L.

1. The sphincter muscle and the pigment epithelium were almost undamaged in the right eye, and they had atrophied in the left eye only on the nasal side (see Fig. 86).

2. No lymphocytic infiltration in the iris stroma of either eye.

5. Male, born 1903. Rotterdam Eye Clinic case.

9– 1–70 intracapsular cataract extraction with iris clip lens implantation OS. There were considerable difficulties with the implantation itself: the anterior superior loop, initially placed behind the iris at 1 o'clock, had to be repositioned immediately when transcorneal manipulation failed to rotate the implant clockwise. Large amount of pigment lost.

12– 1–70 dislocation of the superior loop in front of the iris, and of the inferior loop behind the iris.

16– 1–70 repositioning with a needle knife was only partly successful, because the anterior superior loop had been bent backwards *within* the greater posterior loop.

26– 1–70 visual acuity 0.1, with stenopaeic aperture 0.5. There was some damage to the corneal endothelium infero-temporally.

The eye remained irritated, and secondary glaucoma developed.

10– 7–70 macular oedema?

17– 7–70 acute glaucoma.

18– 7–70 peripheral iridectomy.

224

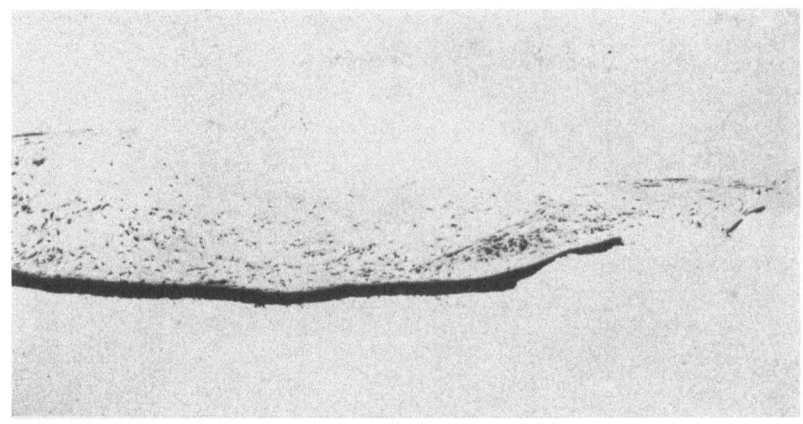

Fig. 86

Case no. 4, left eye. Atrophy of pupillary margin.
O.533 L, c. 3; H.E., × 54. Neg. 26725 (Courtesy w. a. MANSCHOT, M.D.).

24– 7–70 corrected visual acuity 0.25. The intraocular pressure was restored to normal,
  and the eye was quiet.
24– 2–71 visual acuity 0.15. Long-standing oedema at the posterior pole.
 9– 6–71 death of patient.

Histopathology. MANSCHOT, lab. no. O.638.
a) Four deep grooves in the pupillary margin with severe atrophy of the
sphincter muscle.
b) Part of the anterior superior loop was lying within a broad peripheral
anterior synechia of the iris caused by fibrous proliferation from the corneo-
scleral wound.
c) Necrosis of a large part of the superior half of the iris had taken place.
d) The previous site of the partially-dislocated posterior superior loop was in
the centre of the necrotic iris stroma (see Fig. 87).
e) Proliferated fibrous tissue on the inside of DESCEMET's membrane.
f) No pigment deposits in the filtration angle.

6. Male, born 1881. Rotterdam Eye Clinic case.
 5– 5–69 intracapsular cataract extraction with iris clip lens implantation OD.
25– 7–69 corrected visual acuity 0.66.
 2– 9–69 unintentional extracapsular cataract extraction with iris clip lens implantation OS.
  Post-operatively, a choroidal detachment developed which recovered
  spontaneously.

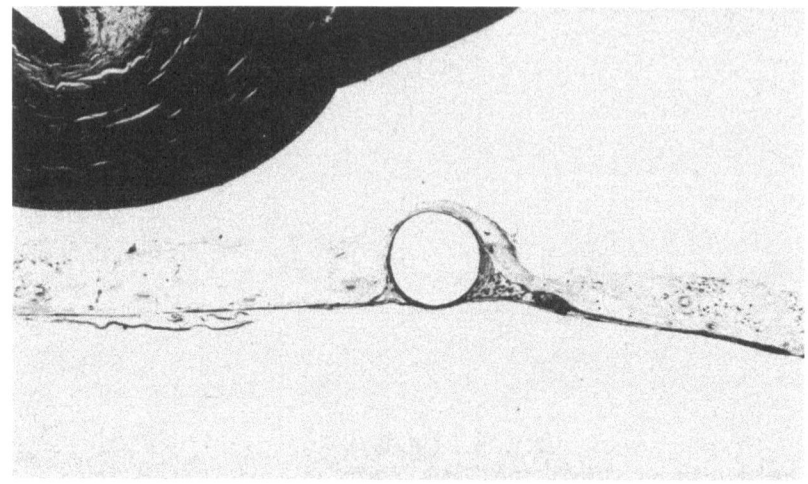

Fig. 87

Case no. 5, left eye. Necrosis of iris. Hiatus is artefact produced by fibrosis around posterior lens loop.

O.638 L, c. 10^9; H.E., ×54. Neg. 26732 (Courtesy W. A. MANSCHOT, M.D.).

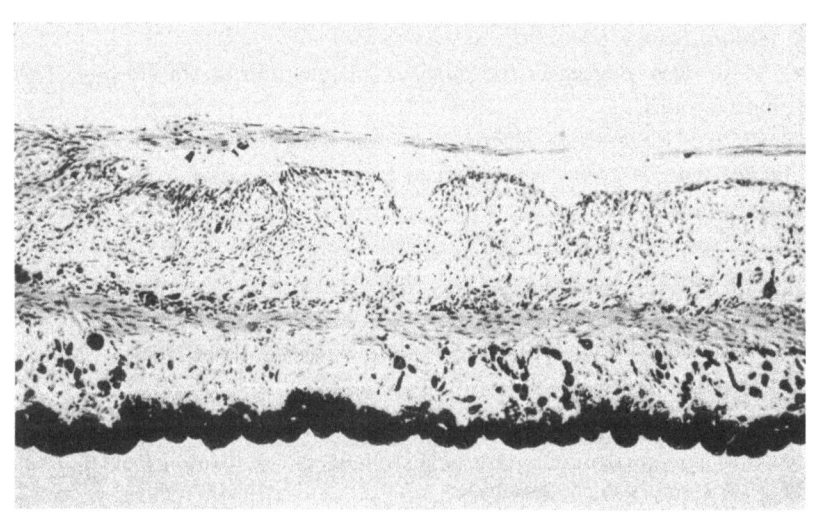

Fig. 88

Case no. 6, right eye. Proliferation of connective tissue over central part of iris.
O.690 R, c. 25; H.E., ×88. Neg. 26731 (Courtesy W. A. MANSCHOT, M.D.).

226

2– 3–70 corrected visual acuity R eye 0.9 and L eye 0.4.

Normal intraocular pressure.

6– 2–72 death of patient.

Histopathology. MANSCHOT, lab. no. O.690 R/L.

a) Four deep grooves in the pupillary margin with severe atrophy of the sphincter muscle in both eyes.

b) Melanophages and melanin granules in the lower part of both chamber angles.

c) Connective tissue had proliferated at the anterior side of the iris of the right eye, temporally near the sphincter muscle (see Fig. 88), and had most probably been caused by mechanical irritation by the wire loops.

d) Local atrophy of the pigment epithelium near the lower pupillary margin of the iris of the left eye.

e) Severe bilateral atrophy of the outer retinal layers and pigment epithelium near the macular region. This was most marked in the left eye.

SUMMARY

The general findings in the 8 post-mortem eyes were as follows:

1. Pressure atrophy of iris tissue, especially in the form of four deep grooves in the pupillary margin due to pressure by the posterior loop attachments, seemed to occur frequently in the iris clip lens cases. This atrophy was less severe in the two post-mortem eyes fitted with an iridocapsular lens, because fixation and centring of the latter type of implant is not effected by sphincter muscle action, but by adhesions in the iridocapsular cleft in which the two loops are embedded.

2. Minor connective tissue proliferation had occurred occasionally on either side of the iris, near the sphincter muscle. Lymphocytic infiltration in the stroma of the iris was found in only one case. It did not cause any discomfort to the patient nor were there any objective signs of inflammation. None of the other cases showed any sign of chronic infiltration.

3. The pigment epithelium regularly displayed local areas of atrophy. These seem to have been caused by mechanical pressure and friction exerted by the wire loops.

4. Pigment was found in the lower part of the filtration angle in one case only.

The findings in the only post-operative case were as follows: a cyclitic membrane, ingrowing connective tissue from the corneo-scleral wound, and a vitreous abscess.

Apart from one eye enucleated seven weeks after a secondary iridocapsular lens implantation, in which the diagnosis of purulent endophthalmitis could be confirmed histopathologically, histopathological examination by MANSCHOT of 8 post-mortem eyes fitted with an iris clip lens or an iridocapsular lens, revealed only mechanical sequelae inherent in the construction of the lens and of little or no clinical importance. Chronic infiltration in the stroma of the iris and some loose pigment in the lower part of the filtration angle, were found in only two separate cases, there had been no clinical symptoms.

Thus MANSCHOT's histopathological study proved the satisfactory tolerance of the eye to BINKHORST lens implants.

However, the severe atrophy of the sphincter muscle in eyes fitted with an iris clip lens was an additional reason for BINKHORST to abandon pupillary fixation in favour of a transiridectomy suture around the superior loops or, in an increasing percentage of cases, in favour of iridocapsular fixation (see Fig. 39 on page 122).

1. THE EFFECT OF PRIMARY BINKHORST LENS IMPLANTATION ON INTRAOCULAR PRESSURE (IOP) AND FACILITY OF OUTFLOW, WITH RESPECT TO THE COLOUR OF THE IRIS.

2. THE EFFECT OF SUPINE AND PRONE POSITION OF THE PATIENT ON THE POSITION OF THE BINKHORST LENS IN THE EYE AFTER INTRACAPSULAR AND EXTRACAPSULAR OPERATION RESPECTIVELY.

3. VISUAL IMPRESSIONS OF PATIENTS, INCLUDING 6 DOCTORS, AFTER A BINKHORST LENS IMPLANT OPERATION.

1. THE EFFECT OF PRIMARY BINKHORST LENS IMPLANTATION ON THE INTRA-OCULAR PRESSURE (IOP) AND FACILITY OF OUTFLOW, WITH RESPECT TO THE COLOUR OF THE IRIS.

In discussions with colleages, the supposition had been put forward that BINKHORST lens implantation would give rise to more loose pigment during and following implantation than a plain cataract extraction, especially in eyes

ophthal-mologist	colour of the iris	number	average age at operation in years	average observation period in days	average difference in IOP in mm Hg; fellow-eyes minus operated eyes	average difference in facility of outflow; fellow-eyes minus operated eyes
Author	brown	20	67.95	553	+1.17	−0.01
	non-brown	26	70.31	435	+3.00	0.00
	total	46	69.28	486	+2.20	0.00
BINKHORST	brown	17	65.76	1613	−0.09	−0.02
	non-brown	29	65.55	1690	+1.34	0.00
	total	46	65.63	1662	+0.82	−0.01

Fig. 89

Averages of the differences in IOP and facility of outflow of the operated eye and the non-operated fellow-eye, in 92 patients fitted with a unilateral primary BINKHORST lens implant, with respect to the colour of the iris.

with a brown iris. Since this pigment would impede the aqueous flow through the trabecular system, an increase in IOP and a decrease in the facility of outflow was to be expected. To test this supposition, ninety-two patients divided into two groups were examined:

1. Forty-six of the author's patients fitted with a unilateral primary iris clip lens implant. Twenty of these patients had brown eyes.

2. Forty-six of BINKHORST's patients fitted with a unilateral primary BINKHORST lens implant: 38 had been fitted with an iris clip lens and 8 with an iridocapsular lens. Seventeen of these patients had brown eyes. In both groups, only unilateral cases that had not undergone further operations of the pseudophakic eye or operations on the fellow-eye were selected.

The IOP was determined in all patients with a SCHIÖTZ tonometer and the facility of outflow with a MUELLER Tonograph Recorder Unit, Model EA. The author used the same instrument on all patients. The data obtained were analysed statistically* by P. VAN LEEUWEN, Head of the Department of Statistics, NIPG-TNO**, Leyden. The averages of the differences between operated eye and non-operated fellow-eye are shown in Fig. 89.

The conclusions based on the statistical evaluation are the following:

1. The difference between the average observation period of the author's patients and those of BINKHORST (486 against 1662 days) is highly significant (p≪0.01). The difference in the average age at operation (69.28 against 65.63 years) is not significant (p<0.10). Further analysis showed that there was no clear relation between observation period and IOP or facility of outflow. Therefore, when analysing the IOP or facility of outflow, it was not necessary to take the length of the observation period into account.

2. Intraocular pressure. The average difference in both groups between non-operated fellow-eyes and operated eyes (+2.20 and +0.82 mm Hg) is not significant (p<0.10).

3. Facility of outflow. The average difference in both groups between non-

---

* To check the hypotheses advanced in this chapter the following tests were used depending on the problem, the nature and the presentation of the data:
To compare two samples: STUDENT t Test, YATES Test.
To test differences in paired observations: STUDENT t Test, Rank Sign Test.
To test relationships: BRAVAIS PEARSON Correlation Coefficients, SPEARMAN Rank Correlations.
Only the p-values obtained from the tests are presented in the text.
** NIPG is the Netherlands Institute of Preventive Medicine.
TNO is the Netherlands Organization for Applied Scientific Research.

operated fellow-eyes and operated eyes (0.00 and –0.01) is not significant (p>0.10).

4. Colour of the iris. The average difference in IOP between non-operated fellow-eyes and operated eyes ($+3.00$ against $+1.17$ mm Hg and $+1.34$ against -0.09 mm Hg) is significantly greater ($p<0.05$) for the non-brown eyes than for the brown eyes. This is related to the fact that the IOP values of the non-operated fellow-eyes are significantly higher ($p<0.01$) for the non-brown eyes than for the brown eyes, whereas the IOP values of the operated eyes are similar.

Conclusion

Primary BINKHORST lens implantation has no significant influence on either IOP or facility of outflow.

The only difference in this respect between eyes with a brown iris and eyes with another colour iris is that the IOP values of the non-operated fellow-eyes are significantly higher in the group of non-brown eyes than in the group of brown eyes, whereas they are similar for the operated eyes.

2. THE EFFECT OF SUPINE AND PRONE POSITION OF THE PATIENT ON THE
POSITION OF THE BINKHORST LENS IN THE EYE AFTER INTRACAPSULAR
AND EXTRACAPSULAR OPERATION RESPECTIVELY.

For the determination of any gravitational antero-posterior movement of a BINKHORST lens, the depth of the anterior chamber had to be measured with the patient's head in supine and prone positions. These measurements were made with the help of an accessory built according to the instructions of C. D. BINK-HORST, which made it possible for a HAAG-STREIT slitlamp no. 900 with depth-measuring attachment II attached to an examination table to be directed either downwards or upwards, as shown in Figs. 90 and 91. All measurements were independently performed by two observers, namely L. H. LOONES, technical assistant of C. D. BINKHORST, and the author. The data obtained were only accepted if both measurements were approximately the same. They were statistically analysed by P. VAN LEEUWEN, Head of the Department of Statistics, NIPG-TNO, Leyden.

a. The results of the measurement of the anterior chamber depth, with the patient's head supine or prone, in 20 intracapsular and 17 extracapsular cases with a BINKHORST lens implant, are shown in Fig. 92.

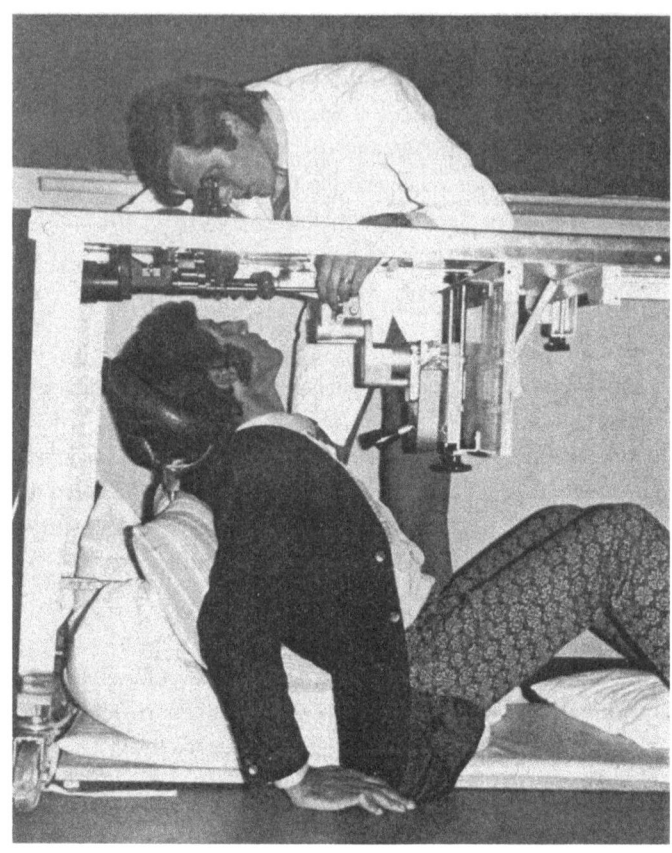

Fig. 90

L. H. LOONES measuring the anterior chamber depth with the patient's head supine.

The conclusions of the statistical evaluation are the following:

1. The average difference of the anterior chamber depth, measured with the patient's head supine or prone, is significantly larger ($p < 0.05$) in the intracapsularly-operated eyes than in the extracapsularly-operated eyes (0.24 against 0.12 mm).

2. The average anterior chamber depth, measured with the patient's head supine, is significantly smaller ($p < 0.05$) in intracapsularly-operated eyes than in extracapsularly-operated eyes (3.31 against 3.52 mm).

3. The average anterior chamber depth, measured with the patient's head

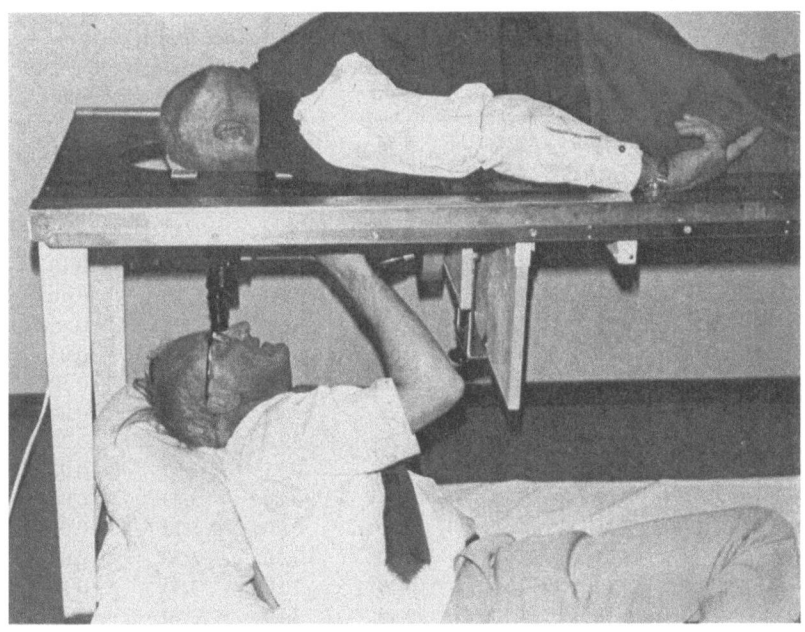

Fig. 91

The author measuring the anterior chamber depth with the patient's head prone.

prone, is also significantly smaller (p<0.05) in intracapsularly-opeıated eyes than in extracapsularly-operated eyes (3.07 against 3.39 mm).

b.   The results of the measurement of the anterior chamber depth, with the patient's head supine oı prone, in 9 eyes after intracapsular implantation and 10 eyes after extracapsular implantation, compared with the values of the non-operated fellow-eyes, are shown in Figs. 93 and 94. These eyes are the same as in Fig. 92, but only those with a normal fellow-eye have been enumerated here.

The conclusions of the statistical evaluation are the following:
1.   In the intracapsularly-operated cases, the differences in measurements in the supine and prone positions for the operated eyes are significantly greater (p = 0.01) than for the non-operated fellow-eyes (0.23 against 0.02 mm). However, this does not apply (p>0.01) to the extracapsularly-operated cases (0.07 against 0.05 mm).
2.   In the intracapsularly-operated cases, the values for the anterior chamber

	intracapsular cases			extracapsular cases		
	supine	prone	difference (mm)	supine	prone	difference (mm)
	3.45	3.20	0.25	3.90	3.85	0.05
	3.50	3.10	0.40	3.30	3.05	0.25
	3.20	2.80	0.40	3.55	3.55	0.00
	3.55	3.30	0.25	3.50	3.50	0.00
	3.35	3.20	0.15	3.80	3.70	0.10
	3.30	3.15	0.15	3.30	2.90	0.40
	3.20	2.90	0.30	3.10	2.75	0.35
	3.40	3.10	0.30	3.00	2.95	0.05
	3.45	3.25	0.20	4.00	3.50	0.50
	3.20	2.95	0.25	3.40	3.40	0.00
	3.50	3.25	0.25	3.10	2.90	0.20
	3.15	3.15	0.00	3.85	3.85	0.00
	3.40	3.25	0.15	3.60	3.60	0.00
	2.65	2.65	0.00	3.70	3.70	0.00
	3.25	2.75	0.50	3.30	3.30	0.00
	3.10	2.90	0.20	3.60	3.50	0.10
	3.50	3.10	0.40	3.80	3.70	0.10
	2.95	2.85	0.10			
	3.80	3.50	0.30			
	3.20	2.95	0.25			
average	3.31	3.07	0.24	3.52	3.39	0.12

Fig. 92

Results of the measurement of the anterior chamber depth with the patient's head supine or prone, in 20 intracapsular (iris clip lenses) and 17 extracapsular (5 iris clip lenses and 12 iridocapsular lenses) cases of BINKHORST lens implantation.

depth measured supinely are significantly higher (p<0.05) than in the non-operated fellow-eyes (3.29 against 3.03 mm). However, this does not apply (p>0.10) to the extracapsularly-operated cases (3.47 against 3.42 mm).

3. In the intracapsularly-operated cases, the values for the anterior chamber depth measured in the prone position do not differ significantly (p>0.10) from those of the non-operated fellow-eyes (3.06 against 3.02 mm). This applies equally (p>0.10) to the extracapsularly-operated cases (3.40 against 3.37 mm).

4. In the non-operated fellow-eyes, the difference in anterior chamber depth measured in the supine and prone positions (0.02 and 0.05 mm) is extremely small (p>0.10).

ophthalmologist	serial number	operated eye			non-operated fellow-eye		
		supine	prone	difference (mm)	supine	prone	difference (mm)
Author	38	3.15	3.15	0.00	2.80	2.80	0.00
Author	77	3.40	3.25	0.15	3.45	3.40	0.05
BINKHORST	280	3.50	3.25	0.25	2.80	2.80	0.00
BINKHORST	462	3.20	2.95	0.25	3.50	3.50	0.00
BINKHORST	474	3.25	2.75	0.50	2.95	2.95	0.00
BINKHORST	488	2.95	2.85	0.10	2.90	2.85	0.05
BINKHORST	506	3.20	2.90	0.30	2.95	2.95	0.00
BINKHORST	543	3.80	3.50	0.30	3.35	3.30	0.05
BINKHORST	568	3.20	2.95	0.25	2.60	2.60	0.00
average of 9 intracapsular cases		3.29	3.06	0.23	3.03	3.02	0.02

Fig. 93

Results of the measurement of the anterior chamber depth, in supine or prone position, of 9 eyes after *intracapsular* cataract extraction and iris clip lens implantation, compared with the values of the non-operated fellow-eyes.

ophthalmologist	serial number	operated eye			non-operated fellow-eye		
		supine	prone	difference (mm)	supine	prone	difference (mm)
BINKHORST	533	3.30	3.05	0.25	3.30	3.30	0.00
BINKHORST	70	3.00	2.95	0.05	3.30	3.30	0.00
BINKHORST	1022	3.40	3.40	0.00	3.40	3.40	0.00
BINKHORST	1025	3.10	2.90	0.20	3.10	3.00	0.10
BINKHORST	1030	3.85	3.85	0.00	3.60	3.60	0.00
BINKHORST	1031	3.60	3.60	0.00	3.70	3.65	0.05
BINKHORST	1036	3.70	3.70	0.00	3.40	3.30	0.10
BINKHORST	1038	3.30	3.30	0.00	3.20	2.95	0.25
BINKHORST	1040	3.60	3.50	0.10	3.50	3.50	0.00
BINKHORST	1041	3.80	3.70	0.10	3.70	3.70	0.00
average of 10 extracapsular cases		3.47	3.40	0.07	3.42	3.37	0.05

Fig. 94

Results of the measurement of the anterior chamber depth, with the patient's head supine or prone, in 10 eyes after *extracapsular* cataract extraction and iridocapsular lens implantation, compared with the values of the non-operated fellow-eyes. Note: the first case is that of an iris clip lens.

From the ophthalmological point of view, it may be concluded that:

1. the anterior chamber depth is significantly larger in the extracapsularly-operated cases than in the intracapsularly-operated cases, in both the supine and prone positions.

The assumption that, after extracapsular extraction, the implanted lens is pushed forward by the thickness of the capsular membrane (BINKHORST, 1967ac, 1969abcd, 1971a) is incorrect. On the contrary, the opposite is true.

2. the difference in the anterior chamber depth in the supine and prone positions is significantly larger in the intracapsularly-operated cases than in the extracapsularly-operated cases.

3. the difference in the anterior chamber depth in the supine and prone positions is significantly larger in the operated eyes than in the non-operated fellow-eyes, but this applies only to the intracapsularly-operated cases.

4. the anterior chamber depth in the supine position is significantly larger in the operated eyes than in the non-operated fellow-eyes, but this applies only to the intracapsularly-operated cases.

Points 1 and 2 indicate that in extracapsularly-operated cases the vitreous is held back. This can only be done by the capsular membrane acting in conjunction with any peripheral lens remnants. This capsular membrane, to which the BINKHORST lens should be fixed in extracapsularly-operated cases, also ensures that in the prone position the lens is, on average, only 0.12 mm nearer to the cornea than in the supine position. In the 4 extracapsularly-operated cases where the lens was 0.25, 0.35, 0.40, and 0.50 mm nearer to the cornea, the author feels it is reasonable to assume that the lens did not become fixed to the capsular membrane or to the peripheral lens remnants, but to the iris by means of synechiae, for example, or that miosis alone was responsible, In the remaining 13 extracapsularly-operated cases the lens moves, on average, only 0.05 mm nearer the cornea.

Although it cannot be proved, this fact may contribute to the decrease in the percentage of ECD occurring after implantation of a BINKHORST lens after intentional *extracapsular* cataract extraction, as well as to the decrease in the percentage of retinal detachments following intentional extracapsular implantation in senile cases (see Figs. 45 and 46 on page 137).

Points 3 and 4 indicate that in cases where the anterior chamber depth differs only a little from that of the non-operated fellow-eye, the BINKHORST lens is moved backwards by a change from the prone to the supine position, but that this only holds good for intracapsularly-operated cases. This means that in intracapsularly-operated cases the aqueous and vitreous allow the lens and the iris diaphragm considerable freedom of movement both forwards and backwards. This is a logical sequence to the absence of zonular fixation of the implanted lens to the ciliary body. However, in cases with extracapsular fixation the posterior displacement is considerably restricted by the capsular membrane.

Conclusion

The range of gravitational antero-posterior movement of a BINKHORST lens in cases with extracapsular fixation, is about as small as that of the crystalline lens; in intracapsular cases it is about 0.2 mm larger, because of the increased freedom of mobility of lens and iris diaphragm in both anterior *and* posterior directions.

3. VISUAL IMPRESSIONS OF PATIENTS, INCLUDING 6 DOCTORS, AFTER A BINKHORST LENS IMPLANT OPERATION.

Patients of BINKHORST and WORST made only occasional mention of the following subjective impressions:

a. photophobia (see also page 29)
    – two patients complained of photophobia (BINKHORST, case 382; WORST, case 380/383).
    – a third patient did not dare to drive a car any longer because it dazzled him to drive from shadow into sun (BINKHORST, case 296/315).
b. colour vision
    – colours appeared more saturated (BINKHORST, cases 1025 and 1053).
    – colours appeared rosier (BINKHORST, cases 233 and 1025), in particular the blue sky (BINKHORST, case 233).
c. miscellaneous
    – observation of 4 specks 'in' the eye. These did not cause any visual disturbance (BINKHORST, case 1053).
    – a sensation as if water were shaking inside the eye (WORST, see case 508 on page 159: iris medallion lens).
    – the image produced by the operated eye rocked about (WORST, case 117).
The author questioned a small group of selected patients about the visual impressions mentioned above. Since doctors may be considered to be trained observers, the author questioned those colleagues who had undergone a BINKHORST lens implant operation. The usual data and results of these doctors' eyes that had been fitted with an implant, are given in Fig. 95.

doctor's initials	sex	year of birth	ophthalmologist	serial number	operation date	L or R eye	latest refraction date	corrected visual acuity
v.O–d.G	♀	1895	OOSTINGH iris clip lens	4	21– 9–70	R	1– 2–73	1.0
				84	14– 9–72	L	1– 2–73	1.0
K	♂	1907	WORST iris clip lens sutured to iris	287	28–10–70	R	3–12–70	1.0
B	♂	1894	WORST iris medallion lens	578	13–10–71	R	30– 1–73	1.0
				887	28– 9–72	L	30– 1–73	0.8
G	♂	1910	BINKHORST iridocapsular lens	IC 141	8–12–71	L	23– 3–73	0.75
				IC 218	18–10–72	R	23– 3–73	1.0
L	♂	1918	BINKHORST iridocapsular lens	IC 175	27– 4–72	R	10–11–72	1.0
				IC 194	28– 6–72	L	10–11–72	0.75
S	♂	1898	Author iris clip lens	115	1–11–73	R	19– 6–74	0.9

Fig. 95
Data and results in the cases of 6 doctors fitted with a BINKHORST lens implant.

These doctors were requested to answer the following written questions:
1. *Question:* Were you bothered by light after the implant operation?

Replies:
  – not bothered (S).
  – less bothered by light (v.O–d.G.).
  – looking at light sources placed high up sometimes produced a halo around the light source, but this did not apply to objects straight ahead (K).
  – light falling on the operated eye produces a very unpleasant sensation. This makes it necessary to wear dark glasses when the light is very bright (B).
  – some trouble with glare when the sun is very bright; oncoming traffic using headlights also causes some bother when not wearing dark glasses (G).
  – bright light, especially from the side, is bothersome because of reflections when driving a car (L).

238

2. *Question:* Did the world appear rosier or bluer to your operated eye after the operation?

Replies:
- unchanged (B).
- the colours became much brighter and more saturated than before, perhaps everything was somewhat bluer (v.O-d.G).
- the world appears to be a somewhat hazy blue, especially during the daytime on a bright day; at night, strong white light sources appear to have a violet tinge (K).
- when I do not protect my eyes during the daytime with dark glasses (40% absorption) I see a rosy image all evening, and white light sources in particular become clearly violet in colour (G).
- initially the blue of the sky was somewhat rosier (L).
- the world is somewhat bluer (S).

3. *Question:* Did you make certain entoptic observations?

Replies:
- no entoptic observations (v.O-d.G, L and S).
- I see the edge of the lens (K).
- until a considerable time after the operation I saw a vibrating thread in the right upper quadrant (B).
- the first few months after the operation I sometimes saw, without any obvious reason, a trap-door in the image within which everything vibrated in a vertical direction. This lasted a few seconds only (G).

4. *Question:* Did you notice anything of the intraocular lens moving when the eye or head was moved?

Replies:
- no movement observed (v.O-d.G, B, G and S).
- during the first year after the operation extra images occurred on looking forward. This gave the impression that the intraocular lens was rocking. This phenomenon disappeared during the past year, which gave me the impression that the lens had become better fixated (K).
- I still don't dare to make sudden movements (L).

5. *Question:* Have you noticed any difference in reading distance in the operated eye, in the supine and prone positions?

Replies:

- no noticeable difference (K, G and L; the latter two had been fitted with an iridocapsular lens).
- the reading distance is a little greater in the supine position (v.O-d.G).
- supine 34 cm, prone 31 cm (S).
- I hardly ever read lying down (B).

Summary

a) Photophobia, especially when light is incident from the side, was present in 4 of the 6 doctors. On questioning patients, PEARCE (1972) encountered this phenomenon to a small extent in 23 of the 72 cases (32%). BINKHORST tried as much as possible to prevent the retina from being overexposed by light. To this end, he reduced the diagonals of the square formed by the posterior loop attachments from 4 to 3 mm in the beginning of 1972. This made it possible for the pupil to assume a diameter of 3 mm (see page 29).

b) Colours appeared to be brighter and more saturated than before. To four of the doctors, the world appeared bluer with the eye that had been operated on. In this respect the pseudophakic eye is no different from the aphakic eye.

KOVAL (1969) investigated the colour discrimination of 13 aphakic, 44 pseudophakic and 68 normal eyes by means of an anomaloscope. The increased sensitivity for violet in the aphakic eye, caused by the absence of the blue, violet, and ultraviolet-absorbing properties of the senile lens, appeared to be reduced when a lens made of Russian perspex was fitted. No difference was encountered in colour discrimination in the red-green region between spectacle lenses and intraocular lenses.

c) Entoptic observations can be manifold. In some cases, apparently, parts of the posterior loops or their attachments are observed, especially if the light is incident from the side.

d) Movements of the image are seldom noticed.

According to PEARCE (1972), 'some of the 72 patients noted lens movement on movement of the head, but this was not a severe complaint'.

e) There is a theoretical explanation for the somewhat greater reading distance in the supine position. It also corresponds with the findings for the intracapsular iris clip lens implants reported on page 232 ff.

The same applies for the reading distances being equal in iridocapsular lens cases.

When calculating the power of the intraocular lens, it was shown that if the distance behind the anterior vertex of the cornea was reduced by approximately 0.3 mm, the power of the implant lens had to be reduced by approximately 0.5 D (see page 12). If this were not done, GULLSTRAND's schematic eye would be $0.68 \times 0.3 = 0.204$ D (see Fig. 3 on page 8) myopic in the anterior focal plane, which would also hold good, approximately, for a vertex distance of 12 mm. This is about equal to the relative myopia of $\dfrac{1}{0.31} - \dfrac{1}{0.34} = 0.28$ D in the case of dr. S. However, this relative myopia is not always noticed by iris clip lens patients in the prone position.

It is the author's experience that patients are, in general, extremely satisfied with their BINKHORST lens.

Conclusion

The complaints that may be caused by a BINKHORST lens implant are few on the whole and can be alleviated in part by sunglasses. They are much less severe than the complaints caused by a spectacle lens correction or a contact lens correction (see Chapter I).

SUMMARY

1. The advantages of implanting a lens made of synthetic material, after a cataract extraction, do not counterbalance the dangers associated with it.
Proposition IX of the thesis by c. h. o. m. von winning, Leyden, 17-12-*1952*.

2. The artificial intraocular lens may be considered to be a great asset to ophthalmology when the indications are carefully considered and the operation technique is adequate.
Proposition 12 of the thesis by a. f. deutman jr., Rotterdam, 13-1-*1971*.

CHAPTER I

COMPARISON OF SPECTACLE LENS, CONTACT LENS AND INTRAOCULAR LENS.
ADVANTAGES AND DISADVANTAGES.

An eye that has become aphakic as a result of cataract extraction, can be opti cally corrected in three ways: by means of a lens placed *in front*, *on*, or *in* the eye.

The lens placed *in front* of the eye, that is in the spectacle frame, has the following disadvantages: magnification of the image by about 25%, spherical aberration, ring scotoma and the associated 'Jack-in-the-box 'and 'welsh' phenomena.

The lens placed *on* the eye, the contact lens, magnifies the image by only some 7% and does not suffer from the other disadvantages of spectacle correction. Moreover, it may result in an optical improvement in the case of a not-too-serious corneal scar. Apart from the general disadvantages of the contact lens, its use is limited because older patients and children experience practical difficulties with insertion and removal. Experience has shown that in the course of time an increasing number of patients stop wearing their contact lenses, especially when there is insufficient motivation as in unilateral aphakia.

The lens placed *in* the eye, the intraocular lens, provides the best optical correction of aphakia by its permanent presence, the absence or only minimal alteration of the image size, and the fact that it can be fitted at any age. In unilaterally aphakic children it simplifies the treatment of amblyopia and increases the chances of restoring binocular vision. It can help unilateral aphakic adults to fulfil the strict conditions of admission to several jobs and professions.

Inequality of the size of the image formed in each eye (aniseikonia) is present to a high degree in unilateral aphakia corrected by spectacles. This inequality is less in contact lens corrections, but is still often too great for binocular vision. In intraocular corrections it may even be eliminated altogether.

Binocular vision is still possible when the image size difference is 5–8 %, but aniseikonia may give rise to complaints even when this percentage is much smaller. In general, the intraocular lens provides the best chance of restoring binocular vision in unilateral aphakia. By taking measurements of both eyes, it is possible to calculate the power of the intraocular lens required to obtain exactly equal image size in the case of the individual patient.

CHAPTER II

HISTORY OF INTRAOCULAR LENS IMPLANTS.

On 29th November 1949, after performing an extracapsular cataract extraction, RIDLEY fitted, for the first time in a human being, an intraocular lens in the posterior chamber of the eye. It was made of perspex, and implanted without fixation and without corneo-scleral sutures. This RIDLEY lens, since fitted in more than a thousand eyes, produced many complications: posterior dislocation in 6 % of the cases, iritis, and secondary glaucoma, necessitating extraction of the implant in 15 % of the cases.

Almost all the types of anterior chamber lenses with fixation in the chamber angle since developed, produced corneal dystrophy in a high percentage of cases. Only the CHOYCE Mark VIII lens did not.

The first anterior chamber lens with iris fixation was the 'collar-stud' lens of EPSTEIN, a modification of the RIDLEY lens.

BINKHORST developed the iris clip lens during the years following 1958. This anterior chamber lens which was fitted for the first time on 11th August 1958, has two anterior and two posterior loops to fixate the optic portion to the iris diaphragm. The iris clip lens was intended to help prevent dislocation *and* corneal dystrophy, which were the major complications in posterior chamber implants and chamber angle-fixated lenses respectively.

The most important modifications to the iris clip lens were placing the anterior and posterior loops at right angles to each other (FEDOROV in 1964), the irido-capsular lens (BINKHORST in 1965) and the iris medallion lens (WORST in 1970). These four lenses are called by the author collectively the BINKHORST lens. The iridocapsular lens has only posterior loops that, after an extracapsular cataract extraction, keep the lens in place through being embedded in the iridocapsular membrane. The iris medallion lens, also without anterior loops, is suspended from the iris by a perlon suture. The advantages and disadvantages of these lenses are discussed.

243

CHAPTER III

TECHNIQUES.

Three aspects are discussed: 1. material used and its sterilisation, 2. surgical techniques, and 3. treatment of the post-operative complications.

Polymethylmethacrylate (perspex), because of its utter inertness, proved to be an extremely suitable material for making an intraocular lens. An intraocular state of irritation originally ascribed to the perspex, turned out to be caused by the fluids used to sterilise the implant. Irritation did not occur when the lens was sterilised with NaOH which was neutralised during the operation by NaHCO₃, after which the lens was rinsed in saline.

The surgical techniques used to fit the implant and the preparation and after-care of patients fitted with an iris clip lens, an iridocapsular lens or an iris medallion lens are discussed for both intracapsular and extracapsular cataract extraction. The most important complications during the fitting of an iris clip lens are: bulging vitreous, incarceration of vitreous between the loops or between the iris and the lens, and vitreous loss. The latter complication is a contra-indication for implantation. Particular cases call for special surgical techniques. Examples are iridencleisis, radial iridotomy, and severe damage to the anterior segment of the eye.

Post-operative complications are classified as occurring early or late, or early and late. Particular mention is made of the treatment of pupillary block, dislocation, and corneal dystrophy.

CHAPTER IV

RESULTS OBTAINED BY C. D. BINKHORST.

The 866 BINKHORST lens implant operations carried out by BINKHORST himself up to 1st January 1972 are divided into iris clip lens implants, iridocapsular lens implants, and the first FEDOROV modification. These three groups are subdivided according to type of cataract, patient's sex, left or right eye, binocular or monocular implant fitted, age at operation, observation period and, finally, visual acuity obtained.

In the group of iris clip lens implant operations (694 eyes), post-operative complications such as dislocation and corneal dystrophy are extensively discussed, and classified according to frequency, cause, prevention, therapy and consequences. The loop length proved to be of paramount importance for the relative frequency of both complications. To prevent dislocation of the implant, regular instillation of pilocarpine or loop suturing were useful. The pre-operative condition of the cornea, especially whether or not FUCHS' dystrophy was present, was an important factor in the rise of corneal dystrophy. During and after the operation it was of importance whether serious complications occurred, and whether there was contact between loop(s) and cornea. The consequences of dislocation were, in general, slight; those of corneal dystrophy, however, were usually very serious: only eyes starting to show corneal dystrophy or threatening to develop it reacted favourably to amputation of the loop(s). In the event of total corneal dystrophy, penetrating keratoplasty sometimes proved to offer the only hope of obtaining an increase of visual acuity. Over the years, the frequency of both dislocation and corneal dystrophy decreased considerably.

In the groups of special cases, glaucoma and diabetes mellitus with or without diabetic retinopathy, did not prove to be contra-indications for iris clip lens implantation.

The group of iridocapsular lens implant operations (170 eyes) was divided up according to the cause of the cataract. Unlike congenital bilateral cataract, congenital unilateral cataract was found to be a contra-indication for operative treatment in view of the other congenital defects that often accompany it. In cases of traumatic cataract, iridocapsular lens implantation proved to produce less satisfactory orthoptic results only if the trauma had occurred before the age of 5 and the patient in question had received treatment too late. In case of complicated cataract, juvenile cataract, cataract of unknown origin, and senile cataract, the results were equally good whether the eye had been fitted with an iridocapsular lens or an iris clip lens.

The percentage of complications after the fitting of an iridocapsular lens is about half that arising after an iris clip lens implantation, and corneal dystrophy is only one-tenth as frequent.

CHAPTER V

RESULTS OBTAINED BY J. G. F. WORST.

The 665 BINKHORST lens implant operations performed by J. G. F. WORST up to 1st January 1972 were treated in the same way as those of BINKHORST in Chapter IV. A direct comparison of the series of BINKHORST and WORST could not easily be made because of the differences in causation of cataract, type of implant used, observation period, and optotypes used to dertermine visual acuity. Nevertheless, WORST's results for visual acuity and complications during and after the operation proved to be comparable to those of BINKHORST provided only the last 400 cases of BINKHORST were taken into consideration.

By suturing the iris clip lens to the iris the percentage of dislocations was reduced from 3.36 to 2.02; however, the percentage for corneal dystrophy increased from 1.68 to 2.83.

In the groups of special cases, glaucoma and diabetes mellitus with or without diabetic retinopathy were once again shown not to constitute contra-indications for iris clip lens implantation.

CHAPTER VI

RESULTS OBTAINED BY THE AUTHOR.

The first 72 iris clip lens implant operations performed by the author on 61 patients of 50 years of age or over, were classified in the same way as those of BINKHORST and WORST. In addition, information about the colour of the iris, corneal astigmatism, stereopsis, intraocular pressure, and the facility of outflow was provided.

Optimal visual acuity was reached 6–8 weeks after the operation in 40 eyes (without complications), in 16 eyes (also without complications) after 4–18 months; in the remaining 16 eyes, the results for visual acuity varied because of temporary or permanent complications.

Stereopsis, direction of the implant, pupil shape, and findings obtained by means of gonioscopy, were all studied separately. Stereopsis was always present unless a reduction of the visual acuity of one eye prevented it. These results were in complete agreement with those determined by the author in a series of 58 patients fitted by BINKHORST with an iris clip lens.

It appeared that the direction of the loops of the implant could subsequently differ from the original vertical position.

Notwithstanding instillation of pilocarpine, the pupils of 13 eyes were not quite square in shape. The causes are discussed.

Gonioscopy revealed no more iris pigment in the chamber angle than after cataract extraction without lens implantation. In 19 eyes, peripheral synechiae were seen to be attached to the wound or to the line of SCHWALBE. Sixteen were on the right-hand side of the eye in question, which was thought to be due to the surgical technique used.

The visual acuity results in this series, and the complications during and after the operation, did not show any great discrepancies compared with those of BINKHORST and WORST.

In the groups of special cases, the loop suture, the combination of synechiolysis, radial iridotomy and loop suture, the overgrowth of an anterior loop by pigmented iris tissue, and diabetes mellitus were discussed. Diabetes mellitus,

246

with or without diabetic retinopathy, proved once again not to be a contra-indication for iris clip lens implantation.

RESULTS OBTAINED IN THE NETHERLANDS WITH BINKHORST LENS IMPLANTS.

The author interviewed all 26 ophthalmologists in the Netherlands who had themselves performed at least 8 BINKHORST lens implant operations before 1st January 1972. In this way he obtained an insight into their motivation, indications, technique, complications, results, and their opinion based on their own experience concerning the contra-indications for implantation. In general, the preparation of the Dutch ophthalmologists had been good. However, the author thought it wrong that 16 of the 26 ophthalmologists interviewed had performed their first implant operation on their own, i.e. without the assistance of a surgeon experienced in lens implant operations. The percentage of dislocation, retinal detachment, implant extraction, and enucleation were, it is true, slightly lower than for those of the other 10 ophthalmologists, but it was just a little larger for corneal dystrophy. The fact that 20 of the ophthalmologists interviewed considered bulging vitreous to constitute the biggest problem immediately prior to implantation, draws attention to the great importance of very good anaesthesia in lens implant surgery.

The incidence of dislocation, corneal dystrophy, retinal detachment, implant extraction, and enucleation, as well as the visual acuity obtained, were compared with the results of BINKHORST and WORST. The most important results agreed with those obtained for the last 494 iris clip lens implant operations of BINK-HORST's series. The percentage of dislocation was smaller for iris clip lenses than for iridocapsular lenses. The percentage of corneal dystrophy was much higher for the iris clip lens than for the iridocapsular lens. The percentage of implant extraction was smaller for the iris clip lens than for the iridocapsular lens; the incidence in general, however, was higher than in the series of BINKHORST and WORST. This may have been due to insufficient experience in repositioning dislocated implants.

In general, the visual acuity results obtained were good. Of the 80 eyes that suffered serious functional damage as a result of approximately 2761 BINKHORST lens implant operations in the Netherlands, all but 8, which had a favourable outcome, were afflicted with total or partial corneal dystrophy. These 80 which formed 2.90% of the total number of cases were distributed as follows: BINK-HORST: 39 (4.50%), WORST: 13 (1.96%) and the remaining Dutch ophthalmologists: 28 (2.28%).

Until results pertaining to a longer period of time become available, the author feels that the future of the BINKHORST *lens and the eyes fitted with it will best be safeguarded by having implantations performed only by ophthalmologists with an interest in and experience of surgery. At the same time, the author does not exclude the possibility that in future the indication for young patients with bilateral cataracts to be fitted with* BINKHORST *lens implants will give ground to an indication for an improved type of contact lens.*

CHAPTER VIII

HISTOPATHOLOGY.

MANSCHOT'S extensive histopathological studies show that the eye tolerates the BINKHORST lens very well. However, all eyes fitted with an iris clip lens showed four deep grooves in the pupillary margin as a result of the pressure exerted by the posterior loop attachments, as well as local atrophy of the pigment epithelium due to pressure by the posterior loops themselves.

The serious pressure atrophy of the sphincter muscle itself was another reason why BINKHORST changed either to fixation by means of a perlon suture around the superior loops of the iris clip lens, or to iridocapsular fixation.

CHAPTER IX

EFFECT OF PRIMARY BINKHORST LENS IMPLANTATION ON INTRAOCULAR PRESSURE AND FACILITY OF OUTFLOW, WITH RESPECT TO THE COLOUR OF THE IRIS.
EFFECT OF SUPINE AND PRONE POSITION OF THE PATIENT ON THE POSITION OF THE BINKHORST LENS IN THE EYE AFTER INTRACAPSULAR AND EXTRACAPSULAR OPERATION RESPECTIVELY.
VISUAL IMPRESSIONS OF PATIENTS, INCLUDING 6 DOCTORS, AFTER A BINKHORST LENS IMPLANT OPERATION.

Intraocular pressure and facility of outflow did not appear to be significantly affected by a BINKHORST lens implant. After the operation no difference was observed between brown eyes and eyes of other colour.

The antero-posterior gravitational movement of a BINKHORST lens in eyes having extracapsular fixation, was about equally small as in normal eyes. It was approximately 0.2 mm greater in eyes having intracapsular fixation, due to the greater freedom of movement of implant and iris diaphragm in the anterior *and* the posterior directions.

The visual impressions of the patients, including 6 doctors, after a BINKHORST lens implant operation, were divided up into photophobia, increased sensitivity to the violet part of the spectrum, entoptic observations of various kinds, movement of the image and differences in reading distance in the supine and prone positions. The most important was photophobia, especially for light incident from the side. In general, the complaints that could be caused by a BINKHORST lens implant operation were slight; in part they could be overcome by means of sunglasses.

EPILOGUE.

HELMHOLTZ has been credited with the remark that he would return to the instrument maker an instrument that was optically as badly designed as the human eye, and that he would refuse to pay the bill. Such a remark is open to criticism. After all, as this thesis shows, numerous investigators have made every endeavour to try to find a satisfactory substitute for the human lens, be it without accommodative properties.

Far from diminishing our appreciation of the optics of the human eye, the history of the development of the intraocular lens implant fills us with ever-increasing admiration for the wonders of Creation.

SAMENVATTING

1. De voordelen van het inbrengen van een lens van synthetisch materiaal na een cataractextractie wegen niet op tegen de gevaren hieraan verbonden.
Stelling IX bij de thesis van C. H. O. M. VON WINNING, Leiden, 17-12-*1952*.

2. Bij voorzichtige indicatiestelling en adequate operatietechniek is de intra-oculaire kunstlens als een grote aanwinst voor de oogheelkunde te beschouwen.
Stelling 12 bij de thesis van A. F. DEUTMAN jr., Rotterdam, 13-1-*1971*.

HOOFDSTUK I

VERGELIJKING VAN BRIL-LENS, CONTACTLENS EN INTRA-OCULAIRE LENS.

VOORDELEN EN NADELEN.

Het door een staaroperatie (cataractextractie) lensloos (afaak) geworden oog kan optisch op drie manieren worden gecorrigeerd: door een lens *vóór*, *op* of *in* het oog.

De lens *vóór* het oog, dus in de bril, heeft de volgende nadelen: vergroting van het beeld met ongeveer 25 %, sferische aberratie, en een ringscotoom met het daarbij behorende 'Jack-in-the-box'-fenomeen en 'WELSH'-fenomeen.

De lens *op* het oog, de contactlens, vergroot het beeld slechts met ongeveer 7 % en mist de nadelen van de brilcorrectie. Zij kan bovendien de optiek verbeteren bij een niet te ernstig hoornvlieslitteken. Afgezien van de nadelen van de contactlens in het algemeen stuit het gebruik echter op praktische moeilijkheden bij het inbrengen en uitnemen door bejaarde patiënten en kinderen. De ervaring heeft geleerd dat in de loop der jaren een toenemend aantal patiënten de contactlens terzijde legt, in het bijzonder bij onvoldoende motivatie, zoals bij eenzijdige afakie.

De lens *in* het oog (intra-oculaire lens) geeft de beste optische correctie van afakie door haar permanente aanwezigheid, de afwezige of slechts minimale verandering van de beeldgrootte en de mogelijkheid, deze lens op alle leeftijden te implanteren. Bij eenzijdig afake kinderen maakt zij de amblyopiebehandeling eenvoudiger en de kans op herstel van het binoculaire zien groter. Bij eenzijdig afake volwassenen kan zij bijdragen tot het voldoen aan de strenge keuringseisen van verschillende beroepen.

Ongelijke grootte van het door ieder oog gevormde beeld (aniseikonie) is in hoge mate aanwezig bij eenzijdige afakie, gecorrigeerd door een bril, in mindere mate – maar voor binoculair zien vaak nog te sterk – bij een contactlens, en niet of bijna niet bij een intra-oculaire lens.

Binoculair zien is nog mogelijk tot een verschil in beeldgrootte van 5–8%, maar klachten door aniseikonie kunnen reeds veel eerder optreden. Bij eenzijdige afakie biedt daarom de intra-oculaire lens in het algemeen de beste kans op herstel van het binoculaire zien. Voor de individuele patiënt bestaat de mogelijkheid, door metingen aan beide ogen de sterkte van de intra-oculaire lens te berekenen, die nodig is voor het verkrijgen van een exact gelijke beeldgrootte.

HOOFDSTUK II

GESCHIEDENIS VAN DE INTRA-OCULAIRE KUNSTLENS.

RIDLEY implanteerde op 29–11–1949, na een extracapsulaire cataractextractie, voor het eerst bij de mens een van perspex gemaakte, intra-oculaire lens in de achterste oogkamer, zonder fixatie en zonder corneosclerale wondhechtingen. Deze RIDLEY-lens, in meer dan duizend ogen geïmplanteerd, gaf veel complicaties: achterwaartse dislocatie in 6% der gevallen, iritis en secundair glaucoom, die extractie van de implant noodzakelijk maakten in 15% der gevallen.

Bijna alle daarna ontwikkelde types voorkamerlens met fixatie in de kamerhoek hebben in een hoog percentage van de geopereerde ogen geleid tot corneadystrofie. Alleen het type Mark VIII van CHOYCE heeft niet tot deze complicatie geleid.

De eerste voorkamerlens met irisfixatie was de 'collar-stud'-lens van EPSTEIN, een modificatie van de RIDLEY-lens.

BINKHORST ontwikkelde de iris-cliplens in de jaren na 1958. Deze voorkamerlens, die voor het eerst werd geïmplanteerd op 11–8–1958, heeft twee voorste en twee achterste supramide lussen ter fixatie van het optische gedeelte aan het irisdiafragma. De bedoeling was, met behulp van de iris-cliplens het ontstaan van dislocatie èn corneadystrofie te vermijden, die de belangrijkste complicaties van achterste resp. voorste oogkamerlens met fixatie in de kamerhoek waren. Als belangrijkste ontwikkelingen van de iris-cliplens ontstonden de modificatie met loodrecht op elkaar geplaatste voorste en achterste lussen (FEDOROV in 1964), de iridocapsulaire lens (BINKHORST in 1965) en de iris-medaillonlens (WORST in 1970), alle vier tezamen door de auteur BINKHORST-lens genoemd. De iridocapsulaire lens heeft slechts twee achterste lussen, die na een extracapsulair verrichte cataractextractie de lens op haar plaats houden door fixatie in de iridocapsulaire membraan. De iris-medaillonlens, eveneens zonder voorste lussen, wordt aan de iris opgehangen met een perlon hechting. De voordelen en nadelen van deze lenstypes worden besproken.

TECHNIEK.

Er worden drie aspecten van de techniek besproken: 1. materiaal en sterilisatie van de implant, 2. operatietechniek, en 3. behandeling van de complicaties na de operatie.

Polymethylmethacrylaat (perspex) bleek door zijn volstrekte inertie uitermate geschikt te zijn als materiaal voor de intra-oculaire lens. Een intra-oculaire prikkelingstoestand, die aanvankelijk aan het perspex werd toegeschreven, bleek veroorzaakt te zijn door vloeistoffen, gebruikt voor sterilisatie van de implant. Irritatie bleef achterwege na sterilisatie van de lens met NaOH, het tijdens de operatie neutraliseren van de vloeistof met $NaHCO_3$ en daarna afspoelen van de lens in fysiologische zoutoplossing.

De operatietechniek van de implantatie en de voor- en nabehandeling worden voor de iris-cliplens, de iridocapsulaire lens en de iris-medaillonlens besproken, zowel na intracapsulaire als na extracapsulaire cataractextractie. De voornaamste verwikkelingen tijdens de implantatie van een iris-cliplens zijn: prominerend glasvocht, inklemming van glasvocht tussen de lussen of tussen iris en lens, en glasvochtverlies. Laatstgenoemde complicatie is een contra-indicatie tot implantatie. Aan de operatietechniek worden in speciale gevallen bijzondere eisen gesteld, bv. bij iridencleisis, bij radiaire iridotomie, en bij ernstige beschadiging van het voorste oogsegment.

De complicaties na de operatie worden verdeeld in complicaties die vroeg, laat of zowel vroeg als laat kunnen optreden. In het bijzonder wordt de behandeling van het pupil-block, van de dislocatie en van de corneadystrofie besproken.

HOOFDSTUK IV

RESULTATEN VAN C. D. BINKHORST.

De 866 BINKHORST-lensimplantaties, tot 1-1-1972 verricht door BINKHORST zelf, werden verdeeld in iris-cliplens, iridocapsulaire lens en de eerste modificatie volgens FEDOROV. Voorts werd ieder type gerubriceerd naar het soort cataract, het geslacht van de patiënt, linker- of rechteroog, binoculaire of monoculaire implantatie, operatieleeftijd, observatieperiode en tenslotte bereikte gezichtsscherpte.

In de groep van iris-cliplensimplantaties (694 ogen) worden van de complicaties na de operatie de dislocatie en de corneadystrofie uitgebreid besproken, ingedeeld naar frequentie, oorzaak, preventie, therapie en consequenties. Het bleek dat de luslengte van overwegende betekenis was voor de frequentieverdeling van beide complicaties. Voor de preventie van dislocatie van de implant was verder geregelde pilocarpine-indruppeling of het maken van een lushechting nuttig. Voor het ontstaan van corneadystrofie was vóór de operatie de conditie van de cornea belangrijk, in het bijzonder het al dan niet vóórkomen van FUCHS-dystrofie, tijdens en na de operatie het ontstaan van ernstige complicaties, en het contact tussen lus(sen) en cornea. De consequenties van dislocatie waren in het algemeen gering, die van corneadystrofie daarentegen meestal zeer ernstig: slechts ogen met een beginnende of dreigende corneadystrofie reageerden gunstig op lusamputatie. Bij totale corneadystrofie bleek perforerende keratoplastiek de enige mogelijkheid om soms een verbetering van de gezichtsscherpte te verkrijgen. De frequentie van zowel dislocatie als corneadystrofie daalde aanzienlijk in de loop der jaren.

In de groepen van speciale gevallen bleken glaucoom en diabetes mellitus met of zonder diabetische retinopathie geen contra-indicatie te vormen tot iriscliplensimplantatie.

In de groep van iridocapsulaire lensimplantaties (170 ogen) werd een indeling gemaakt naar de oorzaak van het cataract. In tegenstelling tot aangeboren beiderzijds cataract bleek aangeboren eenzijdig cataract meestal een contra-indicatie tot operatieve behandeling te vormen door de vaak aanwezige andere aangeboren afwijkingen. Iridocapsulaire lensimplantatie wegens traumatisch cataract bleek alleen dàn minder goede orthoptische resultaten te geven indien het trauma had plaatsgevonden vóór de leeftijd van 5 jaar en de patiënt te laat onder behandeling was gekomen. Bij cataracta complicata, – juvenilis, – e causa ignota en – senilis waren de resultaten na implantatie van een iridocapsulaire lens even goed als na implantatie van een iris-cliplens.

Het percentage complicaties na implantatie van een iridocapsulaire lens is ongeveer de helft van dat na implantatie van een iris-cliplens, bij corneadystrofie zelfs slechts een tiende.

HOOFDSTUK V

RESULTATEN VAN J. G. F. WORST.

De 665 BINKHORST-lensimplantaties, tot 1–1–1972 verricht door J. G. F. WORST, werden op dezelfde wijze gerubriceerd als die van BINKHORST in hoofdstuk IV. Een consequente vergelijking tussen de series van BINKHORST en WORST was niet goed mogelijk door verschillen in oorzaken van het cataract, type van de implant, observatieperiode en optotypen, gebruikt voor de bepaling van de gezichtsscherpte. Toch bleken de resultaten wat gezichtsscherpte en complicaties tijdens en na de operatie betreft, vergelijkbaar met die van BINK-HORST, indien van BINKHORST slechts de laatste 400 implantaties werden beoordeeld.

Door het hechten van de iris-cliplens op de iris daalde het percentage dislocaties van 3,36 tot 2,02; het percentage corneadystrofie steeg echter van 1,68 tot 2,83.

In de groepen van speciale gevallen bleken glaucoom en diabetes mellitus met of zonder diabetische retinopathie wederom geen contra-indicatie te vormen tot iris-cliplensimplantatie.

RESULTATEN VAN DE AUTEUR.

De eerste 72 iris-cliplensimplantaties, verricht door de auteur bij 61 patiënten van 50 jaar en ouder, werden wederom op dezelfde wijze gerubriceerd als die van BINKHORST en WORST, onder toevoeging van de gegevens over kleur van de iris, cornea-astigmatisme, dieptezien, oogdruk en weerstand in de kamerhoek. Optimale gezichtsscherpte werd in 40 ogen (zonder complicaties) 6–8 weken na de implantatie bereikt, in 16 ogen (eveneens zonder complicaties) 4–18 maanden na de implantatie; in de overige 16 ogen wisselde het resultaat betreffende de gezichtsscherpte, door tijdelijke of blijvende complicaties.

Dieptezien, richting van de implant, vorm van de pupil en bevindingen bij gonioscopie werden afzonderlijk bestudeerd. Dieptezien bleek steeds aanwezig te zijn, tenzij vermindering van de gezichtsscherpte van één der ogen dit verhinderde. Deze resultaten waren volkomen in overeenstemming met die welke de auteur vaststelde in een serie van 58 patiënten met iris-cliplensimplantatie, geopereerd door BINKHORST.

De richting van de lussen van de implant bleek na de implantatie te kunnen gaan afwijken van de oorspronkelijke verticale positie.

De vorm van de pupil was ondanks pilocarpine-indruppeling niet volkomen vierkant in 13 ogen. De oorzaken hiervan worden besproken.

Bij gonioscopie werd niet méér irispigment in de kamerhoek gevonden dan na cataractextractie zonder lensimplantatie. In 19 ogen werden perifere synechieën gevonden met de wond of met de lijn van SCHWALBE, waarvan 16 aan de rechterzijde van het desbetreffende oog, hetgeen in verband wordt gebracht met de operatietechniek.

De resultaten met betrekking tot de gezichtsscherpte, en de complicaties tijdens en na de operatie toonden in deze serie geen grote verschillen met die van BINKHORST en WORST.

Bij de groepen van speciale gevallen werden de lushechting, de combinatie van synechiolysis, radiaire iridotomie en lushechting, de overgroeiing van een voorste lus door gepigmenteerd irisweefsel, en diabetes mellitus besproken. Diabetes mellitus met of zonder diabetische retinopathie bleek wederom geen contra-indicatie te vormen tot iris-cliplensimplantatie.

HOOFDSTUK VII

RESULTATEN VAN BINKHORST-LENSIMPLANTATIE IN NEDERLAND.

De auteur had een vraaggesprek met alle 26 oogartsen in Nederland die vóór 1-1-1972 zelf ten minste 8 BINKHORST-lensimplantaties hadden verricht. Daardoor kreeg hij een inzicht in hun motieven, voorbereiding, indicaties, techniek, complicaties, resultaten en hun door ervaring gevormde mening omtrent de contra-indicaties tot deze implantatie.

De voorbereiding van de Nederlandse oogartsen was in het algemeen goed. Het leek de auteur echter onjuist toe, dat 16 van de 26 ondervraagde oogartsen de eerste implantatie alléén verrichtten, d.w.z. zonder assistentie van een ervaren lensimplantatiechirurg. Het percentage voor resp. dislocatie, netvliesloslating, extractie van de implant en enucleatie was bij hun patiënten weliswaar iets kleiner dan bij die van de andere 10 oogartsen, maar juist voor corneadystrofie was het iets groter.

Het feit dat 20 van de ondervraagde oogartsen prominerend glasvocht als het belangrijkste probleem onmiddellijk vóór de implantatie beschouwden, vestigt de aandacht op de grote betekenis van een zeer goede anesthesie bij de lensimplantatiechirurgie.

De frequentie van dislocatie, corneadystrofie, netvliesloslating, extractie van de implant, en enucleatie, alsmede de bereikte gezichtsscherpte werden vergeleken met de resultaten van BINKHORST en WORST. De belangrijkste uitkomsten stemden overeen met die van de laatste 494 iris-cliplensimplantaties in de serie van BINKHORST. Het percentage dislocatie was voor de iris-cliplens iets kleiner dan voor de iridocapsulaire lens. Het percentage corneadystrofie was voor de iris-cliplens veel hoger dan voor de iridocapsulaire lens. Het percentage implantextractie was voor de iris-cliplens kleiner dan voor de iridocapsulaire lens, doch over het geheel genomen groter dan in de series van BINKHORST en WORST, wellicht door onvoldoende ervaring in de repositie van een gedisloceerde implant.

De resultaten betreffende de gezichtsscherpte waren in het algemeen goed. Het aantal ogen dat ten gevolge van ±2761 in Nederland verrichte BINKHORST-

255

lensimplantaties functioneel ernstig werd beschadigd, is, op 8 gunstige uitzonderingen na, gelijk te stellen met het aantal ogen waarin een totale of gedeeltelijke corneadystrofie ontstond: BINKHORST: 39 (4,50%), WORST: 13 (1,96%) en de overige Nederlandse oogartsen: 28 (2,28%), dus in totaal 80 ogen (2,90%).

In afwachting van de resultaten, verkregen over een langere periode, meent de auteur dat de toekomst van de BINKHORST-lens en de hiermee behandelde ogen voorlopig het best gewaarborgd wordt indien uitsluitend oogartsen met chirurgische belangstelling en ervaring de implantatie uitvoeren. Daarbij sluit hij de mogelijkheid niet uit dat in de toekomst voor jonge patiënten met binoculair cataract de indicatie tot BINKHORST-lensimplantatie zal plaatsmaken voor die tot een verbeterde contactlens.

HOOFDSTUK VIII

HISTOPATHOLOGIE.

Uit de uitgebreide histopathologische studie van MANSCHOT is gebleken dat het oog de BINKHORST-lens goed verdraagt. Alle ogen met een iris-cliplens toonden echter zowel vier diepe groeven in de pupilrand als gevolg van druk van de aanhechtingen van de achterste lussen, alsook lokale atrofie van de pigmentepitheellaag door druk van de achterste lussen zelf.

De ernstige drukatrofie van de sphincter pupillae was voor BINKHORST mede aanleiding om over te gaan hetzij tot fixatie door middel van een perlon hechting rondom de bovenste lussen van de iris-cliplens, ofwel tot de iridocapsulaire fixatie.

HOOFDSTUK IX

INVLOED VAN PRIMAIRE BINKHORST-LENSIMPLANTATIE OP DE OOGDRUK EN DE WEERSTAND IN DE KAMERHOEK, MET INACHTNEMING VAN DE KLEUR VAN DE IRIS. INVLOED VAN RUGLIGGING EN BUIKLIGGING VAN DE PATIËNT OP DE POSITIE VAN DE BINKHORST-LENS IN HET OOG, NA INTRACAPSULAIRE RESP. EXTRACAPSULAIRE OPERATIE. VISUELE INDRUKKEN VAN PATIËNTEN, ONDER WIE 6 ARTSEN, NA BINKHORST-LENSIMPLANTATIE.

De oogdruk en de weerstand in de kamerhoek bleken door BINKHORST-lensimplantatie niet significant te worden beinvloed. Er was hierbij na de operatie geen verschil tussen wel en niet bruine ogen.

De door de zwaartekracht veroorzaakte voorachterwaartse beweging van een BINKHORST-lens bleek in ogen met extracapsulaire fixatie ongeveer even klein te zijn als in normale ogen. In ogen met intracapsulaire fixatie was zij ongeveer

0,2 mm groter ten gevolge van de grotere bewegingsvrijheid van implant en irisdiafragma in voorwaartse *en* achterwaartse richting.

De visuele indrukken van patiënten, onder wie 6 artsen, na BINKHORST-lens-implantatie werden verdeeld in lichtschuwheid, verhoogde gevoeligheid in het violette deel van het spectrum, entoptische waarnemingen van verschillende aard, bewegingen van het beeld, en verschil in leesafstand bij resp. rugligging en buikligging. De belangrijkste hiervan was de lichtschuwheid, speciaal voor zijdelings invallend licht. Over het geheel genomen bleken de klachten die het gevolg kunnen zijn van een BINKHORST-lensimplantatie, gering; ze waren deels te verhelpen door een zonnebril.

EPILOOG.

Aan HELMHOLTZ wordt de opmerking toegeschreven dat hij een instrument dat optisch even slecht was als het menselijk oog, zou terugzenden aan de instrumentmaker, en dat hij zou weigeren de rekening te betalen. Een dergelijke opmerking is vatbaar voor kritiek. Immers, talloze onderzoekers hebben zich – zoals uit dit proefschrift blijkt – enorme inspanningen getroost om te trachten, alleen nog maar de menselijke lens zo goed mogelijk te vervangen, en dan nog zonder accommodatievermogen.

Integendeel, het overzicht van de ontwikkeling van de intra-oculaire lensimplantatie vervult ons met een steeds toenemende eerbied voor de Schepping.

REFERENCES

ALLEMAND, H. L' & F. E. ADELSTEIN. Anaesthesie in der Augenheilkunde, in 'Lehrbuch der Anaesthesiologie und Wiederbelebung', chapter 12. Springer Verlag, Berlin, 1971.

ASCHER, K. W. Prosthetophakia two hundred years ago. *Amer. J. Ophthal.* 59 : *445–446* (1965).

ASHTON, N. & D. P. CHOYCE. Pathological examination of a human eye containing an anterior chamber acrylic implant. *Brit. J. Ophthal.* 43 : *577–583* (1959).

—— & J. BOBERG-ANS. Pathology of an aphakic eye containing an anterior chamber implant. *Brit. J. Ophthal.* 45 : *543–549* (1961).

BALEN, A. TH. M. VAN. De implantatie van pseudophakoi volgens Binkhorst bij eenzijdige traumatische cataract. *Ned. T. Geneesk.* 114 : *1883–1884* (1970).

—— Binkhorst's method of implantation of pseudophakoi in unilateral traumatic cataract. *Ophthalmologica* (Basel) 165 : *490–494* (1972a).

—— Four years Binkhorst lens implantation in Rotterdam. Read before joint meeting Irish and Dutch Ophthal. Soc., Dublin, May 1972(b). To be published.

—— Four years' experience with Binkhorst lens implantation. *Amer. J. Ophthal.* 75 : *755–763* (1973).

BARON, A. Tolérance de l'oeil à la matière plastique. Prothèses optiques cornéennes. Prothèses optiques cristalliniennes. *Bull. Soc. Ophtal. Paris* 9 : *982–988* (1953).

—— Prothèses cornéennes et cristalliniennes en matière plastique (présentation d'un film). *Bull. Soc. Franc. Ophtal.* 67 : *386–390* (1954).

BARRAQUER, J. & N. BAILBÉ. Enseignements tirés de notre statistique opératoire dans les cas de remplacement du cristallin cataracté par la lentille de Ridley. *Estud. inform. oftal.* 5 : *13* (1953).

—— Lentilles plastiques dans la chambre antérieure. Indications. Technique. Expérience personnelle sur cent cas. *Bull. Soc. Belge Ophtal.* 114 : *503–516* (1956).

—— Lentilles plastiques dans la chambre antérieure. Facteurs essentiels pour obtenir de bons résultats. *Acta concil. ophthal. Belgica* (Brussels) II: *1709–1711* (1958).

—— Complicaciones de la inclusion segun los diversos tipos de lentes. *An. Inst. Barraquer* III-4 : *588–592* (1962).

BIERLAAGH, J. J. M., A. VAN DER WEE, A. KATS, P. A. M. LÉONARD & C. D. BINKHORST. Technique and perspectives of lens implants (pseudophakoi) in children. Proc. 2nd Int. Orthopt. Congr. Amsterdam (Int. Congr. Series No. 245). Excerpta Med. Found., Amsterdam, 1971.

BIESHEUVEL, K. & A. TH. M. VAN BALEN. Ervaringen met implantatie van artificiële lenzen. *Ned. T. Geneesk.* 114 : *489* (1970).

—— & —— Experience with the implantation of artificial lenses. *Ophthalmologica* (Basel) 163 : *2–7* (1971).

BIETTI, G. B. The present state of the use of plastics in eye surgery. *Acta Ophthal.* (Kbh) 33 : *337–370* (1955).

BINKHORST, C. D. De prognose van de aangeboren en in de eerste levensjaren ontstane staar. *Ned. T. Geneesk.* 87 : *343–350* (1943).

—— Intra-oculaire lensprothese volgens Ridley. Resultaten bij 12 patienten. *Ned. T. Geneesk.* 100 : *3522–3528* (1956a).

—— & F. P. FLU. Sterilization of intra-ocular acrylic lens prostheses with ultra-violet rays. *Brit. J. Ophthal.* 40 : *665–668* (1956b).

—— Ridley's intraocular lens prothesis. The postoperative reaction. Results obtained in 12 cases. *Ophthalmologica (Basel)* 133 : *384–392* (1957).

—— Iris-supported artificial pseudophakia. A new development in intraocular artificial lens surgery (iris clip lens). *Trans. Ophthal. Soc. U.K.* 79 : *569–584* (1959a).

—— De implantatie van kunststoflenzen in het oog. Een nieuwe fixatiemethode: de pupillens of iris-cliplens. *Ned. T. Geneesk.* 103 : *1289–1294* (1959b).

—— Über die endgültige Verträglichkeit künstlicher Augenlinsen bei der Aphakie und deren Verbesserung mittels Fixation der Linse in der Pupille ('Pupillarlinse' oder 'Iris-Clip-Linse'). *Klin. Mbl. Augenheilk.* 134 : *536–543* (1959c).

—— Results of implantation of intraocular lenses in unilateral aphakia. With special reference to the pupillary or iris clip lens – a new method of fixation. *Amer. J. Ophthal.* 49 : *703–710* (1960a).

—— Ervaringen van de implantatie van verschillende typen lens-prothesen bij enkelzijdige afakie; de pupil-lens of iris-cliplens, een nieuwe fixatiemethode. *Ned. T. Geneesk.* 104 : *754–755* (1960b).

—— Indikation und Implantationstechnik der 'Pupillarlinse' oder 'Iris-Clip-Linse' bei der Aphakie. *Klin. Mbl. Augenheilk.* 136 : *35–43* (1960c).

—— Experience with implantation of various types of lens protheses in unilateral aphakia. The pupillary lens or iris clip lens, a new method of fixation. *Ophthalmologica* (Basel) 139 : *500–503* (1960d).

—— Iris clip lens, een door de iris gefixeerde artificiële lens bij afakie (met filmprojectie en demonstratie van patienten). *Ned. T. Geneek.* 105 : *1118–1119* (1961a).

—— The pupillary lens (iris clip lens). An artificial lens for aphakia completely supported by the iris (with film and demonstration of patients). *Ophthalmologica* (Basel) 141 : *479–480* (1961b).

—— Lensimplantatie. *Ned. T. Geneesk.* 106 : *908–912* (1962a).

—— Use of the pupillary lens (iris clip lens) in aphakia. Our experience based on the first fifty implantations. *Brit. J. Ophthal.* 46 : *343–356* (1962b).

—— Aktive und rationelle Behandlung des Altersstars mit der 'iseikonischen' Pupillarlinse (Iris-Klipp-Linse). *Ber. 64. Zus. dtsch. ophthal. Ges. Heidelberg* 1961 : *486–488* (1962c).

—— Artificial pseudophakia. Long-term results obtained with the pupillary lens (iris clip lens) in the first twenty cases of unilateral aphakia. *Brit. J. Ophthal.* 46 *496–502* (1962d).

—— The pupillary lens (iris clip lens). A third method of intraocular artificial lenses in aphakia. *An. Inst. Barraquer* III-4 : *562–569* (1962e).

—— & M. H. M. A. GOBIN. Oogletsels met lenstroebeling bij jonge kinderen. *Ned. T. Geneesk.* 108 : *978–985* (1964a). (Dannheim lens implantations only).

—— & —— Injuries to the eye with lens opacity in young children. *Ophthalmologica* (Basel) 148 : *169–183* (1964b). (Dannheim lens implantations only).

—— B. C. CARDON, R. G. VAN DAMME & H. HOMMERS. The pupillary lens. A substitute for the cataractous crystalline lens. *Med. Radiogr. Photogr.* 42 : *16–23* (1966).

—— Iris-clip and irido-capsular lens implants (pseudophakoi). Personal techniques of pseudophakia. *Brit. J. Ophthal.* 51 : *767–771* (1967a).

—— Lens implants (pseudophakoi) classified according to method of fixation. *Brit. J. Ophthal.* 51 : *772–774* (1967b).

—— Eigene Verfahren der Pseudophakie. Iris-Clip-Pseudophakos und Irido-kapsulärer Pseudophakos. *Klin. Mbl. Augenheilk.* 151 : *21–28* (1967c).

—— & M. H. M. A. GOBIN. Pseudophakia after lens injury in children. *Ophthalmologica* (Basel) 154 : *81–87* (1967d).

—— & P. A. M. LÉONARD. Results in 208 iris-clip pseudophakos implantations. *Amer. J. Ophthal.* 64 : *947–956* (1967e).

—— The fixation of pseudophakoi. *Perspect. Ophthal.* I : *191–194*. Excerpta Med. Found., Amsterdam, 1968(a).

—— & P. A. M. LÉONARD. Implantation of the iris clip pseudophakos. Results in the first 208 cases. *Perspect. Ophthal.* I : *195–214*. Excerpta Med. Found., Amsterdam, (1968b).

—— De bevestiging van pseudophakoi. *Ned. T. Geneesk.* 113 : *2258–2259* (1969a).

—— M. H. M. A. GOBIN & P. A. M. LÉONARD. Posttraumatic pseudophakia in children, in J. François 'Occupational and medicative hazards in ophthalmology'. p. 284–291. Karger, Basel (1969b).

—— —— & —— Posttraumatic artificial lens implants (pseudophakoi) in children. *Brit. J. Ophthal.* 53 : *518–529* (1969c).

—— —— & —— Posttraumatic pseudophakia in children. Proc. Centennial Symp. Manhattan Eye, Ear and Throat Hosp., p. *72–86*, ed. A.I. Turtz. Mosby, St. Louis (1969d).

—— A letter to the editor. *Amer. J. Ophthal.* 70 : *311–312* (1970a).

—— & M. H. M. A. GOBIN. Treatment of congenital and juvenile cataract with intraocular lens implants (pseudophakoi). *Brit. J. Ophthal.* 54 : *759–765* (1970b).

—— The attachment of pseudophakoi. *Ophthalmologica* (Basel) 162 : *205–207* (1971a).

—— & M. H. M. A. GOBIN. Congenitale cataract en lensimplantatie. *Ned. T. Geneesk.* 115 : *822–823* (1971b).

—— Power of the prepupillary pseudophakos. *Brit. J. Ophthal.* 56 : *332–337* (1972a).

—— Praxis und Theorie der 'Iris Klipp Linse' und der 'Irido-Kapsular Linse'. Sitzungsber. 125. Vers. Ver. Rhein.-Westfäl. Augenärzte Bonn. Grafischer Betr. Gebr. Zimmermann, Balve/Sauerland (1972b).

—— Perspektiven der Iris-Klipp-Linse und der Irido-Kapsularlinse. *Klin. Mbl. Augenheilk.* 161 : *477–481* (1972c).

—— & M. H. M. A. GOBIN. Congenital cataract and lens implantation. *Ophthalmologica* (Basel) 164 : *392–397* (1972d).

—— A. KATS & P. A. M. LÉONARD. Extracapsular pseudophakia. Results in 100 two-loop iridocapsular lens implantations. *Amer. J. Ophthal.* 73 : *625–636* (1972e).

—— The iridocapsular (two-loop) lens and the iris clip (four-loop) lens in pseudophakia. *Trans. Amer. Acad. Ophthal. Otolaryngol.* 77 : *589–617* (1973).

—— Twenty years experience with pseudophakia. Some thoughts on the fixation of intraocular lenses. *Docum. Ophthal.* (to be published).

BINKHORST, R. D., G. W. WEINSTEIN & R. C. TROUTMAN. A weightless iseikonic intraocular lens. *Amer. J. Ophthal.* 58 : *73–78* (1964).

BLEEKER, G. M. Variation in depth of the anterior chamber of the eye. Thesis, Amsterdam (1963).

BOBERG-ANS, J. Experience with twelve cases of intraocular anterior chamber implants for aphakia. Two new models of lenses are described. *Brit. J. Ophthal.* 45 : *37–43* (1961).

—— Pathology of an aphakic eye, containing an anterior chamber implant. *An. Inst. Barraquer* III-4 : *585–587* (1962).

—— Simultaneous operation for cataract and glaucoma; report on thirty cases. *Trans. Ophthal. Soc. U.K.* 84 : *113–125* (1964a).

—— Complications from intraocular lenses in aphakia, in 'Complications after cataract surgery', ed. F. H. Theodore, p. *433-448*. Little, Brown & Cy, Boston (1964b).

—— Complications from intraocular lenses in aphakia. *Int. Ophthal. Clin.* 5/1 : *107–122* (1965).

—— Reconstructive surgery in the anterior chamber. *Ophthalmologica* (Basel) Addit. ad 158 : *279–283* (1969a).

—— Reconstructive surgery in the anterior chamber. *Acta Ophthal.* (Kbh.) 47 : *489–497* (1969b).

BOEDER, P. Spectacle correction of aphakia. *Arch. Ophthal.* 68 : *870–874* (1962).

BONNET, R., J. P. GERHARD & M. MASSIN. Les verres de contact. Special issue Bull. Soc. Ophtal. Fr. (1966).

BRESNICK, G. H. Eyes containing anterior chamber acrylic implants. Pathological complications. *Arch. Ophthal.* 82 : *726–737* (1969).

CAUDELL, P. M. The first twelve years of intra-ocular lens construction. *An. Inst. Barraquer* III-4 : *531–542* (1962).

CHEE, P. & D. I. HAMASAKI. The basis for chymotrypsin-induced glaucoma. *Arch. Ophthal.* 85 : *103–105* (1971).

CHOYCE, D. P. Correction of uni-ocular aphakia by means of anterior chamber acrylic implants. *Acta Concil. Ophthal. Belgica* (Brussels) II : *1705–1708* (1958).

—— Correction of uni-ocular aphakia by means of all-acrylic anterior chamber implants. Review of 100 cases. *Brit. Med. J.* 3 : *609–612* (1959).

—— The correction of uniocular aphakia by means of all-acrylic anterior chamber implants. *Amer. J. Ophthal.* 49 : *417–439* (1960).

—— The uses of acrylic anterior chamber implants illustrated by cases shown. *Proc. Royal Soc. Med.* 54 : *849–856* (1961a).

—— All-acrylic anterior-chamber implants in ophthalmic surgery. *Lancet* II : *165–171* (1961b).

—— Anterior-chamber implants with built-in stenopaeic aperture. *Lancet* II : *1233–1234* (1961c).

—— Intra-ocular lenses and implants (adapted from a thesis), 211 pages. H. K. Lewis, London (1964).

—— The Mark VI, Mark VII and Mark VIII Choyce anterior chamber implants. *Proc. Royal Soc. Med.* 58 : *729–731* (1965).

—— Intra-ocular lenses and implants. *E.E.N.T. Digest* 28 : *83–90* (1966a).

—— Intra-cameral and intra-corneal implants. A decade of personal experience. *Trans. Ophthal. Soc. U.K.* 86 : *507–525* (1966b).

—— The present status of intra-cameral and intra-corneal implants. *Canad. J. Ophthal.* 3 : *295–311* (1968).

Long-term tolerance of Choyce Mark I and Mark VIII anterior chamber implants. *Proc. Royal Soc. Med.* 63 : *310–313* (1970a).

—— Intra-ocular implants. Nursing Times 28th May and 4th June. Fisher, Knight & Co. Ltd., St. Albans (1970b).

—— and G. H. BRESNICK. Eyes containing anterior chamber acrylic implants. Correspondence. *Arch. Ophthal.* 84 : *703–704* (1970c).

CHRISTMAN, E. H. Correction of aniseikonia in monocular aphakia. *Arch. Ophthal.* 85 : *148–149* (1971).

COLENBRANDER, M. C. A new test-type. *Ophthalmologica* (Basel) 130 : *219–220* (1955).

—— Contactlenzen. *Ned. T. Geneesk.* 100 : *1308–1312* (1956).

—— Plastic voorkamerlenzen in de oogheelkunde. *Ned. T. Geneesk.* 106 : *278* (1962).

—— Oogheelkunde, 190 pages. A. Oosthoek's Uitg. Mij., Utrecht (1971).

—— Calculation of the power of an iris clip lens for distant vision. *Brit. J. Ophthal.* 57 : *735–740* (1973).

CRONE, R. A. Human cyclofusional response. A letter to the editor. *Vision Res.* 11 : *1357–1358* (1971).

—— & O. M. A. LEURIDAN. Tolerance for aniseikonia. I. Diplopia thresholds in the vertical and horizontal meridians of the visual field. *Alb. v. Graefe's Arch. klin. exp. Ophthal.* 188 : *1–16* (1973a).

—— & —— Tolerance for aniseikonia. II. Determination based on the amplitude of cyclofusion. *Alb. v. Graefe's Arch. klin. exp. Ophthal.* 188 : *17–22* (1973b).

CSAPODY, I. VON. Berufsleben des Augenarztes. Eine ophthalmologische Ethik und Pädagogik. *Suppl. Klin. Mbl. Augenheilk.* 10 (1941).

DALLAS, N. L. Five-year trial of the Binkhorst iris clip lens in aphakia. *Trans. Ophthal. Soc. U.K.* 90 : *725–732* (1970).

DANNHEIM, H. Vorderkammerlinse mit elastischen Halteschlingen. *Ber. dtsch. ophthal. Ges. Heidelberg* 60 : *267–268* (1956).

—— Types of anterior chamber lenses with elastic loops. *An. Inst. Barraquer* III-4 : *570–572* (1962).

DE VOE, A. G. Monocular aphakia and intraocular lenses. Editorial. *Arch. Ophthal.* 72 : *152–153* (1964).

DUKE-ELDER, S. System of Ophthalmology 11, p. 280 and 286. Kimpton, London (1969).

DIJKSTRA, J. G., H. TJASSENS, K. ROSCHAR & J. KAPTEYN. Statistisch onderzoek van de per 1 januari 1954 lopende blijvende renten ex artikel 16 der Ongevallenwet 1921 ter zake van Oogongevallen voorgekomen in de periode 1903–1953. Med.-Statistische mededeling der Soc. Verz. Bank 8 : *29* (1958).

EASTERBROOK, M., P. G. TUFFNELL & J. C. HILL. Bacterial decontamination of polymethylmethacrylate in ophthalmology. *Canad. J. Ophthal.* 4 : *247–257* (1969).

EPSTEIN, E. The Ridley lens implant. *Brit. J. Ophthal.* 41 : *368–376* (1957).

—— Modified Ridley lenses. *Brit. J. Ophthal.* 43 : *29–33* (1959).

—— Experiences with modified Ridley lenses and others. *An. Inst. Barraquer* III-4 : *555–561* (1962).

FASANELLA, R. M. Modern advances in cataract surgery, 216 pages. Pitman, London (1963).

FEDOROV, S. N. Application of intraocular pupillary lenses for aphakia correction (translation). *Vestn. Oftal.* (Mosk.) 78 : *76–83* (1965).

—— Methods employed to fix intraocular lenses (translation). *Vestn. Oftal.* (Mosk.) 82 : *38–43* (1969a).

—— Combined implantations of the intraocular iris clip lens in posttraumatic lens opacifications and secondary cataracts. *Ophthalmologica* (Basel) Addit. ad 158 : *301–302* (1969b).

—— Two case-reports on the correction of unilateral high myopia with intracameral lenses (translation). *Vestn. Oftal.* (Mosk.) 82 : *43–46* (1969c).

—— Implantation of iris-clip-lenses with single stage removal of the crystalline lens through basal coloboma of the iris (translation). *Vestn. Oftal.* (Mosk.) 82 : *58–61* (1969d).

—— (in an interview): Scientific research in behalf of the medical practice (translation). *Nauka i zjiznj (Science and Life)* 8 : *93–95* (1972).

FLOYD, G. Changes in the corneal curvature following cataract extraction. *Amer. J. Ophthal.* 34 : *1525–1533* (1951).

GALIN, M. Intraocular lens implants. *Amer. J. Ophthal.* 65 : *932* (1968).

GASS, J. D. M. & E. W. D. NORTON. Cystoid macular edema and papilledema following cataract extraction. A fluorescein fundoscopic and angiographic study. *Arch. Ophthal.* 76 : *646–661* (1966).

GERNET, H. Oculometriedaten bei Augengesunden. *Ber. 70. Zus. dtsch. ophthal. Ges.*: *598–599* (1969).

—— H. OSTHOLT & H. WERNER. Neue klinische Grundlagen zur Binkhorst-Linsen-einpflanzung bei Altersstar. Ber. 123. Vers. Ver. Rhein.-Westf. Augenärzte. *Klin. Mbl. Augenheilk.* 159 : *135–136* (1971a).

—— —— & —— L'évaluation pré-opératoire des cristallins artificiels intraoculaires. *Bull. Mém. Soc. Fr. Ophtal.* (Paris) 84 : *537–546* (1971b).

—— & —— Augenseitige Optik. Ein neues Gebiet der klinischen Okulometrie. *Ophthalmologica* (Basel) 166 : *120–143* (1973).

GIRARD, L. J., B. FRIEDMAN, C. D. MOORE, R. I. BLAU, C. D. BINKHORST & M. H. M. A. GOBIN. Intraocular implants and contact lenses. *Arch. Ophthal.* 68 : *762–775* (1962).

GOLDBERG, M. F. Hazards of mannitol. Correspondence. *Arch. Ophthal.* 69 : *687* (1963).

GONGGRIJP, F. Dr. Binkhorst vond eindelijk erkenning. Dagblad De Telegraaf, 27th Febr. p. 17, Amsterdam, 1971.

GUERRY, D. Present status of the anterior chamber lens. *Amer. J. Ophthal.* 50 : *250–258* (1960).

—— & W. J. GEERAETS. Complications of anterior chamber lenses. *Amer. J. Ophthal.* 54 : *229–232* (1962).

HEUVEL, J. E. A. VAN DEN and C. D. BINKHORST (open correspondence): Intra-oculaire plastic lenzen. *Ned. Tijdschr. Geneesk.* 108 : *1464–1465, 1728–1729, 2056* (1964).

HIRSCHMAN, H. Intracameral prostheses: experience with 150 pupillary lenses. Read before Amer. Med. Assoc., 21st June, Atlantic City, New Jersey, 1971.

HIRTHE, C. H. Ergebnisse mit künstlichen Vorderkammerlinsen. *Klin. Mbl. Augenheilk.* 153 : *527–530* (1968).

HOFMANN, H. Erfahrungen mit Vorderkammerlinsen. *Klin. Mbl. Augenheilk.* 161 : *481* (1972).

HUSKEN, J. Kijken door een plastic lens. Dagblad De Stem, 14th March p. 9, Breda, (1970).

IRVINE, S. R. A newly defined vitreous syndrome following cataract surgery. *Amer. J. Ophthal.* 36 : *599-619* (1953).

JAFFE, N. S. Current status of intraocular lenses. *E.E.N.T. Monthly* 52 : *290-296* (1972a).

—— Cataract surgery and its complications, 417 pages. C. V. Mosby, St. Louis, (1972b).

JONKERS, G. H. Intra-ocular acrylic lenses. A case report. *Ophthalmologica* (Basel) 126 : *55-57* (1953).

JUNGSCHAEFFER, O. Iris clip lens and retinal detachment. Examination and surgery of three eyes. *Arch. Ophthal.* 88 : *594-595* (1972).

KESSLER, J. Experiments in refilling the lens. *Arch. Ophthal.* 71 : *412-417* (1964).

KING, J. H. & R. A. SKEEHAN. Acrylic lenses in the anterior chamber. Experimental studies in animal eyes. *Arch. Ophthal.* 58 : *392-395* (1957).

KIRSCH, R. E. Glaucoma following cataract extraction associated with use of alphachymotrypsin. *Arch. Ophthal.* 72 : *612-620* (1964).

KOVAL, L. V. The effect on colour perception of an intraocular lens implantation in aphakia (translation). *Vestn. Oftal.* (Mosk.) 82 : *50-54* (1969).

KRAAS, P. Die postoperative Refraktion nach Binkhorst-Linseneinpflanzung. Thesis, Münster (1972).

KRASNOV, M. M. & E. M. ORLOVA. Artificial crystalline lens fixed to the pararadical area of the iris. Extrapupillary iris-lens (translation). *Vestn. Oftal.* (Mosk.) 82 : *46-50* (1969).

KREIBIG, W. Ist die extrakapsuläre Methode der Starausziehung wirklich als veraltet abzulehnen? *Klin. Mbl. Augenheilk.* 160 : *35-40* (1972).

KÜPER, J. Komplikationen nach Implantation von Vorderkammerlinsen. *Klin. Mbl. Augenheilk.* 140 : *639-644* (1962).

LEGRAND, J. État actuel de la question des lentilles intraoculaires dans la correction des aphaquies. *L'Année Thérap. et Clin. en Ophtal.* 16 : *297-306* (1965).

MCLEMORE, C. S. Cadillacs, Volkswagens and aphakic corrections. *Arch. Ophthal.* 70 : *734-735* (1963).

—— Aphakic correction from an aphake's point-of-view. Correspondence. *Arch. Ophthal.* 74 : *443* (1965).

LÉONARD, P. A. M. Cataracte traumatique et lentille intraoculaire. *Bull. Soc. belge Ophtal.* 159 : *701-706* (1971a).

—— & L. EVENS. La vision binoculaire dans l'aphakie unilatérale traumatique. *Bull. Soc. belge Ophtal.* 159 : *697-700* (1971b).

—— Ultrasonographie en lensimplantatie. Read before 167th Ann. Meeting Dutch Ophthal. Soc., Flushing (1972).

—— Lensimplantatie. Geneesk. Gids (Belgium) 1 : *9-16*, 1973.

LEURIDAN, O. M. A. & A. NOORDENBOS. Binocular vision in unilateral aphakia corrected by contact lens. *Perspect. Ophthal.* II : *189-195*. Excerpta Med. Found.,Amsterdam (1970).

LIEB, W. A. & D. GUERRY. Anterior chamber lenses. For refractive correction of unilateral aphakia. *Amer. J. Ophthal.* 44 : *579-598* (1957).

LIEB, W. Rehabilitation Sehbehinderter durch Haftschale und Vorderkammerlinse. *Klin. Mbl. Augenheilk.* 147 : *137* (1965).

LINKSZ, A. Aniseikonia. With Notes on the Jackson-Lancaster Controversy. XV Jackson Memorial Lecture. *Trans. Amer. Acad. Ophthal. Otolaryngol.* 63 : *117-140* (1959).

—— Optical complications of aphakia, in Complications after cataract surgery, p. 597-634, ed. F. H. Theodore. Little & Brown, Boston (1964).

MANN, W. A. Optical correction of aphakia. *Intern. Ophthal. Clin.* 1/3 : *623-648* (1961).

MANSCHOT, W. A. Beiderzijdse cataractextractie. *Ned. T. Geneesk.* 103 : *1087-1088* (1959).

—— Histopathology of eyes with iris clip and iridocapsular lenses. Read before Joint Meeting Irish and Dutch Ophthal. Soc., Dublin, 1972 (to be published).

—— Histopathology of eyes containing Binkhorst lenses. *Amer. J. Ophthal.* 77 : *865-871* (1974).

MARIA, Y., R. BONNET & P. COCHET. L'intervention de Strampelli. *Clin. Ophtal.* 1 : *2-26* (1959).

MAUMENEE, A. E. Obituary Alan Churchill Woods M. D. *Arch. Ophthal.* 69 : *534-537* (1963).

MAXWELL STUBBS, G. The pupillary lens. Some postoperative complications. *Trans. Ophthal. Soc. Australia* 26 : *106-109* (1967).

MILLER, D. & C. H. DOHLMAN. Effect of cataract surgery on the cornea. *Trans. Amer. Acad. Ophthal. Otolaryngol.* 74 : *369-374* (1970).

MORTON GRANT, W. & F. P. ENGLISH. An explanation for so-called consensual pressure drop during tonography. *Arch. Ophthal.* 69 : *314-316* (1963).

MÜLLER, H. & S. PAPASTYLIANOS. 3000 Kataraktextraktionen: Komplikationen und Ergebnisse. *Klin. Mbl. Augenheilk.* 152 : *476-487* (1968).

MÜNCHOW, W. Zur Geschichte der intraokularen Korrektur der Aphakie. *Klin. Mbl. Augenheilk.* 145 : *771-777* (1964).

NAUMANN, G. & R. ORTBAUER. Zur Klinik und Histopathologie nach erfolgreicher Vorderkammerlinsenimplantation. *Ber. dtsch. ophthal. Ges.* 70 : *63-69* (1969).

—— & ——Histopathology after successful implantation of anterior chamber acrylic lenses. *Surv. Ophthal.* 15 : *18-24* (1970).

NORDLOHNE, M. E. Dislocation and endothelial corneal dystrophy (ECD) in patients fitted with BINKHORST lens implants (1958-1972). *Docum. Ophthal.* (to be published).

OGLE, K. N., H. M. BURIAN & R. E. BANNON. On the correction of unilateral aphakia with contact lenses. *Arch. Ophthal.* 59 : *639-652* (1958).

PARRY, T. G. W. Modification in intra-ocular acrylic lens surgery. *Brit. J. Ophthal.* 38 : *616-618* (1954).

PAUFIQUE, L. Faut-il opérer une cataracte unilatérale? *Ann. Oculist.* (Paris) 201 : *1148-1151* (1968).

PEARCE, J. L. Long-term results of the Binkhorst iris clip lens in senile cataract. *Brit. J. Ophthal.* 56 : *319-331* (1972).

PHILPS, A. S. Demonstration of 2 patients at the Joint Clinical Meeting. *Trans. Ophthal. Soc. U.K.* 72 : *669* (1952).

265

REESE, W. S., J. R. FINLAY & H. ROMAINE. Reports on the use of the intraocular acrylic lens (Ridley operation). *Trans. Amer. Acad. Ophthal. Otolaryngol.* 58 : *55–60* (1954).

RIDLEY, F. Safety requirements for acrylic implants, *Brit. J. Ophthal.* 41 : *359–367* (1957).

RIDLEY, H. Intra-ocular acrylic lenses. *Trans. Ophthal. Soc. U.K.* 71 : *617–621* (1951).

—— Intra-ocular acrylic lenses after cataract extraction. *Lancet* I : *118–121* (1952a).

—— Further observations on intraocular acrylic lenses in cataract surgery. *J. Int. Coll. Surg.* 18 : *825–833* (1952b).

—— Intra-ocular acrylic lenses. A recent development in the surgery of cataract. *Brit. J. Ophthal.* 36 : *113–122* (1952c).

—— Further observations on intra-ocular acrylic lenses. *Trans. Ophthal. Soc. U.K.* 72 : *511–514* (1952d).

—— Demonstration of 4 patients at the Joint Clinical Meeting. *Trans. Ophthal. Soc. U.K.* 72 : *669* (1952e).

—— Further observations on intraocular acrylic lenses in cataract surgery. *Amer. J. Ophthal.* 36 : *988* (1953a).

—— Further observations on intraocular acrylic lenses in cataract surgery. *Trans. Amer. Acad. Ophthal. Otolaryngol.* 57 : *98–106* (1953b).

—— Further experiences of intra-ocular acrylic lens surgery. *Brit. J. Ophthal.* 38 : *156–162* (1954).

—— Late surgical results of use of the intraocular acrylic lens. *J. Int. Coll. Surg.* 26 : *335–341* (1956).

—— An anterior chamber lenticular implant. Brit. J. *Ophthal.* 41 : *355–358* (1957).

—— Cataract surgery with particular reference to intra-ocular lenticular implants of various types. *Trans. Ophthal. Soc. U.K.* 78 : *585–592* (1958).

—— Intra-ocular acrylic lenses. 10 years' development. *Brit. J. Ophthal.* 44 : *705–712* (1960).

—— Intra-ocular acrylic lenses. *An. Inst. Barraquer* III-4 : *548–554* (1962).

—— Acrylic implants. Current results. *An. Inst. Barraquer* IX-1/2 : *143–149* (1969).

—— Intraocular acrylic lenses. Improved technique and results. Proceedings of the XXI Intern. Congress. Mexico, 8–14 March 1970. *Intern. Congr. Series* 222 : *771–775*, 1971 (Excerpta Med. Found., Amsterdam).

RINTELEN, F. & G. SAUBERMANN. Pathohistologische Untersuchungen nach Kunststofflinsen-Implantation beim Menschen. *Ophthalmologica* (Basel) 131 : *369–373* (1956).

ROETTH, A. DE. Ridley's cataract operation. *Amer. J. Ophthal.* 36 : *1568–1570* (1953).

RYCROFT, P. V. Acrylic lens implants and keratopathy. *Perspect. Ophthal.* I : *215–218.* Excerpta Med. Found., Amsterdam (1968).

SAUBERMANN, G. Über Resultate nach Kunststofflinsen-Implantation. *Ophthalmologica* (Basel) 129 : *247–252* (1955).

—— Komplikationen nach Vorderkammerlinsen-Implantation. *Ophthalmologica* (Basel) 137 : *178–182* (1959).

SCHARF, J. Demonstration eiener neuartigen Kunststofflinse zur Korrektur der Aphakie, mit Vorstellung operierter Patienten. *Klin. Mbl. Augenheilk.* 128 : *233–235* (1956).

—— Über zweijährige Erfahrungen mit einer Vorderkammerlinse. *Ber. 59. Zus. dtsch. ophthal. Ges. Heidelberg* 1955 : *222–227* (1957).

SCHILLINGER, R. J., R. V. SHEARER & O. R. LEVY. Animal experiments with a new type of intraocular acrylic lens. *Arch. Ophthal.* 59 : *423–434* (1958).

SCHRECK, E. Über ältere und neuere Möglichkeiten zum Ersatz der menschlichen Linse. *Münch. med. Wschr.* 98 : *401–404* (1956a).

—— Erfahrungen mit Vorderkammerlinsen. *Klin. Mbl. Augenheilk.* 129 : *112–113* (1956b).

—— Linsenimplantation nach Staroperation. Augenheilk. in Klinik und Praxis, ed. W. Rohrschneider, p. 151–163. Ferd. Enke Verlag, Stuttgart (1958a).

—— Erfahrungen mit über 150 Vorderkammerlinsen eines eigenen Modells. *Acta Conc. Ophthal. Belgica* (Brussels) II : *1699–1704* (1958b).

SETIAWAN ONG, H. D. Intra-und postoperative Komplikationen bei der Linseneinpflanzung nach Binkhorst. Therapie und Prophylaxe. Ber. 125. Vers. Ver. Rhein.-Westf. Augenärzte Bonn, p. 54–67. Grafischer Betr. Gebr. Zimmermann, Balve/Sauerland (1972).

SLOANE, A. E. Visual function is not a number. *Editorial. Arch. Ophthal.* 68 : *440* (1962).

—— Advice to patients who have cataract surgery in one eye. Correspondence. *Arch. Ophthal.* 79 : *358* (1968).

SMITH, R. Histopathological studies of eyes enucleated after failure of intraocular acrylic lens operations. *Brit. J. Ophthal.* 40 : *473–479* (1956).

STENSTRÖM, S. Untersuchungen über die Variation und Kovariation der optischen Elemente des menschlichen Auges. *Acta Ophthal.* (Kbh.) suppl. XXVI : *59* (1946).

STRAMPELLI, B. Sopportabilità di lenti acriliche in camera anteriore nella afachia e nei vizi di refrazione. *Ann. Ottal.* 80 : *75–82* (1954).

—— Due anni di esperienza con le lenti camerulari. *Atti Soc. Oftal. ital.* 15 : *427–433* (1955).

—— Fissazione di lenti camerulari mediante filo di supramid. *Atti Soc. Oftal. ital.* 17 : *669–682* (1957).

—— Complications de l'opération de Strampelli. *L'Année thérap. Clin. Ophtal.* 9 : *349–370* (1958a).

—— Les lentilles camérulaires après six années d'expérience. *Acta Conc. Ophthal. Belgica* (Brussels) II : *1692–1698* (1958b).

—— Anterior chamber lenses. *Arch. Ophthal.* 66 : *12–17* (1961). Reprinted in: Modern advances in cataract surgery, 216 pages, ed. R. M. Fasanella. J. B. Lippincott Cie, Philadelphia and Montreal, 1963.

—— L'évolution des lentilles plastiques de chambre antérieure. Dernières acquisitions techniques. *An. Inst. Barraquer* III-4 : *519–530* (1962).

—— W. MARCHI & A. VALVO. Lentine in camera anteriore con fissazione esterna (10 anni di esperienza clinica). *Ann. Ottal.* 94 : *9–42* (1968).

TAIEB, A. Des mémoires de Casanova à l'opération de Ridley. *Arch. Ophtal.* (Paris) 15 : *501–503* (1955).

TASSMAN, W. & W. H. ANNESLEY, Jr. Retinal detachment in prosthetophakia. *Arch. Ophthal.* 75 : *179–188* (1966). (Ridley lens implantations only).

THEOBALD, G. D. In regard to the Ridley implant. *Amer. J. Ophthal.* 36 : *1471* (1953).

THEODORE, F. H. ed. Complications after cataract surgery, 672 pages. Little and Brown, Boston (1964).

TÖNJUM, A. M. Intraocular pressure disturbances early after ocular contusion. *Acta Ophthal.* (Kbh.) 46 : *874–885* (1968a).

—— Intraocular pressure and facility of outflow late after ocular contusion. *Acta Ophthal.* (Kbh.) 46 : *886–908* (1968b).

TROUTMAN, R. C. Artiphakia and aniseikonia. *Trans. Amer. Ophthal. Soc.* 60 : *590–658* (1962a).

—— (& 12 others) Discusion lentes plasticas intraoculares. *An. Inst. Barraquer* III-4 : *593–620* (1962b).

—— Correction of unilateral aphakia. The use of intraocular lens implants. *Arch. Ophthal.* 68 : *861–869* (1962c).

—— Artiphakia and aniseikonia. *Amer. J. Ophthal.* 56 : *602–639* (1963a).

—— J. N. GOLDMAN, R. D. BINKHORST, D. E. WILLARD & A. C. CLAHANE. Anterior chamber depth in aphakia. *Trans. Amer. Ophthal. Soc.* 61 : *385–396* (1963b).

—— Intraocular lenses in aphakia. A letter to the editor. *Amer. J. Ophthal.* 68 : *1125–1126* (1969).

—— Reply to Hirschman at meeting Amer. Med. Assoc. 21st June, Atlantic City, New Jersey (1971).

TURTZ, A. I., P. R. MCDONALD, R. CASTROVIEJO & C. D. BINKHORST. Panel discussion. Proc. Centennial Symp. Manhattan Eye, Ear and Throat Hosp., ed. A.I.Turtz, p. 309–314. C. V. Mosby, St. Louis (1969).

URRETS-ZAVALIA Jr. A. Le décollement de la rétine, 713 pages. Masson et Cie, Paris(1968).

VIT, H. & F. TODTER. Ergebnisse nach Einpflanzung von Vorderkammerlinsen. *Ophthalmologica* (Basel) 157 : *76–82* (1969).

VOS, T. A. Cataractchirurgie in de loop der eeuwen. Arts en Wereld, Febr.-Nov., 6 artikelen, 33 pages (1971).

WAGENAAR, J. W. & S. J. VAN DER WAL. Halothaan (fluothane)-narcose bij glaucoom- en cataractoperaties. *Ned. T. Geneesk.* 108 : *1100–1101* (1964).

WEGNER, W. Lentilles intraoculaires de la chambre antérieure. Observations tardives. *An. Inst. Barraquer* III-4 : *573–584* (1962).

WELSH, R. C. Contact lenses in aphakia. *Int. Ophthal. Clin.* 1/2 : *401–440* (1961a).

—— The roving ring scotoma with its Jack-in-the-box phenomenon of strong-plus (aphakic) spectacle lenses. *Amer. J. Ophthal.* 51 : *1277–1281* (1961b).

—— Roving ring scotoma. Letter to the editor and reply from P. BOEDER. *Arch. Ophthal.* 69 : *685–687* (1963a).

—— Ring scotoma. Letter to the editor. *Arch. Ophthal.* 70 : *139* (1963b).

—— Experimental simulation of aphakia. *Brit. J. Ophthal.* 49 : *84–86* (1965).

—— Distressing wound complications from contact lenses for aphakia. Letter to the editor. *Arch. Ophthal.* 79 : *507* (1968).

WOLLENSAK, J. Chemische Einflüsse bei Keratopathia post implantationem (von Vorderkammerlinsen).*Ber. 62. Zus. dtsch. ophthal. Ges. Heidelberg* 1959 : *246–250*(1960).

—— Matières plastiques et lentilles artificielles. *An. Inst. Barraquer* III-4 : *543–547* (1962).

WOODS, A. C. The adjustment to aphakia. *Amer. J. Ophthal.* 35 : *118–122* (1952).

WORST, J. G. F. De uitspoeling van de lens bij congenitaal cataract en traumatisch cataract bij kinderen. *Ned. T. Geneesk.* 111 : *2041–2042* (1967).

—— Removal of the lens by irrigation in congenital cataract and traumatic cataract in children. *Ophthalmologica* (Basel) 156 : *19* (1968).

—— Over fixatie van de 'Binkhorst-lens'. *Ned. T. Geneesk.* 114 : *489* (1970).

—— H. H. H. LUDWIG & R. G. MASSARO. Details of the cryosurgical technique for cataract extraction and its application in a series of 50 implantations of Binkhorst's artificial lens. Proceedings of the XXI Intern. Congress. Mexico, 8–14 March 1970. Intern. Congr. Series 222: *776–780* (1971a). (Excerpta Med. Found., Amsterdam).

—— Note on fixation of the Binkhorst iris clip lens. *Ophthalmologica* (Basel) 163 : *10–11* (1971b).

—— R. G. MASSARO & H. H. H. LUDWIG. Het inbrengen van een kunstmatige lens volgens Binkhorst (met film). *Ned. T. Geneesk.* 115 : *817–822* (1971c).

—— The artificial lens for senile cataract treatment. Past, present and future of artificial lens implantation, as the treatment of choice for senile cataract. *Anais CVI Congr. Brasileiro Oftal.* I : *385–400* (1971d).

—— L'implantation d'un cristallin artificiel (iris clip lens de Binkhorst). *Bull. Mém. Soc. Fr. Ophtal.* (Paris) 84 : *547–562* (1971e).

—— De fixatie van de iris-clip-lens. *Ned. T. Geneesk.* 116 : *811–812* (1972a).

—— R. G. MASSARO & H. H. H. LUDWIG. The introduction of an artificial lens into the eye using Binkhorst's technique. *Ophthalmologica* (Basel) 164 : *387–391* (1972b).

☿ △ ♄

Author's address:
Constantijn Huygenslaan 12,
Vlissingen,
Holland.

Additional information of this book

(The Intraocular Implant Lens Development and Results with Special Reference to the Binkhorst Lens; 978-90-6193-176-8) is provided:

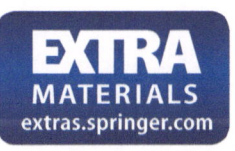

http://Extras.Springer.com

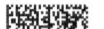